PBC
The Definitive Guide for Patients with Primary Biliary Cholangitis

2nd Edition

Prof David EJ Jones OBE

DEDICATION

This book is dedicated to all the patient groups, and PBC patients, who work so hard to help each other. They are an inspiration. Enormous thanks also go to Vanessa, Matthew and Thomas for all the thoughts and suggestions. I promised Thomas I would find a way of including the word "Coelacanth" somewhere in the book….so here it is.

CONTENTS

THIS GUIDE AND HOW TO USE IT
Second Edition

I have been managing PBC for nearly 33 years now and help run one of the largest clinical services dedicated to the condition in the world, at the Freeman Hospital in Newcastle upon Tyne in the UK. I have had the good fortune to be able to build on the work of two of the true pioneers in the field, Professor Oliver James and Professor Maggie Bassendine. My great interest has always been in the way the disease impacts on the lives of PBC patients. The symptoms and their impact on quality of life (in particular the fatigue that bedevils so many patients). The frustration that many patients feel at the challenge of getting access to up to date treatment in a disease often under-estimated by the general medical community (the more so at a time when treatment options are developing rapidly).

One of my missions, working with the patient groups such as the PBC Foundation and LIVErNORTH who do so much to support patients, has been to help patients and their families understand the disease and the way that it affects them better. A thing that always surprised me was the lack of an easily accessible book explaining the disease aimed at patients and families that I could recommend in the clinic. In 2019 it was easier to buy a PBC T-shirt than a book explaining the disease. After a working lifetime of talking about the disease in ways that people (hopefully) understand I always intended to write that book. In late 2019, on a holiday in the Alps when the snow wouldn't stop falling I finally decided to do it. When the manuscript was half completed the world changed with the onset of the COVID-19 pandemic. Although the PBC patient community did not appear to be particularly disproportionately impacted by COVID itself, there was a more subtle consequence. The needs of the emergency clinical service meant that even the best clinical services struggled to deliver the same level of care as before to their PBC patients. The need for patients to be in control of their own destiny, to be able to understand and manage their disease themselves as much as possible became clear. This made the need for a book like this more pressing than ever. Chapters 9 and 10, which explore living with PBC and speculate about the future were written once the potential long term impacts of COVID-19 became clear and with the need to make PBC care delivery more resilient very much in mind. This first edition of the book was published in June 2020.

Our awareness and understanding of PBC, and the application of this knowledge to the development of better treatments, has, however, increased almost exponentially over the last three years (to the huge advantage of patients, of course). It was always in my mind that a one-off book, no matter how useful at the time, could date quickly, and that updated versions would be needed. This has proved to be the case and led to this second edition being written. There is nothing in the original edition which has proved to be "wrong". However, in some areas it doesn't go far enough into emerging thinking; something that the feedback to the first edition tells me PBC patients are very keen to hear about. In particular, the range of emerging drugs has continued to expand and more detail is now given on these drugs and how we can best use them. There is also new thinking about the causes of fatigue in PBC and how we can potentially treat it. This is one of the most exciting developing areas in the whole field of PBC. There is a further significant change in what has turned out to be a significantly expanded book. To help you identify the areas where thinking and practice have changed (and to help you to make sure you are benefitting from that new thinking) I have included a new chapter explaining how the world of PBC has changed since the publication of the first edition of the book. In writing the first edition I set out to try and answer all the questions I have ever been asked by patients about PBC. Following the publication of the first edition I have had a huge amount of very constructive feedback and a number of suggestions (all of which I have incorporated). One of these was to try and directly answer the most frequently asked questions in a question and answer format, rather than just including the answers in the text chapters. I have therefore included a "frequently asked questions" section as an appendix. I hope you find it useful.

Before starting on the story of PBC, I thought it would be helpful to outline the different ways in which you can approach this book. I wrote it with the intention that people read it as a whole from beginning to end; to tell a story. I have deliberately not referenced specific pieces of the scientific literature as this hinders the readability, and the source material is not readily available to the public. I have, however, included all current thinking. I hope you the reader find it both interesting and helpful. Although the book is mainly aimed at patients I strongly suggest that you get spouses and relatives to also read it. It will help them understand you and the challenges that you face. It will also be helpful to doctors, nurses and researchers who are coming into PBC for the first time. In deciding on my approach, it was very clear that there is a balance to be struck between giving all the information that many people want, and avoiding making the book feel either over technical and daunting or "dumbed down". For this reason, at the beginning or most chapters I have included a **Two Minute Version** which summarises the key information in that chapter. The early chapters introducing the liver and PBC itself provide important background that will help you understand the later chapters that explain how to treat the disease better. Where there is repetition between chapters it is intentional as I am building the story as I go along and it is important to reinforce certain concepts. If a particular chapter is too much for you then please do read its two minute version before moving on.

Alternatively, just reading all the two minute versions in sequence would give you a better knowledge and understanding of PBC than 90% of doctors.

It is said that a medical student learns, in their first year at university, more new words than a foreign language student does. This means that a number of technical terms are used ("medical jargon" if you like). These terms are introduced in the text the first time they are used and are explained in more detail in an appendix which I have called "A Dictionary of PBC". Do keep referring back to this as it will help you to follow the story.

Finally, in the appendix I have also outlined our detailed approach to managing key aspects of PBC. These take the international guidelines for management and expand on them to describe what we actually do in practice. Any doctor could take these and fully replicate our approach to management. Feel free to share them with your doctors.

There is one final, really important, point. The book is designed to be an aid to understanding of the disease. It cannot possibly cover all the scenarios than any individual patient might encounter. It is vital therefore that any decisions about your disease and its management are made following discussion with your doctor or nurse. If reading this book makes those discussions easier to have then I have done my job. The book can't, however, and isn't intended to, replace the management that can be provided by your own doctors who have all the information relating to your condition to hand.

We will be developing online resources and care support opportunities for PBC in 2023 and beyond. We encourage you to keep visiting our new website as it evolves

www.lynup-medica.com

CHAPTER 1: **INTRODUCTION TO THE LIVER**

The 2-Minute Version

- The liver is one of the largest organs in the body, weighing up to 1.5Kg in adult males. It is located in the upper abdomen on the right hand side, tucked under the rib cage which protects it from injury (it is very soft and easily injured by trauma).

- Its structure is simple (millions of identical cells all doing the same thing) but its function is complex (each of those cells does many different things). This complexity of function is why it has proved very difficult to replace it with a machine.

- Amongst the functions of the liver are **processing** nutrients taken up from the bowel after meals, **making** proteins including those that control blood clotting and **cleaning** the blood to remove toxins (including bilirubin and by-products of the body functions). Other functions include **storing** sugar in the form of glycogen and **protecting** the rest of the body against bacteria and other organisms that get out of the bowel and into the blood stream.

- The liver has two types of blood flow into it (the hepatic artery and the portal vein) and one blood flow out (the hepatic vein). It has a second flow out, that of bile, which is made by the liver and drains out of it via the bile duct which eventually drains into the bowel. The bile drainage system allows those things the body wants to get rid of to be drained safely into the bowel. It also carries bile acids (cholesterol-based molecules made by the liver) into the bowel where they play an essential role in making fat in the diet soluble so that the body can handle it.

- The portal vein carries blood from the bowel wall into the liver and is the main route for nutrients from the diet to be taken to the liver for processing.

- The liver can be injured by a number of different things, including infections, drugs and the effects of the immune system. It usually recovers completely as it has an enormous capacity to re-grow after injury.

- If the liver tries to recover whilst injury is still going on scarring can result. If that scarring becomes extensive whilst regrowth is still happening, then the result is cirrhosis. This can limit the ability of the liver to work, and can cause a pressure rise in the portal vein. This is the cause of varices, bleeding from which is an important complication of cirrhosis. Prevention is better than treatment, which is why it is particularly important to try and control the causes of liver disease throughout its course.

- Liver diseases fall into two broad groups. These are disease of the liver cells themselves (the hepatocytes) and diseases of the bile duct (cholestatic diseases). PBC is a disease of reduced bile flow caused by the injury to the small bile ducts in the liver.

Primary biliary cholangitis (universally referred to by the abbreviation PBC, and formerly known as primary biliary cirrhosis) is primarily a disease of the liver. Before you can fully understand the disease it is important to understand a little about the liver, how it is structured, how it works and how it impacts on people when it does not function normally. The clinical features seen in PBC all make sense in the context of how it works (or doesn't work) properly.

THE NORMAL LIVER

The liver is an organ that plays a critical role in the healthy functioning of the body. It is one, however, that people tend to know next to nothing about. A few years ago a survey suggested that over 80% of people didn't even know where the liver was in the body, let alone how it functioned. Unfortunately, the one thing that people do tend to know about the liver is that it is injured by alcohol. This is something that has nothing whatsoever to do with PBC, but which rather plagues the lives of PBC patients! The liver is a large organ which is located in the upper abdomen on the right-hand side. The abdominal cavity is a body cavity that contains many key organs, in particular the bowel (stomach, small bowel and large bowel) and the liver. The abdominal cavity is separated from the chest cavity above it by the diaphragm, a muscular sheet which actively moves up and down as part of the breathing process. The diaphragm is domed in shape, meaning that the abdominal cavity extends higher up in the body than people tend to imagine. This is particularly relevant in the case of the liver, which is normally entirely located within the dome of the diaphragm and covered by the lower ribs. This coverage by the ribs is, presumably, to provide protection against trauma to what is, in practice, a very soft and vascular organ which can bleed profusely if injured. The liver is roughly triangular in shape and can weigh up to 1.5Kg in men.

The anatomy of the liver reflects its key role in metabolism, and the structure that it needs to perform that role. It is made up of millions of identical liver cells (hepatocytes), each of which undertakes all of the key liver functions. It is, in essence, a simple structure made up of repeating identical cells all of which have complex function. This contrasts with the kidney, which has a number of very different cell types performing individual functions, which collectively allow regulation of fluid and salt load in the body (a complex structure performing a simple function). One interesting contrast between the liver and the kidney has been the extent to which function of the organ can be replaced by a mechanical device. Dialysis, in all its forms, is long-established as a replacement therapy for kidney disease. There is, however, no equivalent replacement system for liver disease; something which often surprises both patents and trainee doctors. It is the very complexity of liver function, and the need to replace all missing processes, that means that the liver cannot easily be replaced by anything other than a functioning liver (through recovery of the patient's own liver following failure of the liver or, where needed, transplantation). The, in essence, single function of the kidney makes it far easier to replace with a mechanical system.

The structure of the liver is simple. Blood flows into it and perfuses the hepatocytes which are organised in sheets. Nutrients, oxygen and toxins are then taken up from the blood and processed by the hepatocytes. At the end of the sheets of hepatocytes, the now "cleaned" and de-oxygenated blood leaves the liver via the hepatic vein, joining the inferior vena cava before being returned to the heart for re-oxygenation by the lungs. The liver is unique as an organ in having two sources of blood entering it (in contrast, the kidney has a single blood flow in through the renal artery and a single flow out through the renal vein). These are the hepatic artery and the portal vein. The hepatic artery arises from the celiac artery, thereby sharing blood supply with the upper bowel. It supplies oxygenated blood to the bile duct in its entirety, and contributes to the oxygenation of the liver. The second blood flow into the liver, the portal vein, perfuses the hepatocytes with a blood supply which has drained from the bowel wall. Although partially de-oxygenated (the blood has already perfused the bowel and supplied its necessary oxygen) this flow makes an important contribution to overall liver oxygenation. Critically, however, the outflow from the bowel wall forming the inflow into the liver allows the liver to play its vital role of processing nutritional components absorbed from the bowel.

As well as making, modifying and breaking down molecules taken up from the blood the hepatocytes needs to dispose of residual toxins. This they do by transferring them out of the opposite side of the cell to the one exposed to the blood supply, into spaces called the bile canaliculi. All the bile canaliculi join together to form the small and then large bile ducts (like streams joining together to form a river). The fluid passing through them is called bile. Eventually, ducts from the right and left side of the liver join together to form the common bile duct which joins the bowel in the duodenum (usually just after being joined by the duct draining the pancreas). The by-products of metabolism, and toxins that the body wants to dispose of are, therefore, drained out into the bowel and exit the body in the stool. The small branches of the two blood supplies into the liver (the hepatic artery and portal vein) are bundled together with the branches of the bile duct. This structure, known as the portal tract, is somewhat akin to an electric 3-core cable and acts as a "service network" present throughout the liver. PBC is a disease, fundamentally, of the small bile duct branches (i.e. those present throughout the body of the liver rather than the large bile ducts which drain into the bowel) and the portal tract is therefore a critical site of the injury process.

Bile performs another essential role unrelated to disposal of toxins. Fat in the diet is not water-soluble, meaning that it will not, in its native form, be absorbed from the diet (it forms fat globules amidst the water-based gut fluid). In order to be solubilised it needs to be dispersed by the actions of a detergent. The natural detergents used by the body to solubilise fat are the bile acids; cholesterol based molecules synthesised by the hepatocytes and transported into the bile for drainage into the bowel. The pancreas produces an enzyme, lipase, which breaks down common fats solubilised by bile acids. Lipase is released into the gut in the pancreatic juice via the pancreatic duct, which, as we have discussed, joins the bile duct at the point where the latter joins the bowel in the duodenum. The net result is that fat in the diet is made absorbable by the body. Reduced release of either bile acids or lipase results in a failure of absorption of fat from the diet. This state is called fat malabsorption. Normal absorption of fat from the diet is also important to maintain the levels of a number of key vitamins (vitamin A, vitamin D and vitamin K are fat soluble and pass through the bowel if fat droplets are not dispersed). The effects of fat malabsorption are weight loss, oily and foul smelling stool, and the effects of shortage of fat-soluble vitamins (including night blindness because of vitamin A shortage, bone disease because of vitamin D shortage and clotting abnormality as a result of vitamin K shortage).

One of the critical roles played by the liver is to act as a buffer between the bowel and the circulation. It balances the needs of nutrition with protection of the body as a whole from the effects of toxic substances ingested in the diet, synthesised by the bacteria normally present in the bowel or forming part of the breakdown products of those bacteria. Often not thought of as a part of the immune system the liver is, in fact, an important contributor to protecting against, in particular, bacterial infections. Many disease states, including PBC, result in the bowel wall becoming "leaky", allowing the normally harmless (indeed beneficial) bowel bacteria to get into the portal vein. Unchecked they would get into the wider blood circulation causing sepsis. Enormous numbers of macrophages, cells of the body's protective inflammatory/immune system that "eat" and neutralise bacteria (called, in the context of the liver, Kupffer Cells), are present, aligned to the blood vessels of the liver in a position where they can "consume" any bacteria that get as far as the portal venous inflow into the liver tissue. Where the Kupffer Cells are lost, in the setting of acute liver failure, one of the major risks to life is sepsis because bowel bacteria which get into the portal vein because the bowel wall has become leaky are no longer cleared from the blood.

The liver is essential to clear other toxins and by-products of metabolism produced by the other organs of the body, and to make proteins which are important for body functions. An example of the clearance function is bilirubin, the pigment which, if elevated in the blood, is responsible for jaundice. Bilirubin is a by-product of the breakdown of old red blood cells in the spleen (it is normal for red cells to be recycled after around 150 days, with the iron being re-used by the body and the structure that it normally sits in, the haem group, being converted into bilirubin for disposal by the liver). The disposal is an active process. The bilirubin is conjugated (in essence "tagged for disposal") and then transported out into the bile. If this process is disrupted through a failure to conjugate (or tag) bilirubin, or because of a blockage of the flow of bile, then levels of bilirubin build up in the liver cells and leak back into the blood. The yellow colouring of the bilirubin then gives rise to the clinical appearance of jaundice. Levels of bilirubin in the blood can be measured easily, and are one of the clinical tests that are used to monitor liver diseases. Bilirubin is just one of a number of toxic substances that the liver needs to be able to clear. It is, however, the easiest to see and measure. Best thought of as body "poisons", when they build up in liver failure they can give rise to a toxic state (internal poisoning if you like) which is exemplified by hepatic encephalopathy, a state of brain toxicity beginning with confusion and sleep disturbance and leading eventually to coma. Amongst the other functions of the liver that are essential for healthy life are

- **Conversion of glucose into its storage form glycogen**. This occurs when glucose levels are high in the portal vein after a meal and is in response to insulin released by specialised cells in the pancreas (the Islets of Langerhans). The liver plays a key role in "smoothing out" blood sugar levels from very high peaks after meals to very low in between meals. When the glucose level falls between meals glycogen is broken down again releasing glucose from the liver (and muscle where glycogen is also present) to boost the dietary-derived level. Patients with failure of their liver often have very abnormal blood glucose levels. These are typically very low because such patients often have a low dietary intake.

- **Metabolic function:** In addition to the key metabolic function of glucose regulation many of the body's other key metabolic processes also take place within the hepatocytes. Most of the inborn errors of metabolism, genetic diseases in which specific metabolic processes are abnormal, are thus expressed in the liver. An example is hereditary oxalosis, a genetic disease in which oxalic acid builds up in the blood and causes kidney failure (oxalic acid is also present in high levels in the leaves of rhubarb plants and is the reason why the leaves, in contrast to the stalks, must not be eaten). Although the tissue injury in hyper-oxalosis is entirely to the kidney, the defect causing oxalic acid build up is exclusively expressed in the liver. Kidney transplant is rapidly followed by loss of the new kidney unless accompanied by liver transplant which corrects the underlying abnormality.

- **Protein synthesis:** Almost all of the proteins that the body makes for release into the circulation are produced in part or entirely by the hepatocytes. These include clotting factors (the proteins needed for the blood to clot) and albumin (a blood protein which is essential for the transport of bilirubin etc in the circulation). Albumin in the circulation also plays a key role in regulating tissue fluid levels, exerting oncotic pressure and drawing fluid from the tissues back into circulation. When albumin levels fall in liver disease it is a major contributor to tissue oedema or swelling.

- **Immune/Inflammatory function:** Although seldom thought of as a key part of the body's protection against infection the liver is, as outlined above, a key component of the immune system. In addition to the "filter" role played by the Kupffer Cells it also produces key protective proteins called defensins which are directly anti-bacterial. The liver is also the site of the breakdown of lymphocytes, key white blood cells, after they have performed their typically anti-viral functions. The importance of the liver in infection control is indicated by the high level of infection risk seen in patients with liver failure.

- **Cholesterol and steroid hormone metabolism:** The liver plays a key role in the control of lipid levels in the body; a role that is integral to the pathogenesis of non-alcoholic fatty liver disease (NAFLD) and hepatitis C infection (where the virus gains entry into the hepatocyte through lipoprotein receptors). The liver is responsible for the synthesis of around 80% of the cholesterol made by the body. Something that surprises many people is that the vast majority of our cholesterol is made by the body, and not taken up from the diet. Cholesterol is a completely normal thing to have in the blood and is, indeed, really important for normal body function. This is something which, again, surprises people given the association between high cholesterol and heart disease. A proportion of the cholesterol made in the liver is converted into bile acids, molecules which, as we have discovered, play an integral role in the absorption of fat from the diet and which are also key players in PBC. Bile acids synthesised by the hepatocytes and released into the bile are then taken up again in the ileum (the far end of the small bowel) and returned to the liver via the portal circulation. This "entero-hepatic circulation" means that the vast majority of bile acids are recycled rather than being lost in the stool. It also, however, exposes the bile acid pool to the environment, including the bacteria that normally colonise parts of the bowel. Bile acids can be modified during their passage through the bowel to form secondary and tertiary bile acids with subtly different physical properties to the newly synthesised primary bile acids. The highly complex ecosystem of bile acids, with different properties and levels of toxicity, is, as we will discuss, an important part of the cycle of bile duct damage in PBC.

In addition to cholesterol metabolism the liver also plays a key role in the breakdown of steroid hormones (hormones which are themselves derived from cholesterol, examples of which include cortisol, oestrogen and testosterone). This can have impacts ranging from failure to break down aldosterone (a hormone that regulates salt and fluid levels in the body, build-up of which leads to fluid retention and ascites) to retention of oestrogen which can lead to development of feminine features such as breast development; something seen in particular in people with alcoholic cirrhosis.

LIVER DISEASE: AN OVERVIEW

Disease of the liver is a common and growing problem in all populations. There are two broad forms of liver disease; those in which the target for injury is the hepatocytes themselves (examples include viral hepatitis and alcoholic liver disease), and those where the target for injury is the cells lining the bile duct. These cells are known as the biliary epithelial cells (BEC) or cholangiocytes. PBC is a classic example of the latter disease type; collectively known as the cholestatic liver diseases (from the ancient Greek *chole* (bile) and *stasis* (failure to flow)). Where hepatocytes are the direct target of injury it is easy to understand how failure of liver function arises (direct loss of the cells needed for liver function). In cholestatic diseases, the effect is more subtle. In these conditions the hepatocytes are not initially involved. Instead, damage to the bile ducts leads to a reduction in bile flow. Over time, however, the bile acids, which can no longer exit into the bile because of the downstream blockage, build up in the hepatocytes and cause injury (they can be toxic in some forms). Hepatocyte damage is in many ways, therefore, a consequence of the disease process not a cause. In practice, the hepatocytes initially cope well with the bile acid build up with minimal impact. Eventually, however, they begin to fail to cope and this can lead to a rapid decline; the effect is very much a cliff-edge one. This explains an important distinction between cholestatic and other liver diseases. The former can appear stable for a long period of time and then deteriorate rapidly. In contrast, primary hepatocyte disease tend to progress/deteriorate at quite a predictable rate. What this means in practice is that conditions such as PBC can be somewhat unpredictable. This is the rationale for regular follow-up in the clinic with monitoring of liver function tests, the blood tests used in the clinic to monitor the progress of the disease.

Loss of hepatocyte function (either directly as part of liver injury or indirectly through the effects of build-up of bile in the liver (cholestasis)) is one important component of liver injury and thus liver disease. The other major component is the effects of the body's response to that injury. In practice, the majority of the problems encountered in long-term liver conditions relate more to the nature of this response than to the initial injury process. All initial liver injuries give rise to one or both of two cardinal responses; necrosis of the hepatocytes and apoptosis. Necrosis can be thought of as traumatic, or disorderly form of cell death (a "messy death"). Apoptosis is an orderly form of cell death (a "clean death") in which a cell folds in on itself. It packages itself up for disposal if you like. Necrosis is the type of injury associated with burns or acid injury. Apoptosis is the mechanism of injury seen in response to an immune response (clearance of a cell infected by a virus for example). In both situations, there is a negative consequence from the loss of the cell and, if enough liver cells are lost, liver failure. To this, necrosis (but importantly not apoptosis) adds the negative effects of the cells falling apart, releasing irritant cell contents into the local environment. In a skin burn, where necrosis is a key process, much of the pain and reddening of the skin is a direct result of local inflammation worsened by the effects of necrosed cells. If cell injury continues over a long period of time then a third form of cell injury can come into play; senescence (a "living death"). It is increasingly being appreciated that this is a crucial part of the disease process in PBC. Senescence will be explored in detail in later chapters.

Paradoxically, given that this book is focused on the long-term effects of liver injury, most episodes of such injury actually result in complete recovery. The damaged and dying cells are cleaned-up by the macrophages, and the hepatocytes begin to divide and proliferate to replace the cells that have been lost. This is a property which is unique to the liver amongst solid organs and is quite dramatically effective. If half the liver is removed to treat a cancer, then within 3-6 months the liver will have re-grown to an identical size to that seen before the operation. It is because of the potential to regenerate that the key first part of treating someone with acute liver failure is simply to support them by reducing the impact of injury in order to buy enough time to let the liver recover. Time really is everything. The problem arises if the injury is ongoing, and particularly if necrosis is a prominent component. Where injury is ongoing the "clean-up" process becomes overwhelmed, and the body is continually exposed to injured or dying cells. In all organs, chronic injury ultimately results in the formation of scar tissue (or fibrosis as it is known technically). This represents the body's attempt to "wall off" injured or infected tissues that it can't control or replace. Scar formation ranges in its impact. In the skin it is unsightly and in a joint it can reduce mobility. Important but not life-threatening. In organs, however, it can significantly reduce function. In lung fibrosis oxygen transport into the blood is reduced and in the kidney fibrosis the kidneys malfunction. What about liver fibrosis?

The issues that arise with liver fibrosis depend entirely on the degree, or stage, of the fibrosis. In mild, or early, fibrosis the impact can be minimal or non-existent. The reason for this is the simple structure of the liver compared to other organs. As we have discussed, to function the kidney needs to have a complex structure with all aspects functioning. The basic functional unit of the kidney is called the nephron. This includes a complex structure of cells that first filters fluid out of the blood. This fluid is then concentrated up by kidney tubules before collecting into the ureter. The key thing is that each nephron is formed of thousands of cells and the whole structure needs to be intact for the nephron to work. The liver is very different. The basic unit is a single hepatocyte. Each one can do all the functions of the liver. Provided the liver has enough hepatocytes, they are individually healthy, have an adequate blood supply and can drain bile, then the liver will function. Fibrosis in the liver can, depending on the nature and severity of the liver injury, surround the portal tracts, surround the hepatic vein branches or link (bridge) between the portal tracts. Initially, there is no disruption to hepatocyte numbers, blood flow or bile outflow meaning that in early fibrosis liver function is normal. The issues arise when the architecture around blood supply and bile flow becomes distorted, typically by bridging fibrosis. As hepatocytes become replaced by scar tissue, so the numbers fall to the point where the normal level of reserve function is lost. The tipping point is usually when the bridging becomes complete, resulting in areas of hepatocytes becoming walled off by fibrotic tissue. As outlined above, the liver has the capacity to regenerate when hepatocyte numbers are sensed to be insufficient. Where bridging fibrosis is present, the proliferation takes place within a rigid sphere which puts pressure on the cells and the blood supply. This combination of advanced linking fibrosis and hepatocyte proliferation is known as cirrhosis. Note that cirrhosis does not imply any particular aetiology for liver injury. Any chronic insult to the liver can give rise to cirrhosis. The fact that the general population tends to assume that the word cirrhosis implies alcohol as an aetiology reflects, I am afraid, ignorance.

At present, there are no therapies that can be used in normal clinical practice that are able to remove fibrosis once it is established (although research and trials are ongoing). The management of cirrhosis, therefore, falls into three phases. The first is to attempt to prevent it from developing in the first place by preventing the chronic liver damage that predisposes to fibrosis. This requires effective, and timely, use of therapy to slow, stop and reverse the underlying disease process. There have been major advances in this aspect in a number of liver disease in recent years, most notably viral hepatitis and, yes, PBC. The second phase is, if prevention has not been possible, to manage the complications of cirrhosis that can place the patient at risk. These are outlined in the next section. The third is to consider liver transplantation. Complication management and transplantation have major limitations to them. This means that, for the future, our efforts must be directed at better therapies for underlying disease. If, however, these treatments don't work, or people are only diagnosed with liver disease once cirrhosis is already present (something that happens more frequently than you might imagine) then effective cirrhosis management becomes essential.

CIRRHOSIS AND ITS COMPLICATIONS

Much of the speciality of hepatology used to be focused on identifying, and managing, the complications of cirrhosis. The focus is now shifting to identifying liver disease earlier in its course, and treating the underlying processes to prevent fibrosis and cirrhosis from developing in the first place. There will always, however, be people who have one of the forms of liver disease for which disease modification is not yet available, people who don't respond to treatment and people who present late in the disease when cirrhosis is already established. For this reason, understanding cirrhosis and how to manage it remains of the utmost importance in hepatology.

The clinical complications of cirrhosis reflect a variable combination of two processes. The first of these processes is impaired liver function; an inadequate amount of liver functional capacity to perform the roles that the liver normally performs as a result of the replacement of hepatocytes by fibrotic tissue and the adverse environment within the cirrhotic nodules. The second is portal hypertension; an elevation in the blood pressure within the portal vein because of the impaired flow through the cirrhotic nodules. The specific complications of cirrhosis that we manage in practice are as follows.

Porto-systemic varices: This is the complication of cirrhosis that worries patients and clinicians the most. This is because of the risk of bleeding. Varices arise when the pressure builds up in the portal vein as a result of the obstruction to free flow of portal venous blood through the disrupted structure of a cirrhotic liver; portal hypertension. This must be distinguished from the completely different arterial hypertension which often gets shortened to just "hypertension", which is very common indeed in the population and which has nothing to do with the liver! Increased pressure in the portal vein leads to opening of alternative ways for the blood to flow; typically blood vessels that were open pre-birth (when blood flow patterns are very different) but which normally close soon after birth. They never, however, completely disappear. When they open up as a result of the increase in portal vein pressure they do so with quite thin walls. This, combined with the high pressure in the portal vein, makes them prone to bleeding. They can be found anywhere in the abdominal cavity and bowel wall, but are classically seen at the base of the oesophagus (the gullet) where it meets the stomach. Bleeding from these oesophageal varices is perhaps the archetypal complication of cirrhosis of all aetiologies. Although varices are predominantly a manifestation of portal hypertension, liver failure can complicate the process through reduced production of the clotting factors that the body needs to form clot and stop bleeding. Although in the vast majority of cases portal hypertension arises in cirrhosis because the issues around flow through cirrhotic nodules, it can, in some forms of liver disease, arise in non-cirrhotic disease. PBC is one of those diseases. This means that the presence of varices does not automatically mean liver disease has progressed to cirrhosis (although this is, in practice, usually the case). When varices bleed the flow rate can be very high. This is an out and out medical emergency. The techniques to prevent bleeding in the first place, and to control it when it occurs are, however, very effective and will be discussed in **Chapter 5**.

Ascites: Ascites is the name given for collection of fluid within the peritoneal cavity (the abdominal space). This is another feature of portal hypertension, although, as with varices, liver failure can contribute to the process through reduced protein synthesis. Ascites is made worse if the blood levels of albumin are low as these proteins play a key role in keeping the fluid in the vessels rather than it leaking out into the abdominal space. Lowered albumin levels are a feature of liver disease of all types and the reason why albumin forms part of the liver function blood test panel. Ascites causes two problems for patients. The first is that it can be uncomfortable (as well as unsightly) and can hinder breathing when people lie flat (it wedges the diaphragm which is key for breathing when lying flat). It can also hinder mobility because of the sheer weight of the fluid. The second problem comes from the rare (in PBC ascites at least) complication of ascites becoming infected (spontaneous bacterial peritonitis or SBP). This is usually as a result of gut bacteria finding their way across the bowel wall, typically in patients who are malnourished. SBP causes the ascites to grow in volume quickly, and there can be abdominal pain. It is also a cause for sudden deterioration in liver function tests as the infection places a significant additional strain on the liver.

Hepatocellular carcinoma (HCC): This is a primary cancer of the hepatocytes. It can complicate chronic liver disease of all types. A driver for its development is the proliferation of the hepatocytes seen in cirrhosis. When cells of any type proliferate on a continual basis it leaves them open to "going rogue" and escaping from the body's normal control systems. This is a key predisposing step to the development of cancer. HCC is particularly common in viral hepatitis (especially hepatitis B) because of the additional pro-cancerous effects of the virus. HCC is always commoner in men then in women. HCC is unusual amongst cancers in that we know who is at risk of getting it (patients with cirrhosis). This allows us to watch for it, allowing early treatment. If it is left unchecked, it will progress, growing and metastasising as most cancers do.

Organ failure: Over time, the functional capacity of cirrhotic livers usually deteriorates to the point that there is insufficient function for the needs of the body. This is the clinical state of liver failure. There can, on top of this underlying trend of decline in function over time, be acute deteriorations in liver function as a result of episodes of complication development such as variceal bleeding or SBP, as well as with inter-current illnesses unrelated to the liver; all processes which place additional stress on an already struggling liver. The state of liver failure is indicated by rising bilirubin, the onset of encephalopathy (see next section), falling blood glucose (the liver can no longer buffer sugar) and clotting problems (the liver no longer makes enough clotting factors).

Hepatic encephalopathy: Hepatic encephalopathy is a toxic brain state caused by retention of chemicals by the poorly functioning liver that collect and then impair brain function. It is, perhaps, the archetypal feature of cirrhosis caused by hepatocellular disease. Where it occurs, it is normally as part of a liver failure picture with other features dominating. It is characterised by cloudy thinking and difficulty in concentrating, sleep disturbance and, eventually, coma.

CHAPTER 2: **INTRODUCTION TO PBC**

The 2-Minute Version

- PBC is a disease of reduced bile flow caused by the injury to the small bile ducts in the liver.

- The clinical features of PBC occur as a result of this poor bile flow, with the bile acids which don't drain properly in the bile building up in the liver and causing injury to the liver cells.

- The injury to the bile duct cells can be a result of two different processes. These are apoptosis (an orderly process of cell death where, in essence, the cells fold in on themselves, packaging the dying cells up for disposal) and senescence, a process where cells don't die but enter a "zombie" state.

- There is a significant element of autoimmunity (the development of an immune response directed against the body's own proteins) in PBC, with these aberrant immune responses potentially causing apoptosis in the first place. It is likely, however, that after a while the disease becomes self-sustaining with a cycle of injury to the bile ducts causing bile acid build up and thus more bile duct injury

- Traditionally, it was thought that apoptosis was the main driver for bile duct injury in PBC (i.e. the cells died). More recently, it has become clear that senescence is a major driver (i.e. the cells are alive but not functioning). This may have important implications for treatment as live cells appear to be rescuable even when in a zombie state.

- The bile acids that build up in the liver eventually leak back into the blood stream and circulate around the body contributing to the development of symptoms of PBC such as itch and fatigue.

- PBC can impact on the lives of patients in two distinct ways, through the development of progressive liver injury causing risk to like and through the onset of symptoms such as itch and fatigue. The balance between these two problem sets varies from patient to patient.

The condition we now know as primary biliary cholangitis, commonly referred to as PBC (and previously known as primary biliary cirrhosis), was first described over 170 years ago. Despite its long history, it remains a mystery to most doctors and to far too many patients. Myths abound about what should really be thought of, these days, as a fully treatable disease. This leads, all too often, to patients receiving sub-optimal care in practice. This book is based upon my 30+ years of experience treating patients with PBC, and the insights that that experience can give into how to do things in the best way possible. It is also informed by the, fortunately rare, people in whom the diagnosis of PBC has been missed or made too late, by the people in whom the importance of symptoms is ignored by doctors who focus on blood test, and by the people for whom worry about the disease can blight their lives. If this book helps even one of these people in the future then it will have served its purpose.

PBC is a disease of the liver, although other organs can be involved as part of a disease complex. One of the reasons why the diagnosis of PBC can be missed by doctors and other clinicians is that many of the features that are present early in the disease are rather non-specific in nature. These include fatigue, problems with concentration and itch; none of which instantly make you and your doctor think of liver disease, and all of which can be features of many other conditions. Once an alternative diagnosis has been reached (including skin disease for itch and depression or chronic fatigue syndrome for fatigue) it can be difficult to shake off. Clinical notes tend to reinforce diagnoses, and, over time, it becomes less and less likely that a diagnosis is challenged. Fine if the original diagnosis is correct but potentially harmful if it is not.

LIVER INJURY IN PBC

PBC is a disease primarily of the small bile ducts within the liver; those a little bit downstream of the bile canaliculi at a point where the ducts have begun to have a distinct structure. This structure consists of a smooth lining of biliary epithelial cells, attached to a basement membrane which provides structural integrity. A key factor in the disease process is bile and, in particular, some forms of bile acid which can be toxic to cells if those cells are constantly exposed to high levels because of an abnormality in bile flow. This abnormality in bile flow is known as cholestasis and PBC is, accordingly, normally thought of as one of the "cholestatic liver diseases". The biliary epithelial cell lining of the bile ducts affected in PBC is one cell deep. The affected ducts are positioned in the portal tracts, the structures outlined above which also house the small hepatic artery and portal vein branches which supply the hepatocytes with blood, and the small hepatic vein branches which drain the blood away from the hepatocytes. PBC does not affect the larger bile ducts and the gall-bladder, and, if larger bile duct injury is seen, this is very suggestive of a related but different cholestatic liver disease called primary sclerosing cholangitis (PSC). There are important differences in the risks associated with, and the treatments for, PBC and PSC and it is really important to distinguish the two conditions in practice if management is going to be optimal

The classic lesion seen in PBC is damage to the biliary epithelial cells lining the small bile ducts. Paradoxically, however, this is now only rarely seen in practice as to see it requires a liver biopsy (a technique where a small amount of liver tissue is taken for examination under the microscope) to directly visualise it. Liver biopsy is a technique which is now only rarely used for the diagnosis of PBC because, as will be outlined in **Chapter 4**, the combination of blood tests now available to make that diagnosis are very accurate, and in most cases has eliminated the need for liver biopsy for diagnosis. Biliary epithelial cells initially cope with injury in PBC and proliferate (divide and re-grow) to compensate. Thus, for a long time in early PBC, there can be evidence of biliary epithelial cell injury without any impact on bile flow and/or the development of cholestasis. Eventually, however, the capacity to cope with injury is lost and the bile ducts begin to close down, impacting on bile flow. This is when the disease can begin to progress fast as the hepatocytes are exposed to injury by the bile acids (especially the hydrophobic or water insoluble variants) which are no longer draining efficiently into the bile and which therefore build up within the liver.

The actual mechanism of injury to the biliary epithelial cells in PBC is at the heart of our understanding of PBC. Several processes appear to be at play. The classic view is that the main process is one of apoptosis; a process of programmed cell death where the cells are induced to die by an external signal. The classic model for apoptosis in a disease such is PBC is the action of a "killer" immune cell type (cytotoxic T-cells). These cells arise in immune disease of many types and have been shown, in elegant studies by Eric Gershwin and colleagues, to be present in PBC patients. They infiltrate into the liver and, critically, have the same targeting (or specificity as immunologists term it) as the anti-mitochondrial antibodies (AMA) that are the classic feature in the blood of PBC patients. The presence of such cells, together with the AMA in the blood, the large numbers of immune cells that are found in the portal tracts in PBC, and the fact that PBC patients have a much increased risk of getting other immune diseases (especially autoimmune diseases where the immune system rather than focusing on infectious organisms focus on normal cells that belong to the body), led to the view that PBC is also an immune disease.

There are two facts that slightly complicate this view. The first is that, as outlined in **Chapter 5**, PBC does not normally respond to steroid therapy (or indeed any other of the numerous treatments targeting over-active immune responses that have been tried in the disease). This is in marked contrast to other immune diseases where advanced immune therapy has transformed the outlook for patients. The second fact that challenges the immune model for injury of the biliary epithelial cells is that there is an alternative entirely plausible potential explanation for the apoptosis of these cells. This is the direct action of the toxic, hydrophobic bile acids known to specifically build up in PBC themselves. These disturb the membrane or outer lining of cells such as the biliary epithelial cells and cause direct injury. The resulting injury processes include apoptosis, meaning that the finding of this form of injury in the liver in PBC patients could in fact represent the consequence of PBC (the toxic effect of bile acid build up) rather than the cause (immune injury). If biliary epithelial cell apoptosis is caused by hydrophobic bile acid build-up it does, of course, beg the question as to what causes the bile duct injury that leads to bile acid injury in the first place?

There is a further complication to our understanding of why and how biliary epithelial cells are injured in PBC. There is emerging evidence to suggest that there is an additional mechanism at play; cellular senescence. Our understanding of the fate of injured cells has increased significantly over recent years. The simplest mechanism to understand is necrosis ("messy death") in which the cell is ruptured, killed and its contents are spilled. This, as we have discussed, is the type of cell death seen with external traumatic events such as burns. The body tries to avoid this process at all costs as the mess can have knock-on effects on otherwise uninjured cells, spreading damage. Apoptosis, also outlined earlier, is a mechanism for unhealthy cells to undergo a "clean death". The cell is given a signal to die by the immune system or by chemical signals and, in essence, commits suicide. Its structures fold in on themselves reducing the potential for damage to other cell types. The remains of the dead cell are then cleaned up by the macrophages and other scavenger cells of the immune/inflammatory system. We now, however, understand a further fate which can befall cells which is senescence ("living death"). Senescent cells enter a state in between normal function and death where they are still alive but unable to function normally. The term "zombie cell" has been used and it is not a bad description. Senescence occurs as a consequence of cell oxidative stress (a consequence of inflammation) and as an end step of proliferation (where cells have exhausted their capacity to divide and proliferate because of the number of times they have already divided). It is now clear that senescence of biliary epithelial cells occurs and contributes to the loss of function of the bile ducts in PBC. Indeed, bile duct senescence appears to be a particularly aggressive process when seen in PBC. To complicate the picture further (as if it needed complicating further!), senescence is not a passive process. Senescent cells release large quantities of cytokines (proteins that activate the immune system) which further activate the existing autoimmune responses which are themselves part of the process of injury in PBC.

Biliary epithelial cell injury in PBC appears, therefore, to be a complex and multi-directional interplay between three processes, necrosis, apoptosis and senescence. The balance between these processes and, critically, the order in which they occur, is not just of arcane interest to scientists. As we will explore later in this book this issue lies at the very heart of the question as to how we can most effectively reverse PBC in the future and attain the ultimate goal; that of disease cure.

One of the cardinal features of PBC is its long-term nature, with bile duct injury continuing, typically, over many years. Whilst many patients tolerate this very well (many more PBC patients will die **with** PBC than die **from** the disease) it can cause injury in two ways that give rise to long-term patient impacts. The first is through the progressive loss of bile ducts altogether. A subgroup of PBC patients, often the younger ones, appear to get a more aggressive form of bile duct damage which leads eventually to almost complete loss. Harm in this group comes from hepatocyte dysfunction resulting from the very high levels of toxic bile acids retained in the liver because of the extreme bile duct loss. In simple terms the toxic bile acids can't get out of the liver. This group of patients can go on to need liver transplant without ever developing cirrhosis. The other impact seen in this group of people with very aggressive loss of the bile ducts (termed ductopenia) is prominent itch. As we will explore in **Chapter 7,** itch in PBC is closely related to, if not directly a result of, retained bile acids leaking back into the peripheral circulation, meaning that this group of patients, who have the highest degree of bile acid retention, typically have the highest level of itch.

The second result of chronic liver damage in PBC is, as is the case with all forms of liver disease, the development of fibrosis and, ultimately, cirrhosis. As we will keep returning to, the term cirrhosis in PBC has caused many issues over the year and is, in many ways, an inaccurate word to include in the disease name. Cirrhosis can, and does, develop, however, in the end stages of PBC in some patients (albeit with a rather unique form to it termed biliary cirrhosis). As discussed in the previous chapter fibrosis or scar formation is a natural process in the body when injury has occurred, and the body cannot fully heal the injured tissue restoring its normal integrity. Any injury present over a long time can predispose to fibrosis in any organ meaning that the process is by no means unique to the liver. Long term injury in PBC therefore, as in other forms of chronic liver disease, gives rise to fibrosis around the affected portal tracts and, eventually, between the tracts. Ultimately, this gives rise to a liver-wide matrix of scarring. Although fibrosis per se is not unique to the liver there is a specific property of the liver which, when combined with scarring, gives rise to the unique process of cirrhosis.

Although cirrhosis and its complications have, as outlined previously, long been thought of as the defining issue in chronic liver disease their impact is, paradoxically relatively limited in PBC. Progression to cirrhosis does not occur in most people (especially if they have been treated early and effectively) and when it does occur it develops slowly and is well tolerated. Cirrhosis needs to be thought of, looked for, and managed effectively, but there are more important issues for PBC patients. In many ways the impact of bile duct injury and ductopenia are far greater and represent the direct focus for treatment. In terms of numbers of patients impacted it is the symptoms of PBC that give rise to the greatest burden. This introduces, rather well, the concept of looking at PBC in terms of the problems it causes. This approach will naturally lead us on to the solutions to those problems which is the focus of most of the rest of the book.

THE IMPACT OF PBC ON PATIENTS

There are three broad ways in which PBC impacts on patients, and understanding and approaching these is the focus of much of this book. There is a significant degree of misunderstanding about disease impact, however, amongst both patients and clinicians and it is helpful to take an overview before exploring the detail.

Impact through chronic disease and risk to life: Historically, the main (indeed essentially only) focus of management in PBC, as with all liver diseases, was to reduce the rate of progression of liver injury in order to avoid the development of the complications of cirrhosis with their risk to life. These included varices, ascites, HCC, hepatic encephalopathy as well, of course, as liver failure. As outlined above, there is, in the case of PBC, the additional important aspect to disease progression of ductopenia or bile duct loss.

Compared to most of the other, commoner forms of chronic liver disease, where the hepatocyte is the principle target for injury, cirrhosis in PBC is relatively uncommon and has a lower degree of impact. Portal hypertension occurs and varices can represent a significant bleeding risk. Ascites is, however, relatively uncommon. Hepatocellular function remains good until very late in the disease and hepatic encephalopathy (the toxic brain state which occurs when the liver cannot clear toxins which then impact on the brain) is very uncommon indeed. Hepatocellular carcinoma is also uncommon, particularly in female PBC patients, and typically only occurs after many years of disease.

Ductopenic disease can lead to progressive failure of the liver. Its greatest impact is, however, through the development of itch as described in the next section.

Impact through symptoms and impaired quality of life: Whereas the problems associated with cirrhosis development impact on a minority of patients at any one time (only those with advanced disease) the majority of patients at any one time will experience one or more of the symptoms of the disease. Perhaps the biggest mistake that clinicians make in the management of PBC is the failure to appreciate that the symptoms of PBC occur throughout the disease course and are **not** just a feature of advanced disease. A result of this is the failure to appreciate that they are, typically, the main problem for patients. The two symptoms with the greatest impact are itch and fatigue (in a variety of forms). The causes and treatments of the symptoms of PBC are discussed in detail in **Chapter 7**. An important concept in understanding the impact of symptoms on patients with PBC, as with any disease, is that of Health Related Quality of Life (HRQoL); the extent to which health states impact on that aspect of life quality determined by health. In simple terms, this is a case of understanding the nature of the problem in order to attempt to find a solution. PBC is one of the first liver diseases in which HRQoL has been studied in detail (perhaps reflecting the holistic view of the clinicians and patient groups in the field), although even then it does not have the widespread level of understanding that it warrants. It is important, in the setting of symptoms, to think in terms of the cumulative impact of all symptoms on quality of life rather than to focus on a single symptom, no matter how seemingly important that individual symptom is. Improvement in a single symptom will not typically improve life for patients if others are left untreated. Even worse, over-focus on a single symptom can lead to the use of treatments that improve that symptom whilst making others worse. The classic example of this is the use of anti-histamines to treat itch in PBC; drugs which make fatigue worse, typically to a degree that makes the benefit to itch not worth it.

Impact through having a chronic rare disease: There is a further impact of PBC that I am very familiar with after working with patients for several decades. This is the burden resulting from having a chronic liver disease for many years that is both rare and poorly understood. PBC is a disease that very few people have heard of. There are no celebrity champions for the disease and no one wears PBC ribbons (as they do for HIV and breast cancer). This can make patients feel isolated. Ignorance also comes to the fore with the negative perceptions around liver disease in general, and the erroneous association with alcohol in particular. In the case of PBC, as outlined in the next section, this motivated PBC patients to go as far as to successfully campaign to change the name. Almost no patients will come to the Newcastle clinic for a first visit without a tale to tell about being questioned (often repeatedly) about how much alcohol they drink. A further impact that patients frequently describe is one of being questioned as to how ill they really are. "You look normal" is a frequent comment. It is one of the paradoxes of cholestatic liver diseases such as PBC that the damage can be all internal with no external signs as to the degree of injury. One of my reasons for writing this book is to provide a resource to help patients better understand their disease and take ownership of its management. Another, however, is to create something that patients can give to their family members and loved ones to better help everyone understand this disease.

PBC: WHAT'S IN A NAME?

From the 1940s onwards, when the disease was "re-discovered" (having first been described in the 1850s), this disease was known as primary biliary cirrhosis, with the abbreviation PBC entering widespread use. It is worth reflecting on what the phrase means, and the problems that have resulted from the use of this name. "Primary" refers to the fact that, at the time the phrase was coined, the reasons for the disease developing were unknown (secondary biliary cirrhosis is when a similar disease process of biliary epithelial cell injury arises as a consequence of physical obstruction to the bile duct; a rare complication of gall stones or bile duct surgery). "Biliary" refers to the main target of injury namely the bile duct. It is the third word "cirrhosis" that causes the problem. As outlined previously, cirrhosis represents the end-consequence of a combination of tissue injury, fibrosis formation and regeneration of the liver. This leads to a nodular appearance with areas of near normal liver tissue constrained within a network of scar tissue. In PBC, cirrhosis is a very late stage in the disease process (Stage IV) and at any one time the vast majority of patients being managed in our clinic do not have cirrhosis (they are in Stages I-III). The term is therefore incorrect, and worrying, for the majority of patients.

There is, however, another issue with the term cirrhosis. In the eyes of the public and media this is synonymous with alcoholic liver disease. This use of the terminology is, of course, completely erroneous (a significant proportion of people with alcoholic liver disease don't have cirrhosis and worldwide the majority of people with cirrhosis have a cause of liver disease which is unrelated to alcohol (this, of course, includes PBC patients)). Ignorance amongst the broader population and, regrettably, even amongst some health care professionals can lead to stigmatisation of PBC patients. The inaccuracy, for most patients, of the term primary biliary cirrhosis, and the stigmatisation around the word cirrhosis, led to a world-wide, patient-led campaign to change the same. This was highly effective and the term primary biliary cholangitis is now in widespread use. Although not perfect (to an extent the words biliary and cholangitis are duplicative) the term more accurately describes the disease process seen in most patients and avoids the use of the word cirrhosis. It also retains the abbreviation PBC which is in universal use. The name change in PBC represents a landmark example of patient advocacy supported by the clinical and academic community.

CHAPTER 3: **THE CAUSES OF PBC**

The 2-Minute Version

- There are two aspects to the question "what causes PBC?" These are **aetiology** and **pathogenesis**. The question of the aetiology of any disease is about why you got it rather than someone else. Pathogenesis is the process by which the disease caused injury to your body and caused the symptoms and complications you are experiencing. Understanding aetiology can help prevent a disease. Understanding pathogenesis can help treat it once it is established.

- The aetiology of PBC is an interaction of genetic risk factors and environmental triggers. In this sense, it is typical of most chronic diseases.

- The genetic factors in the aetiology of PBC are a combination of very many small risk factors, none of which are abnormal (i.e. they are variants of normal). All appear to act on the immune system. There is no "PBC gene" as such, meaning that genetic testing isn't helpful in diagnosis of the disease or understanding the risk in family members.

- We know much less about the triggers that activate the disease in people whose gene "mix" puts them at risk. This means that, at present, there is nothing we can do to prevent PBC in people.

- PBC family members have an increased risk of developing the disease compared to the general population. The overall risk to any family member is, however, low (under 1 in 100) and we do not normally recommend family screening. The increased risk in families could represent shared genes or a disease trigger in a shared environment (i.e. amongst family members who live together).

- There are two key pathogenetic processes in PBC and understanding how they come about and how they relate to each other is at the heart of understanding the disease (so that we can treat it better).

- The defining process in PBC is damage to the cells lining the small bile ducts which drain bile out of the liver. Eventually the bile ducts can be lost, resulting in a state known as ductopenia. When bile flow is interrupted, the bile acids (molecules normally forming an important part of bile) build up in the liver causing damage to the liver cells. This damage can result in scarring and, eventually, cirrhosis.

- The critical question is why does damage to the bile ducts occur?. It is almost certain that the damage is, in part at least, a result of the immune system incorrectly targeting some of the body's own healthy cells (autoimmunity). One theory is that the genetic part of PBC aetiology makes these autoimmune responses more likely to happen in the first place, and an environmental trigger sets them off.

- Once injury to the bile duct begins, it starts an ongoing cycle of self-perpetuating injury. In this cycle, the bile acids that cannot drain from the liver cause more injury to the bile ducts and further reduce the flow of bile. Breaking, or even reversing, this cycle of injury is the focus of treatment in PBC.

When doctors and scientists think about the causes of any disease they split them into two aspects. Aetiology and pathogenesis. You will hear these terms used frequently (and often incorrectly). **Aetiology** refers to the true cause of the disease. Why did it develop in you as opposed to someone else, and why did it develop at the time that it did rather than at some other time? **Pathogenesis** refers to the pathways by which the aetiology of disease results in tissue damage and the clinical features of the disease. The "how" as opposed to the "why". Patients frequently ask me in the clinic what causes PBC. I strongly suspect that this question is actually a combination of 2 rather more focused questions

1) "How can you treat the disease?" This requires understanding of disease **pathogenesis**

2) "Will my daughter or son get it and can you prevent it?" This requires understanding of **aetiology**

I suspect there is often a third question set that is in the background. This is "did I cause it by something that I did and will I be the cause of it in my daughter or son". These questions reflect an element of guilt that I think patients sometimes feel. They are quickly answered by **no** and **no**!

THE AETIOLOGY OF PBC

PBC is thought to arise through a combination of genetic and environmental factors. This combination is widely accepted to underpin the vast majority of chronic diseases. This is especially the case in the large family of autoimmune diseases of which PBC is conventionally thought to be a member. This has traditionally always been explained as the "ploughed field and the seed". The genetic aspect is the underpinning environment, the way in which a person is "built", without which you will never get the diseases. The "seed" is the trigger that converts one of the many people in the population who are in theory genetically susceptible into the small number who actually develop the disease. The way I explain this to patients in the clinic is about the risk of banging your head on the doorframe! Only the very tallest people will bang their head on the doorframe as they pass through it. Height is largely genetically determined and is predictable from the height of a person's parents. The height of the door frame clearly plays a role though, and clearly has nothing to do with an individual or their genetic make-up. The genetics of height, and the environment of the door frame therefore combine to put a small proportion of the population at risk of developing a bruise on their forehead!

As with many diseases such as PBC, much more is known about the genetic aspect of disease risk than the environmental, although clearly the latter would be much more amenable to intervention to change risk ("you can't change your parents"!).

The Genetic Basis of PBC: The study of the genetic basis of disease has increased exponentially in recent years, with the advent of new genotyping technologies following on from the Human Genome Project. This will undergo a further expansion in the next few years as whole genome sequencing becomes an easily accessible tool, potentially reaching into routine clinical practice. Sequencing a whole genome, which took years and billions of dollars in the Human Genome Project, is now available for $1000 and can now be done literally overnight (although the analysis of the large amount of resulting data can take a lot longer!). The easy availability of genetic data in a disease such as PBC can lead to the perception that genetic factors play a dominant role in aetiology. This is, in fact, probably not the case, with environmental factors probably predominating

There are several strands of evidence pointing to a genetic component to PBC aetiology. The first, and most traditionally important, is the concordance rate in mono-zygotic (identical) and di-zygotic (non-identical) twins. Identical twins are, as the name suggests, identical in terms of their inherited gene set. They also, typically, share the same environment (they usually live together throughout childhood when a lot of key disease risk factor exposure occurs). Non-identical twins share the same environment, and a proportion of their genetic make up, but this is only to the same degree would be the case for non-twin brothers and sisters. If the disease rate is the same in both identical and non-identical twins, and that rate is higher than in the normal population, it points to an environmental factor in disease aetiology. In contrast, if the disease rate is higher in identical twins than non-identical it suggests that the shared genetic make-up is the pre-dominant factor. There are relatively few twin pairs in PBC (especially identical) so the data are limited. What data there are suggest a high concordance rate (increased likelihood that if one identical twin has the disease so does the other compared to non-identical) suggesting a genetic effect. The concordance rate is not 100%, however, meaning that there must be at least a component of environmental triggering that is also necessary.

Although twin pairs with PBC are relatively few and far between, families with more than one affected member are much more common. The increased risk is statistically significant (there are more affected family members than there "should be" based on the population frequency for the disease). The sibling relative risk in the North-East of England (the increased risk you run of getting PBC if you have a brother or sister with the disease) is around 10-fold; the mother/daughter relative risk is slightly higher at 35-fold. There are two important points to make about these figures. The first is that although they have been interpreted as confirming a genetic component to disease they could, of course, also support an environmental factor as siblings and mother/daughter pairs tend to spend a number of years living in the same environment. The second important point is that these figures sound more worrying than they should do. Although the increased risk of PBC in siblings where one has the disease is 10 fold, the prevalence of the disease (number of people in the population living with the disease at any one time) is only 35/100,000 in North-England. This means that the absolute risk for the sibling of a PBC patient is 350/100,000 or 0.35%. This means that the vast majority of the siblings of a PBC patient will **not** develop the disease. Even in mother daughter pairs, the most affected relationship, the absolute risk to the daughter of a mother with PBC is only around 1%.

In recent years, the precise nature of the genetic risk of PBC has begun to be understood in detail. This has occurred with the advent of modern genetics tools. PBC has been studied extensively using Genome Wide Association Study (GWAS) in very large cohorts of patients across the world, indeed many of the people reading this book will have taken part in these studies. The basis of the GWAS approach is that throughout the genome (the name for the whole genetic sequence that we all have divided into 23 pairs of chromosomes) there are areas where there is predictable variation. This acts as a map of "co-ordinates" throughout the genome. These "co-ordinates" link to variations in the genes, the parts of the genome that are translated into the proteins that go to make up the body. Mapping the "co-ordinates" therefore allows us to build up a picture of the gene variations that each of us have. It is important to realise that what is mapped in these studies is not abnormal gene variants (the single disordered genes that give rise to conditions such as cystic fibrosis) but variations in normal that, combined together for all genes, make us all different (unless we have an identical twin). There isn't, therefore, a genetic "cause" for PBC as such rather there is a genetic "explanation".

The GWAS studies in PBC have given rise to two broad conclusions that increase our understanding of the disease. The first is that it is not the case that one or a small number of genes make a significant contribution to PBC. Rather, the risk appears to be because of the cumulative impact of a very large number of small effects. This finding is in keeping with all autoimmune diseases studied to date, and mirrors personal traits such as height. As we have discovered earlier (remember the door frame?) height is to a significant degree genetically determined (nutrition also plays a role). There is not, however, a "height gene". Instead, multiple variations in normal genes combine to have the effect. The second is that, in essence, all genes shown to be associated with PBC to date are ones that control the development and expression of immune responses. They are all immune genes, focusing, in particular, on the way in which the immune system "sees" foreign protein and activates immune responses to that protein. They also appear to be genes that play a role in the nature of that immune response. **What this finding tells us is that whatever other processes are playing**

a part in PBC, the building blocks of the immune system appear to play a fundamental role in determining who gets the disease.

The next stage of the study of the genetic basis of PBC will be to use whole genome sequencing. This is the approach of determining the entire code for the genome from beginning to end. This is an increasingly available technique (the price continues to fall dramatically) and has the advantage that it doesn't miss gaps between the "co-ordinates" and the actual genes which can be an issue in the GWAS approach. Perhaps its biggest challenge is the scale of the data that it generates, which, when undertaking a study involving a number of people, requires advanced computing technology simply to be able to cope with it!

Paradoxically, the study of the genetic basis of PBC does not give rise to the one thing that everyone expects it to which is a genetic test to determine who is at risk of disease. Patients ask about this very frequently because of the familial risk of disease, and the desire to work out who within a family might be at the greatest risk. The reason why there is not a genetic risk predictor is precisely the same one as to why PBC is not a genetic disease. Genetic tests require there to be a single gene (or very small number of genes) which are very strongly associated with the disease. As we have seen, in PBC the genetic component of risk comes from the cumulative impact of a very large number of genetic variants, the individual contribution of which is very small. It would be theoretically possible to combine a large number of these variations into a composite genetic score that gave a high degree of certainty of the disease in people that had all of them. The challenge would be that the vast majority of people who actually went on to develop the disease would not have all of them. The test would, therefore, be of very limited use clinically.

The Environmental Basis of PBC: In comparison to the genetic basis of PBC, the environment triggering process, presumed to be responsible for conversion of risk of developing disease into overt disease, has been less well studied. This is largely because it is a very challenging thing to do. The theory is that a genetically "at risk" person, who is likely to be one of many such people in the population (the majority of whom statistically, of course will not go on to develop PBC), is exposed to something (as yet unknown) which triggers the disease. The challenge is that it is very likely that any such triggering event will have occurred a very long time before the disease becomes clinically apparent (after what we call a latent period). We therefore do not know what the trigger is that we are looking for, and we don't know when in someone's life we are looking for it! One of my colleagues memorably described this as being "like looking for a needle in a haystack when you don't know what a needle looks like and you aren't sure about a haystack"!

There are two broad approaches to studying potential environmental triggers in any disease setting; geo-epidemiology and the case control approach. In geo-epidemiology studies the basic approach is to identify all the patients with the disease that you are interested in living within a defined geographical area and look for disease clustering that co-maps with potential risk exposures. Disease clustering is where there are more people with the disease in a defined geographical area than there should be based on the population frequency of disease. There are, naturally, more people with any disease per square mile in areas of high population density so these figures must be corrected for overall population density. Even when corrected in this way there appear to be areas where PBC is quite heavily clustered. This has been interpreted as suggesting a shared environmental exposure that triggers the disease. This may well be the case, but we just need to be cautious as in close-knit communities family members frequently live close to each other. In this setting clustering could reflect a genetic influence as well as an environmental one.

The first modern geo-epidemiology study in PBC was done in Sheffield in the UK. In this study, PBC patients were approximately 10 times more likely than the population as a whole to get their domestic water supply from a single reservoir, the Rivelin. When the quality of the water was explored there didn't appear to be any characteristic pattern or abnormality. The study was carried out in the 1980s, however, meaning that the analytical technology available to examine the water was relatively limited. The examination for potentially toxic levels of chemicals (which weren't seen) also assumes that the trigger might be a direct toxic effect. The potential for a toxin to be concentrated within the body through long-term exposure, or because it is concentrated in one particular tissue or organ (highly relevant in PBC because bile is concentrated as it flows down the bile duct), was not explored in the study.

A further study was carried out in New York, looking at the frequency of PBC in relation to Federal waste dumps where toxic waste was disposed of. PBC patients were significantly more likely to live near one of these waste dumps. There were, however, no follow-up studies to try to identify what it might be in the environment around these dumps that was linked to PBC.

Perhaps the most detailed PBC geo-epidemiology programme has been carried out in the North-East of England, with detailed mapping of all patients (a really important aspect if these studies are to be accurate and useful). There are distinct clusters of patients, which appear to have been stable over time (the areas that had clusters of PBC 30 years ago still have them today, even if the actual people within the cluster have changed as older patients have died and new patients developed the disease). Across the whole region, the frequency of PBC has increased, although whether this is as a result of greater awareness of the disease, with more doctors testing for it, or a true increase in the disease rate, isn't clear. There is also a striking association between PBC frequency and previous coal mining activity, especially where the mines were open in the 1960s and 1970s. It is interesting to note that Sheffield in South Yorkshire, and Swansea in South Wales, both areas where the frequency of PBC appears to be high, also have a long and defining history of coal mining. The most recent Newcastle studies have begun to explore what it might be about mining activity that links to PBC. They have suggested a possible role for the metal cadmium, which is well known to be disturbed by mining activity, and to, as a result be present at greater levels in the water and soil in mining areas. Interestingly in the light of the New York study, the Newcastle study looked at rubbish and waste tips and showed no association with PBC.

The second broad approach to studying potential environmental triggers is the case control study. In this approach, ideas about things that might cause the disease are developed into a questionnaire that asks whether people have been exposed to them. A frequency of exposure figure on its own means nothing, of course, so a control group of people are needed who are as identical as possible to the study population save for PBC (i.e. same sex, same age, same area of residence). This approach has suggested interesting associations, but has some significant limitations. The first is, obviously, it requires us to have ideas as to what the cause might be. A classic example is the story of *helicobacter pylori*, the bacterial infection of the stomach now known to be the cause of peptic ulcers. Before its discovery there were many case control studies to look at the cause of ulcers that found many potential associations (smoking, stress at work, blood group etc). None of these studies, however, asked about the true cause, which we now know to be infection with helicobacter! The second limitation is that these studies are exquisitely sensitive to matching of the study and control group. Perhaps paradoxically, the challenge in study recruitment can often be around the right controls or comparator people. They don't have the condition and therefore don't have a vested interest in taking part in the research. The final limitation of the approach is around recollection bias. Patients with a condition such as PBC have often thought long and hard about why they might have developed the disease. This can sometimes lead to them being more familiar with past events and exposures. It is my observation, for example, that PBC patients tend to be much more familiar with their record of vaccinations than people without PBC. This doesn't mean that vaccinations cause PBC, just that it is a not-illogical possibility that a lot of patients have thought of themselves.

Significant case control studies have been carried out in Europe and the USA, with a consistency to their findings. Based on these studies, it is now widely accepted that PBC patients are significantly more likely to be (or to have been) cigarette smokers, to have a history of chronic urinary infections and to have used hair colouring or perming products. They are also significantly more likely to have another autoimmune condition (such as thyroid disease and rheumatoid arthritis) in either their own medical history or their family history. The associations with smoking, urinary tract infection and autoimmune disease risk factor into our thinking in the clinic when we approach the all-round management of patients.

There is one further limitation to all studies that have looked for disease triggers in PBC (as is, indeed, also the case for such studies in other diseases). Association is not causation. What this means is that all these studies show that some factors are more common in PBC patients than in non-PBC patients. This does not mean that they cause PBC, however. They could be a consequence of PBC or simply an association. Take the observations around waste-tips in New York and around urinary tract infection. It could be that each of these is a cause of PBC (although it might be difficult to think of the link). It could also be, however, that PBC patients in New York struggle with the symptoms of PBC or the consequences of disease progression, meaning that they either cannot work, or they end up taking a part-time or lower paid job. This may mean that they cannot afford a house in a nice neighbourhood and end up living somewhere where house prices and rents are cheaper. Areas next to a rubbish tip perhaps. Similarly, women with PBC often have low levels of oestrogen. This can lead the lining of the urinary tract to thin, making it more susceptible to infection. Chronic urinary tract infection could therefore be a consequence rather than a cause of PBC.

Does any of this matter to PBC patients, beyond the possible satisfaction that might come from understanding their disease better? The answer is possibly, but it remains too early to know. In autoimmune hepatitis (AIH), another autoimmune liver disease, it is now recognised that 2 antibiotics can trigger the disease (minocycline and nitrofurantoin). Avoiding these antibiotics can reduce the likelihood of getting AIH (although it doesn't eliminate it as there are probably multiple other triggers). Identifying the disease trigger or triggers in PBC may, in the future, help us to begin to develop disease prevention strategies through trigger factor avoidance. These would be most useful in people with an enhanced risk of developing the disease such as the relatives of patients with PBC. It is likely, however, to be a very long time until this approach reaches the clinic.

THE PATHOGENESIS OF PBC

What is probably much more important to patients is what the mechanism is by which the liver actually comes to be injured in PBC. This matters, of course, because it links directly to how we can treat the disease effectively. In understanding the pathogenesis of PBC, we need to understand, and link, the two cardinal features of the disease; damage to the small bile ducts within the liver and the development of characteristic anti-mitochondrial and anti-nuclear antibodies that react with the body's own proteins (autoantibodies). The development of fibrosis and eventually cirrhosis are the downstream consequences of these two processes.

Bile duct injury in PBC: The actual process by which the cells lining the small bile ducts (the biliary epithelial cells or BEC) are damaged is increasingly well understood. As I outlined in **Chapter 2**, two processes predominate. The first is apoptosis or programmed cell death, and the other in senescence.

To recap, apoptosis is a process by which a cell is given a signal to die by an external or internal process. A classic example is the killer cell of the immune response, the cytotoxic T-cell, eliminating a cell infected with a virus. As the cell is acting as a breeding ground for the virus, it is in the interests of the body to eliminate it. It is also, of course, advantageous for the body not to allow the cell to simply fall apart as this would release the virus allowing it to infect other cells. Cytotoxic T-cells, therefore, after recognising the infected cell via a receptor on the surface (the T-cell receptor) that can identify proteins from the virus processed to make them visible to the immune system, gives a signal to the cell to fold in on itself; dying whilst neatly packaging up the potentially harmful virus. The apoptosed cell remnants are then cleaned up by the scavenger cells of the immune system such as the macrophages. Apoptosis is also a natural part of human development when tissues remodel themselves. An example is the webbing between our fingers. In utero, developing humans have webbing between their fingers and toes that is a little like a duck's foot. By the time they are born this has disappeared. The cells of the webbing have been programmed to disappear through apoptosis.

Apoptosis of the biliary epithelial cells in PBC undoubtedly occurs. We can see the cells undergoing apoptosis in liver biopsies when we use the right detection approach. Does this mean, therefore, that they are being targeted by the killer cells of the immune system, perhaps because they are infected by a virus? There is certainly good evidence to suggest that cytotoxic T-cells do target the biliary epithelial cells (albeit probably recognising the body's own proteins rather than a virus (see the next section on autoimmunity)). It is not, however, as simple as that. There are other potential mechanisms for apoptosis in PBC, in particular the actions of toxic bile acids (which can certainly cause cells to undergo apoptosis in laboratory experiments and which are retained in the liver in PBC).

Bile acids are, as explained earlier, there to allow fat to be absorbed from the diet. They are a complex family of cholesterol-based molecules that are, to a greater or lesser degree, irritant to the cells of the body. These vulnerable cells include the biliary epithelial cells. Bile duct damage in PBC caused by biliary epithelial cell injury can lead to retention of irritant bile acids in the liver and bile duct, causing further injury to the biliary epithelial cells through apoptosis. This gives rise to a vicious cycle of progressive injury. It also means that it is difficult to know, from the presence of apoptosis of biliary epithelial cells on biopsy alone, whether this is a feature of an underlying process causing the disease (the immune system) or a consequence of bile duct injury and the retention of bile acids. Whatever the mechanisms, apoptosis appears to be an important part of the disease process, and one of the ways in which ursodeoxycholic acid (UDCA, the standard first line treatment for PBC which I will discuss in **Chapter 5**) works is to reduce the impact of apoptosis on the bile duct cells.

The second, and highly intriguing, mechanism for biliary epithelial cell injury in PBC, is senescence. Senescence probably arises as an end-result of a failed attempt by the biliary epithelial cells to cope with injury by apoptosis. Where bile duct injury occurs, a process of bile duct proliferation frequently accompanies it where the bile duct cells divide to increase the numbers of cells and attempt, we think, to replace the lost bile ducts. The issue is that all almost cells in the body are limited in terms of the numbers of times that they can divide. This is certainly the case with the hepatocytes and biliary epithelial cells. Exceptions to this rule are the so-called stem cells. The best example of these are bone marrow cells which need to be able to continue to divide to stock the blood with new cells to replace those that are broken down at the end of their life. In non-stem cells, restriction on the number of divisions a cell can undertake is probably a protective mechanism to prevent un-regulated division and, thus, cell immortality; the hallmark, of course, of cancer.

In PBC, therefore, bile duct senescence probably occurs because of the chronic bile duct injury and the body's response to it. When cells become senescent, they enter a state of limbo where they can neither proliferate any more, nor function properly, yet remain alive. The term "zombie" cells has been used in the popular press and is actually not a bad term. We know that senescence of bile duct cells occurs in PBC (we can detect it under the microscope). We also know that its development is a bad sign. The presence of senescence is seen much more commonly in people with aggressive disease who are on their way to losing their bile ducts. We also know that, as is the case with the zombies we see in films, zombie cells are not benign. They appear to produce lots of cytokines, the chemicals that activate the immune system, and chemokines, the chemicals that attract the cells of the immune system into tissues. This is probably a natural mechanism to promote the elimination of senescent cells which are no longer useful to the body. The problem is that if you get rid of senescent biliary epithelial cells, and there is no longer any way to replace them, you run out of bile ducts! The immune-system stimulation by senescent cells probably explains why interface hepatitis (the inflammation around the portal tract seen in high risk PBC) and biliary epithelial cell senescence go together and are both features of high-risk disease with a reduced likelihood of response to treatment.

Two further intriguing aspects to the story of cellular senescence in PBC have emerged recently. The first relates to the complex symptoms of PBC. There is now evidence to suggest that mice that are made to become cholestatic develop clinical features such as loss of short term memory and ability to concentrate that are highly reminiscent of the fatigue-related symptoms that we see commonly in PBC. When you look at the livers of these mice they have exactly the same process of senescence happening to their bile duct cells as happens in PBC patients. The intriguing new finding is that exactly the same process of senescence is occurring in the brains of the mice. This suggests the possibility that senescence in PBC isn't limited to the liver and in fact occurs in other parts of the body. If it occurs in brain cells it may be contributing to fatigue.

The second aspect that has emerged recently has enormous potential for better treatment of PBC. When I wrote the first edition of this book I hinted at the possibility that cell senescence in PBC (at that point restricted to the liver as at that stage we had no sense that senescence might be a more broadly-based phenomenon) could in theory be reversible. Apoptotic cells are dead and gone. They might be replaceable but they certainly aren't recoverable. Senescent cells are still alive, albeit not functioning. That means they have to be, in theory at least, recoverable. The problem was that at the time of the first edition it was just that, a theory. We didn't have any drugs able to reverse senescence. What we now know is that senescence is indeed reversible and the drug that reverses it is obeticholic acid (Ocaliva, one of the drugs already used for second-line therapy in PBC). Intriguingly, obeticholic acid seems to reverse senescence of both bile duct cells and brain cells. Importantly, neither ursdeoxycholic acid nor bezafibrate, the two other drugs routinely used to treat PBC (as first line therapy and as a second-line therapy option respectively) have any anti-senescent action. Indeed, bezafibrate appears to, in mice at least, make senescence worse....What implications does this new information hold for treatment of PBC. At the moment we are using obeticholic acid late in the disease after UDCA failure. Senescence appears to become established, in both high risk PBC patients and in mice, early in the disease. This raises the possibility that we may at the moment be using obeticholic acid too late in the disease in PBC to benefit from its anti-senescent properties. Trials to look at the benefit of obeticholic acid for fatigue and "brain fog" in PBC and reversing early disease are already under way in the UK.

Autoimmunity in PBC: The second cardinal feature of PBC is the development of the autoantibodies (antibodies that react against the body's own proteins) that are so important for disease diagnosis. These autoantibodies are part of a broader breakdown of the mechanisms by which the body distinguishes "self" (the proteins that form part of its own tissues and organs) and "non-self" (proteins that come from infectious organisms such as bacteria and viruses).

Antibodies are one of the body's key tools for fighting infection. They are proteins with very characteristic patterns, and structures, which allow them to recognise and stick to proteins and other molecules from infectious organisms, thereby neutralising them and preventing them from causing harm within the body. Autoantibodies arise when the immune system, for a variety of reasons, falsely identifies the body's own proteins as being foreign and a threat. They are relatively common in the population as a whole, suggesting that the immune system is, to an extent, leaky. They certainly do not automatically suggest the presence of autoimmune disease (although, as discussed in the next chapter, the link between the presence of autoantibodies and of active disease is stronger for PBC than for almost all other autoimmune diseases).

The characteristic anti-mitochondrial antibodies (AMA) seen in over 95% of PBC are, as their name suggests, directed at the mitochondria; structures within cells that are responsible for energy generation. The actual target for most of them is an energy generating enzyme called pyruvate dehydrogenase complex (abbreviated, confusingly to both PDC and PDH, both of which, to add further confusion sound a lot like PBC (a total co-incidence)) and, in particular, its enzyme-2 (or E2) component. We use the term AMA in clinical practice because it so accurately describes what we see in the laboratory. In the scientific study of PBC the terms anti-PDC, anti-PDH, anti-PDC-E2, anti-PDH-E2 and anti-M2 are all used. The important thing to remember, if you come across these terms, is that they all mean the same as AMA! Around 25% of PBC patients also get autoantibodies directed at structures in the nucleus of cells (the part of the cell that contains the chromosomes). These anti-nuclear antibodies or ANA (which can present a real diagnostic challenge) are directed at protein structures that are essential for the function of the nucleus, especially pore structures that allow molecules into and out of the nucleus.

Although autoantibodies are the part of the immune system which is easiest to study in PBC it is important to remember that other aspects of the immune system, for example the cytotoxic T-cells, also recognise the same proteins as the autoantibodies and play an equal, if not greater role in the damage to the biliary epithelial cells. The striking shared characteristic of all the proteins that PBC autoantibodies and T-cells recognise is that they are directed against proteins which play a really fundamental role in how a cell functions. As we shall see, this gives rise to some interesting questions as to how and why an immune response is "allowed" by the body to develop to them.

The immune system has no prior "knowledge" as to the potential infections that the body might encounter in the future. How does it, therefore "know" how to create antibodies that will react with an unknown future infection? The short answer is that it doesn't. It uses a different approach entirely. The process by which antibodies and T-cells react with any particular protein includes, in essence, random sequence generation, in which limitless random protein sequences are generated from the amino acid building blocks that are linked together to generate all proteins. This limitless approach means that the potential to bind to any foreign organism is inbuilt into the system. When an organism is encountered, the T-cell or B-cell (the cell that produces an antibody that binds to it) is activated. Each B-cell, as it matures, ends up expressing a single antibody specificity and a "sample" is expressed on the cell surface where it can bind passing organism; this results in the B-cell being given a signal to begin to divide, thereby increasing exponentially the number of B-cells expressing the "selected" antibody. Clearly, such a random mechanism will give rise to the potential for antibodies that react with the body's own proteins and other molecules, as well as "foreign" proteins present in infectious organism. If the system has no prior knowledge of what belongs to the body, and what doesn't, the potential for continual recognition of, and damage to, healthy tissues is obvious. In the early days of our understanding of the immune system the pioneer Paul Ehrlich coined the expression "horror autotoxicus" to describe this potential state of chaos.

Although autoimmunity (the development of a harmful immune response to the body's own tissues) clearly occurs, and PBC is one example of many diseases where it is part of the disease process, it is perhaps surprising, given the all-encompassing potential reactivity of the immune system, that it doesn't happen all the time. Only around 5% of the population will develop a clinically significant autoimmune diseases at some point in life. How is this balance between universal reactivity potential to ensure the immune system achieves its primary goal which is to protect us from infection, and self-protection, achieved? There are two key aspects which I have termed negative selection and context regulation.

Negative Selection: The vast majority of developing antibodies and T-cells that could recognise the body's normal tissues are, in practice, deleted from the immune repertoire (the term for the totality of possible available immune responses) before they can ever cause problems. The mechanism for this is too high a degree of recognition. The immune system is "hard-wired" to treat an antibody on the surface of the B-cell (or indeed a T-cell surface receptor) that reacts too effectively with a protein or other target molecule as being potentially harmful (especially if not "seen" in the context of a risk signal (see below)). Stimulation of the cell through the surface antibody or T-cell receptor which is too strong results not in a signal for the cell to divide and multiply (the normal response when a harmful protein to which mounting an immune response would be beneficial is encountered), but in a signal for the B-cell or T-cell to die (through our old friend, the process of apoptosis). I always describe this as being a little bit like Goldilocks and the 3 bears' porridge. If an antibody or T-cell doesn't recognise a protein then it is not useful (the porridge is too cold). However, if it recognises it too well it will over-activate the immune system causing an inappropriate response (the porridge is too hot). What is needed is a middle level of recognition (neither too hot nor too cold). Negative selection is about removing immune responses that are "too hot". The vast majority of such negative selection takes places in the very earliest stages of the development of the immune system in utero or early after birth.

Context regulation: A critical factor in regulating the expression of immune responses is to require the context in which a protein is "seen" by the immune system to be appropriate in order to permit activation of a response. There are several layers to this contextualisation. Furthermore, control of immune responses is funnelled through the actions of "helper" T-cells (lymphocytes that express two proteins called CD3 and CD4 on their surface). An immune response requires the function of these cells reacting to a specific protein. Without such help, immune responses are turned off rather than turned on. Activation of the "helper" T-cells requires them to be activated by cells of the inflammatory system termed "antigen presenting cells". They are only functional when themselves activated by local inflammation. Inflammation is the process by which the body reacts (non-specifically) to local irritants. These can, importantly, include components of bacteria such as the coating that bacteria express. Local bacteria, therefore, irritate the tissue, attracting and switching on antigen presenting cells. These sample the local environment, including the bacterial proteins, and process and present components of the bacteria to the "helper" T-cells. Because the bacterial proteins are not present in the body whilst the immune system is developing its profile of possible responses, potential to respond has not been negatively selected, and the helper T-cell is activated to help the immune response and then eliminate the bacteria. Two check-points have been overcome. The presence of inflammation provides a context suggestive of infection which triggers activation of the antigen presenting cell, and the "foreign-ness" of the bacterial protein means that the immune response has retained the capacity to respond to it. In contrast, although one of the body's own proteins (say a protein present in the biliary epithelial cells) will be perfectly visible to the immune system it will be in a context in which there is no inflammation and the capacity to respond to it will have been removed by negative selection. The 2 check-points have combined to prevent an inappropriate immune response to the body's own protein.

A final and subtle element to context comes in the form of route of exposure to a protein. The immune system has very powerful mechanisms to promote tolerance (non-response immunologically) to foreign proteins encountered in the bowel and via the portal vein. This is for the obvious reason that a foreign protein encountered in this setting is very likely to be from the diet. Celiac disease demonstrates the issues that can arise when immune responses arise to dietary protein. The liver sits at the interface between the vascular system draining the gut (where it is advantageous to be able to limit response to new proteins that are encountered because of the probability that they are a part of the diet) and the general circulation where new proteins are likely to be from an infection. It therefore has a particular complexity to its context regulation. It appears to be highly sensitive to swings in context regulation, going from high levels of tolerance to foreign proteins to high levels of immune reactivity.

What is happening in PBC? The fact that breakdown of immune regulation or tolerance to the body's own mitochondrial and nuclear proteins clearly occurs in PBC means that the checks and balances in the system have broken down or been bypassed in some way. How may this be happening? A major focus has been on a process of "molecular mimicry" that allows negative selection to be bypassed. Pyruvate dehydrogenase complex is present in all cells (other than red blood cells) in all animals and is almost identical in all these species. It goes further than that. It is also present in all bacteria. The reason this has arisen is that the role it plays is fundamental to life, and its structure is essential if it is to work effectively. When we have an infection with a bacterium containing pyruvate dehydrogenase complex, however, one of the immune responses almost universally is to that pyruvate dehydrogenase. The immune system, therefore, has to distinguish between the two proteins, even though the similarity between them is very substantial. A challenge for negative selection. The "dilemma" for the immune system (although of course it isn't a dilemma as the immune system doesn't "think" about what it does) is that to stop the capacity to respond to pyruvate dehydrogenase from bacteria is to lose an aspect of the immune response to that bacterium which could be life-saving. On the other hand, to allow it to occur unchecked would potentially lead to damage to an energy-generating enzyme which is critical for life. The immune response, therefore, treads a fine line. Sometimes, however, it seems that it can deviate from that line, allowing a response to be developed against bacterial pyruvate dehydrogenase which cross-reacts with human. In this model, the bacterial infection which was exposing the body to pyruvate dehydrogenase complex would also provide the inflammatory context to activate the immune system.

There is another intriguing potential possibility in PBC. Pyruvate dehydrogenase complex is very unusual in that although it is a large protein it needs another small molecule to be attached to it (called lipoic acid) to allow it to function generating energy. Without the lipoic acid attachment it doesn't work. The final structure for pyruvate dehydrogenase complex, therefore, is a protein which is coded for by genes, giving it a pre-determined, fixed structure, and another small molecule added on afterwards. Lipoic acid appears to be both important for function and for the immune response to pyruvate dehydrogenase. It is the part of pyruvate dehydrogenase complex which the immune response seems to focus on. Potentially importantly, the process for adding lipoic acid to pyruvate dehydrogenase can be inaccurate. In the laboratory at least, other molecules can be added in place of lipoic acid. These molecule differences can be enough to allow the immune response to recognise the adulterated pyruvate dehydrogenase and mount a response that then reacts with the natural human protein. If this chemical, as opposed to infectious, route to bypassing immune tolerance were to be important it would still need an inflammatory context to allow the response to be expressed. There is an additional element to the disease process that may play a role here. There is now good evidence to suggest that the bowel wall is leaky in PBC, allowing bacteria to get into the portal vein. Many years ago it was shown that the livers for PBC patients had bacterial components present within them which we presume reflects this process. It could be, therefore, that a chemical change in the lipoic acid attachment in PBC bypasses negative selection, whilst portal vein bacteria generating inflammation provide a permissive context. At present, however, this, like all theories as to how the immune responses arise in PBC, remains just that; a theory.

How might all this thinking about the immune pathogenesis relate back to the earlier discussion about aetiology? In terms of the genetic factors identified in our study of aetiology the link is likely to be simple. All the genetic factors identified to date relate to check points and controls in the immune response. It is likely, therefore, that the genetic profile in PBC makes context creation easier, and facilitates the bypass of negative selection. The potential environmental models are tantalising. Does the increased risk of urinary tract infection suggest a route for bacterial cross-reactivity with pyruvate dehydrogenase? Potentially even more excitingly, does the association between PBC and rubbish tips and mining areas suggest leakage into the environment of a chemical that can find its way into the lipoic acid attachment process giving rise to a form of pyruvate dehydrogenase that is chemically different enough to allow the immune system to recognise it? Time will tell.

The Chicken and the Egg in PBC: There is a fascinating further possibility in PBC, and one that has potentially huge implications for our approach to treatment. Implicit in all the discussion to date (and in all conventional models of the disease) is the concept that PBC is an autoimmune disease. In the autoimmune model, immune responses arise through one or more of the mechanisms outlined above, and these responses end up targeting the biliary epithelial cells. These cells are damaged, and the bile ducts begin to malfunction. Bile acids build up causing further biliary epithelial cell damage and eventually bile duct loss (through the combined processes of apoptosis and senescence). The toxic environment then leads to scar formation, fibrosis and eventually cirrhosis.

I have spent my working life exploring this "classical" model for the disease. There are two big questions that it gives rise to though

1) Why, if the immune response is the big driver for the disease, has no immune-system targeting therapy been shown to be effective. As we will discuss in **Chapter 5**, all the effective therapies in PBC to date target the bile acid-driven bile duct injury process. All the therapies targeting the immune response have been shown to be ineffective. The conventional answer has been that immune therapies are being used too late in the disease, but it feels like it is unlikely this could be the case for everybody and every treatment.

2) Given that pyruvate dehydrogenase complex is present in every cell in the body, why is the injury in PBC restricted to the biliary epithelial cells in the liver? Again, this is potentially explainable. Perhaps the chemical that replaces lipoic acid or alters pyruvate dehydrogenase complex in some other way is concentrated in the bile and therefore exerts its effect there, triggering an immune response there which is then directed back there.

In recent years a radical alternative hypothesis has been proposed. The implication of this is that we have got the model completely the wrong way round. In the new model for the disease, the initial injury is directly to the bile duct, but it is not immune in origin. The biliary epithelial cells normally have a sophisticated mechanism for protecting themselves from toxic injury (remember bile is almost always irritant). A protective layer is formed across them using molecules transported into the bile for that specific purpose. In PBC, for reasons unknown, this protective layer is either lost or loses function. This exposes the biliary epithelial cells to injury. As part of the "toxic" bile duct injury pyruvate dehydrogenase complex is changed chemically. This bypasses the normal negative selection protection against an immune response to a self-protein allowing the immune response to pyruvate dehydrogenase to develop and be expressed. This further injures the cells (the immune response in this model "turbo-boosts" the original toxic injury). This model would explain the targeting of the bile ducts (the injury begins there), and the lack of response to immune therapy (this is only a later part of the process and treating it therefore only removes part of the injury). It would also fit with the environmental risk data (the environmental trigger could be being concentrated in the bile and causing the very initial biliary epithelial cell injury. The model would also help us to understand the relatively low impact of the genetic risk factors related to immune control (they are controlling the secondary process).

Understanding which of these models is correct matters hugely to patients because of the implications for treatment. If the new model is correct, then understanding the very initial injury process is fundamentally important. If everything follows from this (bile acid driven apoptosis, senescence, immune injury and beyond) then it will be critical for us to be able to identify this process and treat it as early as possible. It may even be the case that if the driver for initial injury is an environmental factor we can prevent or reduce exposure to it preventing PBC. Perhaps the most obvious implication is that although immunotherapy may be important to give complete control of PBC it can never be enough on its own.

After a career focused on the traditional model, where the immune response is the first step in PBC and all the bile duct injury is a consequence, I am becoming increasingly convinced by the new model, in which the immune response is a consequence of the initial injury and an amplifier for the eventual injury pattern.

CHAPTER 4: **DIAGNOSING & MONITORING PBC**

The 2-Minute Version

- Diagnosing PBC is easy **but needs doctors to have thought about it** if they are going to order the right tests to confirm it! Increasing awareness about PBC is, therefore, critical for making sure that all patients are diagnosed in a timely fashion.

- The diagnosis is made using three different test types. If two or more of these are abnormal then this is enough to make the diagnosis with confidence. This approach is over 95% accurate. Once the diagnosis has been made these diagnosing tests don't need to be repeated.

- The first of these tests is for specific antibodies which are unique to PBC. Anti-mitochondrial antibody (or AMA) is present in 95% of PBC patients, and is almost never seen in people who don't have PBC. A smaller percentage of PBC patients also have a particular type of anti-nuclear antibody (or ANA).

- The second is blood tests looking at the biochemical function of the liver (known as liver function tests or LFTs). The characteristic feature in PBC is elevation of one of these tests called alkaline phosphatase (ALP). This is the one test that is repeated in PBC, as it is an important part of how we check on the response to treatment.

- The third test is a liver biopsy, when a small fragment of liver is taken using a needle, and looked at under the microscope. This allows us to see the characteristic pattern of damage to the bile ducts directly. A liver biopsy can also give important information about the degree of scarring and the presence (or not) of cirrhosis. It is also a vital test when it is thought that overlap could be present.

- The combined accuracy of LFT and antibody testing means that biopsy is rarely needed to diagnose PBC, and it is no longer used routinely for this purpose. There are also better, and safer, ways of checking for scarring (such as Fibroscan which is a non-invasive ultrasound-based test). Biopsy does still have an important role in working out the best treatment regimen where patients have aggressive disease and it is a safe and usually painless procedure.

- Once PBC has been diagnosed and treated, it is important for it to be monitored. The mainstays of monitoring are LFTs, which can assess both the severity of the disease and the response to treatment (these are the blood tests that are done whenever you go to the clinic) and Fibroscan which can assess progression of scarring in the liver (and predicts the risk of complications). A recent international study on nearly 4000 patients in 12 countries has shown that the information that comes from Fibroscan adds significantly to the information that comes from blood tests and that optimal follow-up involves both tests being done.

- Where cirrhosis is present, or strongly suspected, additional screening needs to be carried out. This includes with endoscopy ("telescope test") to check for varices, and ultrasound (along with an additional blood test call alpha-fetoprotein (AFP)) to look for liver cancer.

If you have reached this far in the book then it is likely that you or your loved one will already have been diagnosed with PBC. This is important as the biggest risk in PBC is faced by people in whom the disease hasn't been diagnosed, and therefore can't be treated. Please read on, however, as understanding how a diagnosis of PBC is made could help you help someone else, perhaps someone in your family, who is less fortunate than you are.

There are two broad routes to a diagnosis of PBC being made. These are diagnosis following clinical suspicion and diagnosis through screening. In the former, the possibility of PBC, or some other form of liver disease, has been suspected by a clinician based on symptoms or other clinical features. This has led to tests being ordered which have been interpreted as suggesting PBC. In the latter, tests potentially suggestive of PBC have arisen in the context of a clinical screening event (such as perhaps hypertension follow up or "well woman" screening). The route to diagnosis does not matter as long as the diagnosis is not missed. My experience is that diagnosis through screening is sometimes slower than as a result of clinical suspicion. The moral, perhaps, should be that whenever anyone has screening tests (blood tests, x-rays etc) they should find out the results of all the tests and ask about the significance of any abnormalities.

SUSPECTING PBC

Although a rare condition (rarity in medical terms is defined as fewer than 500 people with the disease per million of the population and PBC is thought to affect 400 per million) its distribution is very skewed, with nine women affected for every man. It is also a disease which is commoner in the over 40s (although there is an important group of younger patients, who often have a more aggressive form of the disease and in whom the diagnosis is frequently delayed or missed precisely because of perceptions as to the affected age group). The net result is that PBC can affect up to 1 in 700 women over the age of 40, making it far from uncommon in this group. Given also the extent to which PBC is now treatable (in contrast to a number of other chronic liver diseases), and the importance of early diagnosis, the possibility of PBC should be actively considered in anyone showing clinical features compatible with the diagnosis. PBC should then be suspected and tested for

In people with suggestive blood tests: This typically happens in two settings. The first is people found to have an elevated alkaline phosphatase (ALP) or gamma-glutamyl-transferase (GGT) (see **Table 1**). These are routine blood biochemistry tests which form part of a routine panel of tests ("liver function tests" or LFTs) done in numerous clinical settings, including monitoring people with diabetes, high blood pressure and high cholesterol. When a high alkaline phosphatase or gamma-glutamyl transferase is found it is almost never because the clinician ordering the test suspects that the patient has PBC. This means that the connection between test elevation and possible PBC needs to be made after the test abnormality has been found. This is where lack of awareness on the part of clinicians can be a real problem. The possibility of PBC should be considered in **everyone** demonstrating this blood test pattern.

The second setting is people found to have anti-mitochondrial antibody (AMA) or one of the other autoantibody patterns that are highly suggestive of PBC (**Table 1**). It sounds somewhat paradoxical that people should be found to have an autoantibody that was not expected (if it was not expected why was it tested for?). It is important to remember, however, that autoantibodies in many countries (including the UK) are ordered as panels. This means that if you were ordering a test to look for, say, thyroid antibodies because of suspicion of thyroid disease, or rheumatoid factor in the setting of suspected rheumatoid arthritis, the resulting panel would include the PBC-specific autoantibodies. A positive PBC autoantibody test is just as positive, and just as important, if it is a chance finding as if it was a test ordered specifically to look for PBC!

When a chance elevation of alkaline phosphatase, gamma-glutamyl transferase or AMA (or other PBC autoantibody test) is encountered, the automatic first step must be to order the other test type. This means measuring autoantibody levels if alkaline phosphatase is elevated and alkaline phosphatase if PBC autoantibodies are found. Positivity of both tests lies at the heart of the PBC diagnosis.

In people with suggestive symptoms: One of the characteristics of symptoms in liver disease is that, for the majority of the disease course, they have no characteristic features (odd as it might sound). This is particularly the case in PBC. People tend to think of jaundice and ascites as being the characteristic features of liver disease. In practice in PBC, they are very rare, only being seen in a tiny group of patients with very advanced disease. The reason why they have become rare is one of the success stories of PBC over the last couple of decades; we have become much better at diagnosing it, treating it early and, where necessary, moving to liver transplant in a timely fashion. Very occasionally, patients will first present with jaundice or ascites from PBC. This is usually in people who have had no other symptoms to alert doctors, and who do not have any screening blood tests done. The key point is that if doctors expect a PBC patient to be jaundiced they will miss the vast majority of PBC patients, and will miss the opportunity to treat them effectively. The symptoms that should particularly alert a clinician to the possibility of PBC are itch, fatigue and dryness of the eyes and mouth.

Itch is in many ways the classical symptom of PBC and its assessment and management are described in detail in **Chapter 7**. The trap for the unwary is, of course, that unless you are aware of the link with PBC there is no reason to suspect that someone whose only symptom is itching has significant liver disease. It is usually the case that people with PBC itch have had the symptom ascribed to allergy, hives or some other form of skin disease. The two features that should make a clinician think that there is a potential liver cause are the absence of any rash (with the exception of skin damage caused by scratching) and the characteristics of the itch. In PBC, itch is typically a deep sensation with the irritation feeling like it is underneath the skin (people often describe it as being like "creepy-crawlies" under the skin). The other clue to a PBC cause can be the distribution of the itch. The palms of the hands and soles of the feet are often involved, as well as the scalp; all areas where itch of other causes is unusual.

Although itch is the classic symptom of PBC, fatigue is in fact the commonest symptom and, across the patient population the one with the greatest overall impact on life quality (**Chapter 7**). Experience suggests that it is also the easiest symptom to have its significance missed. The challenge is, of course, the multiple causes of fatigue ranging from physical medical problems (diabetes, thyroid disease and anaemia are collectively very common in the typical PBC population age group and are all characterised by fatigue) to mental health problems (fatigue is a big issue in depression) and life-style issues (working too hard or partying too hard!). There is also the very large group of individuals given the diagnosis of chronic fatigue syndrome (CFS/ME). Given that the diagnosis of CFS/ME is largely a negative one (it is made by excluding other causes for fatigue) it is easy to see how a clinician who doesn't know that PBC causes fatigue, and therefore doesn't test for it, can end up giving a fatigued PBC patient the diagnosis of CFS/ME. The frequency of PBC in the population, the impact that fatigue can have in the condition, and the availability of effective treatments (for the disease itself if not yet at least fatigue) mean that I strongly believe that looking for PBC should be included in the screening protocol for chronic fatigue. The autoantibody and alkaline phosphatase tests needed to diagnose PBC are both very cheap and easily available.

The other symptom set that should make a clinician think about PBC is the presence of dry eyes and dry mouth. These features are not directly part of PBC but are the classic features of Sjogren's Syndrome; an autoimmune disease that affects the tear and salivary glands causing them to dry up. This can lead to dry and "gritty" eyes that are prone to conjunctivitis, and a dry mouth that can lead to an increased risk of mouth infections and difficulty in swallowing dry food in particular. Although Sjogren's Syndrome is a distinct condition to PBC the association is very strong indeed (over 70% of PBC patients will have at least some Sjogren's-like clinical features).

Whenever a patient has any of these symptom types as a presenting feature they should be assessed for the presence of PBC. In the first instance this should be through the combination of autoantibody screening (looking for AMA and/or the characteristic anti-nuclear antibodies of PBC) and liver function test assessment (looking for elevation of the liver biochemical tests particularly associated with PBC namely elevation in alkaline phosphatase or gamma-glutamyl transferase). This is particularly the case in people who have a family history of PBC or a personal or family history of another autoimmune disease. In each case, the previous history significantly increases the likelihood of PBC as a diagnosis.

DIAGNOSING PBC

Once the possibility of PBC has been considered then diagnosis is usually relatively straightforward. The criteria for diagnosis were established in Newcastle around 30 years ago. This was initially to aid with research into PBC, but the criteria have entered widespread clinical use and are recommended by all clinical guidelines for the disease. There are 3 test types used in making the diagnosis of PBC

Liver biochemistry ("liver function tests" or "LFT"): These are a panel of blood tests that are very commonly done in many clinical settings (hence the discovery of unexpected LFT abnormality as a route to suspicion of PBC). Within the panel of tests there are two that are key for PBC diagnosis. *Alkaline Phosphatase (ALP)* is a protein enzyme released from stressed or injured biliary epithelial cells. This process of cell stress is an integral part of the disease in PBC and ALP elevation is universal in the disease (at least prior to treatment; it can return to normal with effective therapy). ALP elevation is therefore a cardinal feature of the disease. A second enzyme (*Gamma-Glutamyl Transferase (GGT)* can also be released by injured bile duct cells and is a useful confirmatory test. The LFT profile also includes additional protein enzymes called the transaminase. These are released by the hepatocytes primarily, meaning that elevation in them suggests hepatocyte rather than bile duct injury. These are *Alanine Transaminase (ALT)* and *Aspartate Transaminase (AST).* Although medical students are taught that elevation in ALP indicates a cholestatic or bile duct related liver disease, and ALT or AST a hepatocyte or hepatitic disease things are rarely as clear cut as this. In most liver diseases both are elevated to some degree. It is the relative elevation of the individual enzymes which is suggestive of the disease type (in PBC as a cholestatic liver disease it is typically ALP which is disproportionately elevated, although ALT elevation can also be seen, albeit typically with a lesser degree of elevation).

Paradoxically, although ALP, ALT and AST are conventionally described as "liver function tests" they do not of course, as I have described them, measure liver function. They in fact measure liver injury. The conventional LFT panel includes two further tests which do measure function of the liver (although both are not pure measures of liver function either and can be abnormal in other clinical situations). These are *bilirubin* and *albumin*. Bilirubin is a by-product of the breakdown of haemoglobin. Red blood cells have a normal life span of around 150 days. After this, they begin to lose their shape and function and they are replaced by newly maturing red cells produced in the bone marrow. The old red blood cells are broken down in the spleen. At the core of haemoglobin is a chemical group called a haem group which contains the iron essential for oxygen transfer from the lungs to the tissues (the essential function of red blood cells). When the red blood cell is broken down the iron is extracted from the haem group and recycled. The rest of the haem group cannot be used and is disposed of. It is converted to bilirubin which is transported to the liver by albumin molecules, taken up by the liver cells and conjugated ("tagged") for transport out into the bile duct and thence the bowel, allowing disposal from the body. Jaundice, a common feature of liver disease, is a state of elevation of bilirubin. This can occur, in the context of disease of the liver, when the liver is either unable to take up and "tag" the bilirubin molecule because the hepatocytes are injured or unable to transport it out into the bile. It can also occur if there is a block to bile flow causing back pressure of bilirubin into the hepatocyte and leakage back into the blood. In PBC, the loss of cross-sectional area of the small bile ducts gives rise to elevated bilirubin. This, however, occurs very late in the disease. Because bilirubin excretion requires normal hepatocyte function the bilirubin level is a true liver function test, albeit one that is not that useful in most patients with PBC.

Perhaps the commonest trap with regard to bilirubin in PBC, and indeed any chronic liver disease, is Gilberts Syndrome. This is a relatively common genetic abnormality in the UGT1A1 gene which encodes one of the enzymes that "tags" (conjugates) bilirubin for transport out into the bile. This abnormality, perhaps better thought of as a variation in normal, leads to people running a naturally higher bilirubin level than normal individuals. The elevation in bilirubin is with unconjugated ("untagged") bilirubin. The issue with Gilberts Syndrome is not the problems it causes (it probably doesn't cause any, although some people have suggested that it can cause fatigue) but the fact that around 4% of the population have the change. This includes 4% of PBC patients, as the variant is neither commoner nor rarer in PBC patients than in the rest of the population. This means that 4% of PBC patients can have a bilirubin value **which is normal for them** of up to 50μmol/litre compared to the upper limit of normal of 17-20 (the range depends on the laboratory; be really careful with bilirubin values as it is one of the tests where results are expressed differently in different countries (the USA uses a measure of mg/decilitre which has an upper limit of normal of 1.0-1.2)). The difference between 17 and 50 does not sound like a large one but a value of 50 would be enough to worry a PBC clinician and to begin to think about discussing liver transplantation. One of the important messages we give to people training in PBC management is to look at the patient and all their tests as a whole. If the bilirubin value appears to be too high in the context of the other clinical features and tests, think about Gilberts Syndrome. Testing for its likely presence is easy. It requires a conjugated and unconjugated bilirubin split (normally the laboratory will give a single value for the total bilirubin but on request will split this into the conjugated and unconjugated ("tagged" and "untagged") components). If the elevation is from unconjugated bilirubin it is likely that Gilberts Syndrome is the cause. If it is conjugated it is likely to be the PBC. Gilbert's Syndrome has one additional trick to play on the unwary. The bilirubin elevation is variable and is normally more marked when people are under stress or feeling unwell. It is very common for people with Gilberts to get a more marked bilirubin elevation (and to become clinically jaundiced) when they have a cold or the flu. The combination of feeling unwell and worsening jaundice can lead to obvious concern that they both result from a worsening of PBC. This is why it is so important to, if Gilbert's Syndrome is present, know about it, record it in the clinical notes and tell the patient so that they can warn future clinicians. This may all feel a little over-emphasised but I have come across more than one patient referred for liver transplantation on the basis of their bilirubin rise after an operation when it was simply Gilbert's Syndrome! When told that they have nothing wrong with them other than mild PBC and Gilbert's Syndrome they were amongst the happiest patients I have encountered…….

Albumin is, in contrast, a protein which is produced by the hepatocytes and released into the circulation. Hepatocyte dysfunction is, therefore, associated with reduced albumin level. Although a marker of hepatocyte function, albumin is also dependent on dietary intake of protein and can, accordingly, be low in chronic poor nutrition states or with malabsorption; a process seen at increased frequency in PBC because of the association with pancreatic dysfunction and celiac diseases (**Chapter 8**). Albumin can also be lost into the bowel ("protein losing enteropathy") and from the kidney ("nephrotic syndrome) in conditions unrelated to PBC.

Autoantibodies: The autoantibodies of PBC, introduced in **Chapters 2** and **3**, provide less of an insight into disease pathogenesis than might be perhaps anticipated. The role they play in diagnosis is, in contrast, fundamentally important. Anti-mitochondrial antibodies (AMA) are 95% sensitive and specific for PBC. What this means is that 95% of patients have them, and 95% of people in the population with AMA will have PBC. Even the group with AMA who appear to not have PBC (their LFTs are normal) probably have an early or evolving form of the disease. To an approximation, therefore, AMA=PBC.

I am frequently asked two questions about AMA. The first is does the level matter, and, in particular, does a higher level suggest worse disease.

The short answer is no! There is a minimum level AMA needs to reach to be significant (because serum can be naturally "sticky" giving false positive tests). In most countries this is a titre of more than 1:40. This way of expressing antibody concentrations can be confusing. It comes from the approach taken in the lab, which is to serially dilute serum and re-test it to find the point at which the test becomes negative. Neat serum, fresh from a patient is 1. If that is diluted with an equal volume of non-serum it is 1:2. If that is diluted again with an equal volume it is 1:4 and so on. In each dilution the proportion of original patient serum, and thus the amount of antibody, is reduced. Eventually it will no longer be detectable. The last detectable level is the level recorded. Most laboratories stop diluting at 1:640 or 1:1280, largely because the test is, by that point, so significantly positive that it makes no difference. Beyond the minimum level (above 1:40) the AMA level appears to have no prognostic significance (patients with very high levels have disease that is neither better nor worse than anyone else). Fluctuations over time also don't mean anything, with the result that once someone has had a diagnosis of PBC made there is little point in repeating the AMA test.

The second question I am asked is does it matter which test is used. Again, the short answer is no. There are a number of different approaches, and therefore different names, for the test (AMA, anti-PDC-E2, anti-M2 etc). All are measuring the same thing (albeit in different ways), and if one of them is positive then you have AMA and there is no reason to use a second test. There are very occasional people whose AMA will be detected, for technical reasons beyond the scope of this book, by one test but not another. For this reason, if someone really did look like they had PBC, but the AMA test used as first-line was negative, we would repeat the measurement using a different test.

The anti-nuclear antibodies (ANA) of PBC are more complex. These are reactive with sub-structures in the nucleus; in particular pore proteins that facilitate the nuclear entry and exit of molecules. These have characteristic distributions on the standard immuno-fluorescence test of multiple nuclear dot or nuclear rim. These too have alternative approaches to detection (anti-Gp210 and anti-sp100) and, again, the technique used to detect them does not matter, as long as they are tested for! Where one of these antibodies is present in the absence of AMA it carries just the same significance for diagnosis as AMA would. As with AMA, the level of antibody has no clinical significance once it has been detected. PBC-specific ANA are seen less frequently than AMA (in around 20% of patients in the UK). There is some evidence to suggest that when they are present the disease can follow a more aggressive course. At present, however, detection of PBC-specific ANA does not lead to an alternative approach to treatment.

In identifying PBC-specific ANA it is really important to distinguish them from the ANA seen in other autoimmune conditions such as SLE ("lupus") and, of particular relevance to PBC patients, autoimmune hepatitis (AIH). AIH is, of course, relevant because a number of PBC patients have AIH-like features and the two diseases are best thought of as being related. It is important to distinguish PBC, AIH and PBC with AIH-like features (so called PBC-AIH overlap (**Chapter 5**)) as the treatment approaches are different. The ANA seen in AIH has a diffuse nuclear staining pattern, covering the whole nucleus. If this is seen in a patient who is also AMA positive it is strongly suggesting of PBC-AIH overlap. The two alternative types of ANA that can be seen in PBC make it particularly important for clinicians to determine the pattern of the antibody staining (the standard result that we get just has the level of the antibody not the pattern). Failure to understand PBC-specific ANA, and the assumption that ANA is therefore an AIH feature, is one of the reasons why PBC-AIH overlap has probably been significantly over-diagnosed in the past.

In addition to AMA and PBC-specific ANA, PBC patients can sometimes also express additional antibodies against cellular structures (such as the centromeres). The significance of these antibodies is, at the moment, not clear and they do not form part of the standard diagnostic set

Liver Biopsy and Histology: The third cardinal test is liver biopsy, a procedure where a very small amount of liver tissue is taken for examination under a microscope by a pathologist. The sampling is either done through the skin, usually under ultrasound direction ("percutaneous liver biopsy" or through the neck vein via a tube that is a passed through and down until it lies in the liver and can access tissue ("trans-jugular liver biopsy"). Although people worry about liver biopsy it is, in fact, a safe and usually non-painful procedure. Much less frequently performed than in the past, it is still a very valuable test where there is diagnostic doubt. The biopsy pattern also helps us make sense of the clinical pattern of the disease. There are three components to the picture of tissue damage in the liver in PBC. These are

- **Damage to the small intra-hepatic bile ducts themselves**. Initially subtle, this becomes more pronounced as the disease progresses until, eventually, the bile ducts become obliterated (a state known as ductopenia). Between damage and destruction, the biliary epithelial cells appear to enter into a phase of attempted recovery through proliferation (the cells split to create more cells in an attempt to regenerate the bile duct). As outlined in **Chapters 2** and **3** the initial injury to the biliary epithelial cells appears to be through apoptosis, with later bile duct loss being driven by senescence. This is now thought to be the end-result of the attempted proliferation when the cells run out of the capacity to divide anymore and enter the senescent "zombie" state.

- **Inflammation.** This is initially contained within the portal tracts (the structures containing the small bile duct as well as the branches of the hepatic artery and portal vein), eventually spilling out into the peri-portal areas (the areas around the portal tract). Granulomas can form (bigger structures formed from the fusion of several inflammatory cells) and are characteristic, sometimes helping to distinguish PBC from other diseases. In some patients the inflammation can appear to "break out" into the hepatocyte structures. This so-called "interface hepatitis" has traditionally been thought of, in the setting of autoimmune liver disease, as a feature of AIH. It is now clear, however, that interface hepatitis can also be seen in aggressive PBC without PBC-AIH overlap. Failure to appreciate this possibility is another reason why overlap has been over-diagnosed in the past (**Chapter 5**).

- **Fibrosis.** Fibrosis, or scarring, is the end-result of any process of chronic injury in the body and represents at attempt by the body to at least limit the impact of injury if it can't heal the tissues. Fibrosis can occur in any liver disease and PBC is no exception. The pattern seen in PBC is slightly different to liver diseases that impact primarily upon the hepatocytes. It starts in the areas around the portal tract and eventually begins to "reach across" from portal tract to portal tract (so called "bridging fibrosis"). Eventually, this lattice work of scar tissue becomes fully linked up. When the liver cells begin to proliferate in response to the injury, to maintain the amount of functioning liver tissue, is the point when the process of cirrhosis has begun. The term cirrhosis refers to the combination of extensive fibrosis and hepatocyte proliferation and **does not** imply any particular disease aetiology, despite what popular opinion might think.

Historically, the biopsy findings in PBC have been integrated into a 4 stage scale and this concept has entered into widespread use. Slightly different variants exist, but the stages are basically the same across the different systems

Stage 1 – Portal Stage: Normal sized portal; portal inflammation, subtle bile duct damage. Granulomas are often detected in this stage.

Stage 2 – Periportal Stage: Enlarged portal tracts; periportal fibrosis and/or inflammation. Typically characterized by the finding of a proliferation of small bile ducts.

Stage 3 – Septal Stage: Active and/or passive fibrous septa linking the portal tracts.

Stage 4 – Biliary Cirrhosis: Nodules present.

There is one final, important, aspect to liver biopsy in PBC. The disease is frequently very patchy in nature, meaning that the relevance of what one small portion in the biopsy shows can be limited. This, more than any other reason, is why liver biopsy has fallen out of favour in PBC.

Making the Diagnosis in Practice: The diagnosis of PBC is made based on combinations of the three cardinal test types outlined above
DEFINITE PBC is diagnosed when all three of the test abnormalities are present

- Alkaline phosphatase above the upper limit of normal
- AMA or PBC-specific ANA at a titre of greater than 1/40
- Compatible or diagnostic liver biopsy changes

PROBABLE PBC is diagnosed when two out of the three abnormalities are present. The terminology "probable" can be interpreted as suggesting a lower degree of certainty about the diagnosis. This is a throw-back to the origin of these criteria in research. In practice, most people with PBC are now diagnosed on the basis of raised ALP and significant AMA titre. This combination is over 95% accurate for the diagnosis of PBC and the addition of liver biopsy adds nothing in terms of overall accuracy (because of the impact of disease patchiness). Liver biopsy has fallen out of fashion for diagnosis as discussed below. Obviously, the necessary two positive tests cannot be reached in people who are AMA and ANA negative without a biopsy.

AMA POSITIVITY WITH NORMAL LIVER FUNCTION TESTS

One of the commonest referrals we receive is of patients with AMA but no abnormality in LFT. The question we are asked is what does this mean and what further investigation and treatment is needed? This group consists of three sub-groups.

The first group is people with very early PBC who are on their way to developing LFT abnormality, but in whom their AMA has been found before the LFT abnormality has occurred. A study carried out on the 1980s in Newcastle suggested that the majority of people with AMA but normal LFT were in this group, and went on to develop the classical disease (albeit in a very mild form). More recent data suggest that the combination of AMA and normal LFT may be more common than originally thought, and that only around 25% will go on to get true PBC.

The second group are people who appear to be AMA positive long-term, but who do not develop the disease. This is probably now the majority. Stable long-term AMA without overt PBC is a highly interesting clinical state. It suggests, as discussed in **Chapter 3**, that AMA probably does not play a direct role in causing liver damage but is, instead, a marker of the disease. We presume that the AMA positive normal LFT group develop the upstream disease process that gives rise to AMA, but lack the, probably genetic, risk that this upstream process goes on to cause liver injury.

The third type of patients are the rarest, and ones that tend not to be talked about in text books. However, I have seen a number of people in this group over my career. These are people who develop AMA which then disappears. This usually follows an acute illness seemingly unrelated to the liver, and which is typically flu- or pneumonia-like in nature. In these individuals, AMA can be present for up to a year before eventually disappearing. My suspicion is that this is an infectious triggering event breaking down immune tolerance as discussed in **Chapter 3**. My personal theory (and it is just a theory) is that this is caused by infection with mycoplasma, a primitive bacterial-like organism that can cause an atypical pneumonia. Where AMA are lost, the risk of future PBC development decreases substantially.

Our approach to people who are AMA positive but with normal LFT is to explain, to reassure and to plan follow-up. Reassurance is important and appropriate. Even where this group go on to develop PBC the risk of disease progression to cirrhosis is very low indeed, meaning that the overall risk from PBC is minimal. There is some risk of developing overt disease, and treatment is more effective when given early in the disease, so it is correct to follow up with annual LFTs. This can either be done in the community or in the hospital setting. It is just important someone does it, is aware of the results, and acts on them if they change. When someone in this group develops LFT abnormality, thereby achieving the 2 diagnostic criteria necessary for probable PBC, our practice is to immediately start them on UDCA therapy. We would almost never suggest a liver biopsy in this scenario.

One final questions about the AMA positive normal LFT group is a tricky one. Do they ever develop the characteristic symptoms of PBC without having first progressed to full PBC? One view is that they don't and can't (they don't have PBC) and that perception of symptoms is a result of people becoming aware of them because of the concern being raised about PBC (a form of placebo effect if you like). My view is different. Over the years I have seen a number of people who were found to be AMA positive only **after** they were investigated for a symptom (usually fatigue, but sometimes itch). Given that they had the symptom before the presence of AMA was known about, awareness of AMA cannot possibly have contributed to symptom perception. In the original Newcastle study of AMA positive normal LFT patients, biopsy was carried out (something that makes this study unique). The majority of patients had some degree of mild PBC change in their liver. Given that we know (and will discuss in **Chapter 7**) that symptom severity is unrelated to disease activity or severity in PBC it is perfectly plausible to me that this mild PBC change is sufficient to lead to symptoms. My personal approach is, therefore, to discuss UDCA therapy in the symptomatic AMA positive normal LFT group, the logic being that the presence of symptoms is acting as a "fourth diagnostic criterion". There is no evidence as to whether this approach is beneficial. There is also, however, no evidence that it isn't!

WHAT ELSE COULD IT BE? THE DIFFERENTIAL DIAGNOSIS

When doctors are training they are taught to think of "short-lists" for potential diagnoses which are then narrowed down to make the actual diagnosis. This is a fail-safe approach because it makes you actively consider and exclude the other likely, and frequently important, possible diagnoses. In PBC, the accuracy of autoantibodies such as AMA for the diagnosis, when seen in combination with raised ALP and/or GGT, makes diagnosis straightforward (indeed there is really no excuse for missing the diagnosis in patients with these features). The challenge comes in the small group of patients who are autoantibody negative. This is where important mistakes can be made if doctors are unwary.

The single biggest mistake that is made, in my experience, is to fail to distinguish between PBC and the related, but distinct, autoimmune cholestatic liver disease **Primary Sclerosing Cholangitis (PSC)**. PSC is, like PBC, a disease where damage to the bile ducts occurs. Although damage can occur to the intra-hepatic bile ducts as in PBC ("small duct PSC"), it is more typical for the larger bile ducts to be involved. This can be anywhere throughout the bile duct, including the large extra-hepatic bile ducts. Although small duct disease can be diagnosed on liver biopsy (as for PBC), large duct disease requires specialised imaging, most usually with magnetic resonance imaging (MRI) in the form of magnetic resonance cholangio-pancreatography (MRCP) where the findings of duct structuring are diagnostic. Given that this test will always be normal in PBC the two diagnoses should never really be confused. Still, however, it happens. The reason why distinguishing the 2 diseases matters is not because the drug treatments are different (ursodeoxycholic acid is used in both, although the evidence to suggest it is effective in PSC is quite a lot weaker than for PBC), but because of a very specific risk associated with PSC (but **not** PBC). This is risk of colon cancer and bile duct cancer (cholangio-carcinoma). PSC, but not PBC, patients need to undergo regular bowel and bile duct surveillance to identify these cancers at a stage when they are hopefully still treatable. Diagnosis of PSC when the disease is in fact PBC gives rise to un-needed tests (and concern). The reverse, a diagnosis of PBC when the disease is in fact PSC can lead to missed cancer and a disaster for the patient. When in doubt treat as PSC!

The conditions other than PSC that can be mistaken for PBC are all rare and rarely give rise to diagnostic problems. They split into two groups, the conditions that look like PBC on a liver biopsy and conditions that can give rise to clinical features that mimic PBC. The biliary epithelial cells lining the small bile ducts appear to be a cell type that are particularly prone to injury. Whether this is because of the nature of the immune response in the liver, or because of the toxic environment which they have to cope with (even healthy bile is irritant), is not clear. Whatever the reason, injury to the bile duct cells with eventual duct loss accompanied by a portal tract inflammatory response is a feature of a number of disease processes. Critically, however, most are in the context of another clear disease process and none are associated with AMA or PBC-specific ANA. The differential diagnosis is always, therefore, AMA negative/antibody negative PBC emphasising, yet again, the caution that should be taken in diagnosing AMA negative disease. Amongst the conditions that can be characterised by bile duct cell loss are

Sarcoidosis: A multi-system chronic inflammatory disease of unknown origin. Although lung disease is the most common manifestation, liver inflammation with bile duct injury can occur. Of this group of PBC-mimicking conditions it is the only one in which granulomas (structures formed by the accumulation of inflammatory cells called macrophages), a feature of PBC, are also seen. Historically, hepatic sarcoid patients have been treated with low dose prednisolone although there is no real evidence that it is needed or works.

Graft versus Host Disease (GVHD): In the setting of transplantation, in particular bone marrow transplant, immune cells in the donor graft can begin to react against the host. This effect is termed graft versus host and is the opposite to the more familiar effect in which the host immune system attempts to eliminate the graft (rejection). A number of tissues can be involved, including the skin with characteristic rashes and the bowel with loss of the lining and diarrhoea. The liver can also be involved with immune injury against the bile duct cells giving a very PBC-like appearance. Prior history of transplant could raise the possibility, but in the absence of transplant GVH cannot occur, meaning that this differential diagnosis should never cause problems.

Ductopenic Rejection: In liver transplantation, chronic rejection of the organ takes the form of bile duct injury. Again, the prior history of liver transplantation makes this diagnosis easy.

Secondary Biliary Cirrhosis: This is a rare process that arises as a result of obstruction to the bile duct causing injury to the bile duct cells "upstream" of the blockage, probably through a combination of pressure effects and the toxic properties of bile. This most commonly occurs after surgical injury to the bile duct (usually in the setting of laparoscopic gallbladder removal). It can also occur, however, as a result of chronic bile duct stricture arising as a rare complication of gallstones in the common bile duct (i.e. gallstones that have migrated from the gallbladder into the bile duct and become lodged causing obstruction). Gallstones are seen at an increased frequency in PBC making a hybrid of secondary biliary damage and PBC theoretically possible. I have never, however, seen the combination. All guidelines recommend imaging the bile duct at the point of diagnosis of PBC (with ultrasound followed by an MRCP if the ultrasound shows abnormality) to ensure that there isn't an element of bile duct injury confounding the clinical picture of PBC.

Vanishing Bile Duct Syndrome: To complicate the picture even further, occasional people are seen in whom loss of the bile ducts appears to be a spontaneous process without any apparent cause. This usually occurs without the other liver biopsy features such as portal tract infiltrate and granulomas. The relationship between this and AMA negative PBC is far from clear. Given that UDCA therapy would appear to be a logical approach to protecting the bile ducts in all ductopenic diseases, including vanishing bile duct syndrome, the differentiating of this condition from mild PBC may be more of a semantic issue than anything else.

The functional mimics of PBC are more complex and may be under-diagnosed. In essence, they all represent variations on a theme of transporter abnormality. The body's epithelial layers (the layers of cells that form the linings of the body (the skin, lung lining, bowel lining, bile duct etc) are designed, by their very nature, to be a barrier to things getting into or out of the body (to be "leak proof" in simple terms). You only have to look at the problems encountered in people with burns, such as significant fluid loss and risk of entry of bacteria into the circulation, to understand the issues that arise when this barrier function is lost. This poses a problem, of course, when it comes to chemicals that the body wants to get rid of because they have reached the end of their usefulness or are potentially harmful. An impervious barrier would keep them in. A controlled system is needed to allow such chemicals to be specifically transported out of the body. We have, therefore, evolved families of transporter molecules which cross the cell membranes (the linings of cells) of the epithelial cells which can transport chemicals into them and then out of the far side of the cell. This allows these chemicals to be transported, in the case of say bilirubin, into the hepatocyte where they are conjugated ("tagged") and then carried out of the far side into the bile canaliculus (the beginnings of the bile duct). Where these transporters fail to function normally there will be a failure in normal bile production. Clinically, this can have a very similar appearance to conditions where there is a physical blockage of bile flow, with build-up of bilirubin and jaundice as well as itch. There are four main settings where transporter dysfunction is seen

Drug Side Effects: A number of commonly used drugs can impact on the function of bile transporters. These include

- Oestrogens and progesterones as used in the oral contraceptive pill and hormone replacement therapy
- Some antibiotics, including in particular flucloxacillin, and anti-fungals (e.g. terbinafine used for nail fungal infections)
- Anti-psychotic and related drugs such as chlorpromazine
- Anabolic steroids

In some cases, this can evolve into a directly PBC-mimicking process with actual bile duct injury (presumably for the same reasons of cyclical injury as apply in PBC). Drug effects should be thought of in everyone presenting with clinical features suggestive of PBC (as they should be in everyone with liver disease) and if in doubt the drug should be stopped, at which point the liver injury will resolve if the drug is to blame. The recovery process can actually take some time.

Sepsis: Bile transporters can sometimes become "stunned" and fail to work normally when people have septicaemia (an active bacterial infection in the blood). This represents one of the reasons why very sick people can develop LFT abnormality. It resolves as the infection is controlled and shouldn't really give rise to confusion in diagnosis as the features of sepsis will usually be obvious. It is, however, one of the traps that unwary doctors can fall into; assuming that someone who is very sick and is jaundiced must be sick because they have severe liver disease. Sometimes it is just the sickness state that causes temporary liver injury.

Genetic Cholestasis: One of the most challenging differential diagnoses for PBC is genetic cholestasis. Genetic abnormalities occur in many, if not all, the transporters that are key for the transport of bile acids into the bile ducts, as well as protectant molecules such as bicarbonate and phosphatidylcholine which are essential for the health of the biliary epithelial cells. These give rise to a number of conditions such as Alagille's syndrome, Benign Recurrent Intra-Hepatic Cholestasis (BRIC) and Progressive Familial Intra-Hepatic Cholestasis (PFIC). This is a complex area and a detailed discussion is not relevant to this book. There are, however, a number of important points about these conditions. The first is that these are traditionally thought of as severe disease states, running in families and often presenting in childhood. The overlap with PBC would therefore appear, at first sight, limited. It is increasingly clear, however, that milder variants of a number of these conditions can occur, typically in adults and usually presenting with liver biochemistry abnormality and itch; features that do look like PBC. The second point is that the obvious test to look for them in potential patients, namely genetic testing, is costly and often not easily available out with the severe, more obviously familial cases. A positive diagnosis is therefore frequently difficult in practice. As with the other functional cholestasis states, the key feature if there is a genetic basis to disease is the absence of autoantibodies. This emphasises, once again, the importance of autoantibodies in making a positive diagnosis in PBC and the care that must be taken in diagnosing AMA/ANA negative disease. Genetic testing should be actively considered in autoantibody-negative patients with cholestasis and no alternative positive diagnostic history or tests.

Cholestasis in Pregnancy: Intrahepatic cholestasis of pregnancy (ICP) is a relatively common condition characterised by the onset of cholestasis towards the end of pregnancy. It can be associated with significant itch in the mother, with characteristics very similar to PBC itch. LFT abnormality and, in particular, elevation of serum bile acids (a test not frequently done in PBC but which is very commonly done in pregnancy–related liver disease settings) are common test findings. The main clinical significance of ICP is in the risk it poses to the baby towards the very end of pregnancy. For this reason, it is normal for the baby to be delivered one or two weeks early. ICP is thought to arise through the combined effects of high levels of oestrogen (with a mechanism therefore related to the oral contraceptive and HRT effect outlined earlier), and variations or abnormalities in transporter molecules. It can, accordingly, be thought of as a hybrid of drug-type and genetic-type cholestasis. The relevant history is, clearly, pregnancy. Furthermore, the mother will not have PBC autoantibodies. Distinguishing ICP and PBC should therefore be straightforward. It has been suggested that PBC patients are more likely to have a history of itching in pregnancy suggestive of the possibility of ICP. This may be recollection bias of the type described in **Chapter 3**. It may also be that this represents an early expression of PBC, perhaps made more overt because of the high oestrogen levels, which then settles after delivery. The disease then returns to its previous slower trajectory not re-emerging until several years later.

TO BIOPSY OR NOT BIOPSY?

This is one of the most contentious questions in the management of PBC. Historically, biopsy confirmation of the disease was seen as essential. The advent of the 3 diagnostic criteria, and the reliability of a diagnosis of "probable disease" based on the combination of AMA or PBC-ANA in the context of raised ALP, means that this is no longer the case. In fact, there is now a perception that biopsy is "no longer needed". Therefore, we have gone from a situation where everyone was biopsied to one where very few potential PBC patients have biopsy investigation of the disease. Where does the truth lie in terms of the need for biopsy? The following are my own thoughts on the issues around liver biopsy in PBC and a summary of my own practice.

- For the majority of patients, typically older, with mild elevation of ALP and clear-cut AMA a biopsy is not necessary for diagnosis. If the biopsy is positive for the disease you will treat with UDCA. If the biopsy comes back as normal, however, the patient will still have liver abnormality based on blood tests and will still have AMA. You will, therefore, still treat with UDCA. Ergo the biopsy has not changed your management.

- A normal biopsy despite blood tests suggestive of PBC is not as uncommon as you might think. PBC is, as we have discussed, a notoriously patchy disease with different areas of the liver involved to different degrees. It is not uncommon for a cirrhotic liver removed at transplant to be found to have areas of either normal liver tissue or very early disease. A biopsy is a small sample from one area of the organ. Is that area representative? The analogy I use is of picking one person from the crowd at a big football match and expecting them to be representative of the crowd as a whole. They could be an archetypal football supporter. However, they could be someone's 10 year old son. If it was the 10 year old son you picked you wouldn't use the information to assume that all football crowds were made up of 10 year olds……..

- The starting point for writing this book was, however, the fact that PBC is, in practice, often not managed as well as it could or should be. It is a disease that still kills people, or means they need a liver transplant. To argue for less diagnostic testing is therefore slightly counter-intuitive. The argument should be for better, smarter testing not simply more or less.

- If in doubt, biopsy is always the right thing to do. There are also certain situations when it is essential

    a) *Autoantibody negative disease*. If there are no autoantibodies then it is impossible to achieve the 2 diagnostic tests needed without a biopsy. The possibility of PSC weighs heavily here

    b) *Alternative additional diagnoses*. We are increasingly seeing patients with both PBC features and those of other chronic liver diseases such as non-alcoholic fatty liver disease (NAFLD). Where more than one potential diagnosis is present the only way to understand what is driving the disease is biopsy

    c) *Potential overlap disease*. If overlap is present then the treatment approach is likely to be different, involving steroids (an approach I would never use for simple PBC).

Because of the side effects and implications I would never start steroids for overlap without biopsy confirmation

d) *High risk disease.* The direction of travel in PBC is towards better treatment given earlier for people with high-risk disease. It is now clear that we can identify high-risk disease at the beginning of the disease process (younger patients, higher levels of biochemical abnormality etc) and the future focus will be towards a personalised approach to therapy. Confirmation of high risk disease, and identification of optimal treatment approaches, will increasingly require the information on disease process that only biopsy-based approaches can provide.

- The risks and discomfort associated with biopsy have been, perhaps, a little over-stated. Modern practice, where biopsy is done using "biopsy guns" under ultra-sound control, or via the jugular vein gaining direct access to the liver are very safe and with minimal discomfort associated.

MONITORING PBC

Once PBC has been diagnosed, and treatment has been started, we move to the monitoring phase of the disease. PBC can fluctuate and progress meaning that it needs to be watched carefully, typically on a life-long basis. The advent of current, more dynamic, management approaches means that ongoing assessment as to whether treatment is optimal is now more important than it has ever been. The approach to monitoring is described in detail in the next chapter. It matters, however, less who does the monitoring and, to a certain extent, what form the monitoring takes than that **someone does it and acts on the results**. In my experience, where opportunities to manage PBC better have been missed it is usually the case that the disease was monitored fine, but that the worsening results hadn't been acted upon. Recent data suggests that the most accurate prediction of future risk in PBC comes from a combination of blood tests and Fibroscan. Crucially, these test approaches give complementary information. Blood tests (especially alkaline phosphatase) focus very much on the degree of liver injury that is currently taking place (and which can be improved with treatment). Fibroscan focuses on the degree of scarring that is present as a result of previous injury and thus the risk of the complications of cirrhosis developing.

Table 1: Blood tests used in the diagnosis and assessment of PBC

Alkaline Phosphatase (ALP)	An enzyme (a form of protein) that is released by injured cells. Where levels are elevated it suggests that there is an increased level of cell injury. ALP is particularly produced by the cells lining the bile duct so elevation is suggestive of cholestatic disease such as PBC. It can also be produced by other organs (especially by growing or diseased bone) so ALP elevation on its own does not automatically mean liver disease is present. Liver disease is suggested if elevated ALP is accompanied by elevation in another liver enzyme Gamma-GT (below) or if an additional tests shows the ALP is of liver origin. In a woman over the age of 40 the commonest cause of an elevated ALP of liver origin is PBC and antibody testing (below should always follow its discovery).
Gamma-Glutamyl Transferase (Gamma-GT, GGT)	Another enzyme typically released by injured bile duct cells and measurable in a blood test. It can fluctuate more than ALP making it a less reliable test. In a PBC clinic it is largely used to confirm that elevated ALP is of liver origin. Many doctors believe that GGT elevation suggests high alcohol consumption. It doesn't and this is one of the sources of the fallacy about alcohol excess in PBC patients.
Bilirubin	By-product of the breakdown of the haem group of red blood cells (the molecule that contains the iron essential for haemoglobin function). It is produced in the spleen, carried to the liver by albumin, taken up by the hepatocytes and conjugated (attached to another molecule to allow its ejection out into the bile). Any failure in this pathway (increased breakdown of red cells, disordered transport to the liver, decreased conjugation capacity or blockage to bile flow) can lead to bilirubin elevation in the blood. This can be measured as a blood test and, if high enough, is visible as a yellowing of the skin (jaundice). The whites

	of the eyes (sclerae) are the part of the body where this can be most readily visible. In PBC, elevation of bilirubin is a relatively late feature and one that should always cause concern. Rising bilirubin is used clinically to decide if, and when, liver transplantation is appropriate.
Albumin	A serum protein produced at high levels by the liver. It plays a key role as a transporter molecule in the serum and, through the osmotic effect (a natural process whereby more concentrated solutions draw fluid into themselves to dilute their concentration), in controlling tissue fluid flux. It is reduced when hepatocellular function is decreased, as well as in malnutrition states (including those caused by abnormality in absorption of food from the diet). In keeping with other synthetic function measures in PBC it remains normal until very late indeed in the disease.
Prothrombin Time (PT)	This is one of the measures of the clotting function of the blood. It is very sensitive to reduced liver synthetic function of protein clotting factors, and also levels of the fat soluble vitamin K which is essential for clotting factor activation. Prolongation (beyond the normal time of 12 seconds), occurs within 30 minutes of the onset of liver failure making the test a highly useful one in monitoring acute liver functional status. In PBC prolongation is almost always because of vitamin K deficiency and "true" prolongation (i.e. even after vitamin K supplementation) is a rare and very late disease feature. In the population as a whole the commonest cause of PT prolongation is treatment with warfarin which acts through blockade of vitamin K function!
Immunoglobulin G and M (IgG and IgM)	Antibodies produced by the immune system in response to an infection or vaccination are immunoglobulins. Total immunoglobulin levels of two types are useful additional tests in PBC. The M fraction (IgM) is almost always elevated in PBC (although the level of

	elevation is not associated with disease severity). Occasionally, although it is not one of the classic diagnostic tests in PBC high IgM can help in making a diagnosis when other tests are inconclusive as there are few other causes of IgM elevation. The IgG fraction is elevated, in the setting of liver disease, in autoimmune hepatitis (AIH, a related but distinct autoimmune liver disease to PBC). PBC patients, importantly, sometimes also have an element of AIH (as discussed in **Chapter 4**) and this needs to be identified and managed as part of the disease spectrum if effective control is to be achieved. Elevated IgG is a useful marker to suggest that this overlap between PBC and AIH may be present.
Autoantibodies	Autoantibodies (antibodies produced by the immune system that react with the body's own structures) are almost universal in PBC and are an important feature for effective and, critically, early diagnosis. One of the reasons that autoantibodies are such a useful diagnostic test in PBC is that the pattern seen in the condition is an unusual and very specific one that occurs in no other diseases. The classic PBC autoantibody is ***Anti-Mitochondrial Antibody (AMA)*** which is present in over 95% of patients and if seen with abnormal liver biochemistry is diagnostic of the disease. Other test types are available ("anti-M2", "anti-PDC-E2" etc), however these are just technical alternatives to measuring the same antibody used by different laboratories and there is no significance between any of them in terms of meaning. PBC patients can also get very specific antibodies directed at the nucleus of cells (***Anti-Nuclear Antibody (ANA)***). ANA are more complicated than AMA and come in a number of different types. The commonest type, and one NOT associated with PBC other than in people with AIH overlap is a diffuse

	staining pattern across the nucleus. This is classically seen in Lupus (SLE) and AIH. The PBC ANA have characteristic staining patterns of multiple nuclear dots (MND) and nuclear rim (NR). Again other test varieties are available (anti-Sp100 and anti-gp210 respectively and, as with AMA, the difference between the findings with different tests are not clinically meaningful. ANA are not as common in PBC as AMA with, in the UK, around 20-30% of patients showing positivity. Occasional patients are AMA negative and ANA positive. Provided the ANA are PBC-specific as discussed above these antibodies are as diagnostic for PBC as AMA are.

CHAPTER 5: **TREATING PBC**

The 2-Minute Version

- PBC should be thought of as being **fully treatable.** It is increasingly clear that failure to get complete control of the condition is more related to failure of doctors to make a timely diagnosis and to use the treatment options that are now available than it is to lack of effectiveness of those treatments.

- Most people are diagnosed when the disease is early, and the goals of treatment are to prevent progression to cirrhosis and to treat symptoms.

- If cirrhosis is already present, or develops despite treatment, it is still important to treat PBC to protect the remaining liver, although some of the newer drugs should be used only cautiously in people with more advanced cirrhosis. It is also important to look for, and treat, the complications of cirrhosis (such as varices) which can pose a direct risk. Where significant complications of cirrhosis have occurred the potential value of transplantation should be considered (**Chapter 6**).

- The initial treatment for all patients with PBC, at all stages of the disease, is **Ursodeoxycholic Acid** (UDCA or "urso") at a dose of 13-15mg/Kg body weight (83-96mg/stone body weight). This gives a typical dose of between 600 and 1200 mg per day. UDCA is less effective if the dose is too low so it is important to get it right.

- Most people can take UDCA fine. Sometimes it causes nausea, in which case reduce the dose at first and build it up slowly. We recommend people take the whole dose in the evening. If you are taking cholestyramine ("Questran") for itch it is important to space it away from UDCA. UDCA does not reverse PBC, just controls it, and should therefore continue life-long.

- For many people, UDCA is the only treatment they need and with this treatment their life-expectancy returns to normal. In some people additional therapy is also needed to get better control of the disease. The need for additional treatment is decided on liver blood tests done after a minimum of 12 months of UDCA. People identified as needing additional treatment are conventionally called "UDCA non-responders" although in reality even they are getting some response to UDCA; just not enough.

- The main, and the only licensed, second-line therapy (in 2023) is **obeticholic acid (OCA)** which is approved for use in PBC patients showing an inadequate response to UDCA, or who cannot tolerate UDCA. It is normally taken along with UDCA. It can often have dramatic effects on liver biochemistry within a short period of time. The starting dose is 5mg per day (unlike UDCA it is not adjusted by body weight) with the dose increased to 10mg if it is tolerated well and the desired improvement in tests is not seen with the lower dose. The starting dose must be reduced in people with more advanced cirrhosis (to 5mg once per week). If cirrhosis is too advanced with, for example the development of varices or jaundice, OCA should be avoided completely.

- OCA is usually well tolerated. In some people itch can be made worse by OCA but this typically responds to the usual treatments used for PBC itch (**Chapter 7**). Bezafibrate (or fenofibrate in the USA) is not licensed for use in PBC but can be a useful alternative to OCA when itch is an ongoing problem. Kidney and liver toxicity can be seen and it should, as with OCA, be used really carefully in cirrhosis. The combination of OCA and bezafibrate along with UDCA is under evaluation in a clinical trial. This combination is, however, already in use in specialist centres. The addition of bezafibrate to OCA appears to both increase effectiveness compared to either agent alone and seems to mitigate any itch caused by OCA.

- A number of further drug options are currently being evaluated as alternative second-line therapies. Results look promising. Clinical trials are ongoing and the opportunity to take part in such trials should be considered as an option for UDCA non-responders.

- A small number of PBC patients also have features of autoimmune hepatitis and are described as having "overlap". Where this is really the case steroids and other immune therapies can be useful. Overlap has been over-diagnosed in the past, however, and many people treated with steroids who do not really need them now we understand more about high risk PBC and the role of drugs such as OCA. All past diagnoses of overlap should be re-considered in the light of current advances in PBC.

- Treating symptoms is an integral part of treating PBC and is covered in **Chapter 7.**

Once PBC has been diagnosed it is crucial to move on to effective management. There are two aspects to the management of any chronic disease. The first is the specific treatments that are used (drugs, operations etc) to improve the clinical outcome in the disease. The second, and equally important aspect, is the framework in which that treatment is given and monitored, and in which the patient is supported. There can be a tendency for doctors to focus on the former and to put less emphasis on the latter. Living with PBC, and making sure that life quality is as close to normal as is possible, requires, however, both aspects of management to be as high quality as possible. Emerging data from the UK and other countries suggests that there are limitations in the effectiveness of treatment for PBC in practice across large parts of the country. If, after reading this book, you feel that you aren't getting the treatment you should be ask why not!!

TREATING THE DISEASE ITSELF

PBC should be thought of, in 2023, as an (almost) completely treatable disease. Too often, however, patients end up putting up with second best treatment given in a haphazard way. Patients themselves, working with the patient groups, have a major role to play in ensuing that each individual gets access to the same very high quality care. One of the mantras that patients coming to my clinic are familiar with is one of "owning the problem and owning the solution". By this I mean accepting the diagnosis and its implications, and playing an active role in making sure that you get the best possible treatment to live the longest and best life that you can.

The aims of treatment: It may seem strange to talk in terms of the aims of treating PBC. Is the answer not obvious? In fact, it is a little bit more complex than clinicians often think and this can lead to missed treatment opportunities. There are two broad aims to treatment. The first is to make life span as close to normal as is possible. The second is to make the quality of that life as high as we can. The critical point is that these two goals are, to a significant degree, independent. Many clinicians assume that if you achieve the former the latter will naturally follow. This is frequently not the case. Disease risk obviously warrants being a major focus of treatment. The symptoms of disease that impact on quality of life, however, should be thought of as equally important and need effective treatment in their own right.

Treatment aimed at lengthening life in PBC is, in the first instance, targeted at slowing progression of the disease to either liver failure or the development of cirrhosis with its associated complications. As outlined in **Chapter 3** there are two advanced disease risk processes in PBC; the development of cirrhosis as with all chronic liver diseases (albeit with a different pattern because of the biliary nature of the disease) and the development of significant ductopenia. The division is, to an extent, arbitrary, as the approach to treatment is largely the same (at least at present). Once cirrhosis has developed there are specific approaches which need to be taken to reduce the risk of complications. These are outlined later in this chapter. Where advanced liver disease has developed, liver transplant may be an important treatment option. In this chapter we will explore the things that would make us think that transplant might be appropriate. Transplant itself will be considered in **Chapter 6**. Symptom management will be considered in detail in **Chapter 7**.

Standard practice has evolved in PBC is recent years. We now use first line therapy, assess response, and where needed, move to adding a second agent. I will consider both, as well as the complex question of overlap between PBC and AIH and what it means for treatment.

First-line treatment for PBC: Ursodeoxycholic Acid (UDCA, frequently referred to by patients as "urso") is standard first line therapy and should be offered to all patients. The standard dose is 13 to 15 mg/Kg of body weight and it needs to be adjusted up or down if body weight changes. The first observations that UDCA is a useful drug for PBC came in the 1980s, with a number of important trials carried out in the 1990s. Although these weren't without controversy (the true extent of the benefit with UDCA in these trials was argued about for a long time) long-term follow up studies such as UK-PBC and the Global PBC study have demonstrated, beyond any doubt, that UDCA slows progression to cirrhosis and reduces the risk of death or need for transplant. There is also evidence to suggest that UDCA reduces the risk of bleeding from varices. UDCA is, therefore, regarded as the bedrock of treatment for PBC. PBC patients started on UDCA typically see a reasonably rapid improvement in their liver function tests. In some patients these tests normalise. In the majority, however, they improve but fail to return completely to normal. It is very unusual for patients to show no improvement with UDCA. If UDCA is discontinued for any reason tests will typically revert back to their starting point as the drug controls the disease rather than having a more profound curative or reversing effect. This means that once started it should be regarded as a life-long therapy.

Perhaps surprisingly, given that it has been in widespread use in PBC for so long, we still don't completely understand the mode of action of UDCA. It is itself a bile acid with a hydrophilic structure (meaning that it dissolves in water) thereby contrasting with the bile acids that typically build up in PBC which are hydrophobic (i.e. don't dissolve in water) in nature and are, in contrast to UDCA, toxic to the liver and bile duct cells. Mechanisms of action for UDCA, all of which may be beneficial in PBC include

- Displacement of hydrophobic bile acids within the bile acid pool. Because UDCA is a bile acid it is taken up from the bowel and enters the entero-hepatic circulation, being returned to the liver and then transported back into the bile. This results in a less irritant bile pool reducing cholestatic damage. Patients taking a standard dose of UDCA can end up with UDCA making up over 50% of their bile acid pool.

- Anti-apoptotic actions. Apoptosis of the biliary epithelial cells is a key disease process and UDCA may protect against this.

- Antioxidant effects. Oxidant stress (the damage caused by the release of free-radicals in tissue) is a big part of the disease process in PBC. UDCA is one of the agents that can reduce this effect, reducing tissue damage.

UDCA is normally very well tolerated by patients, although some people can struggle with sickliness. Where this is an issue, two things are worth trying. The first is to split the dose. We usually recommend that UDCA is taken as a single dose last thing at night. It is sometimes easier to tolerate if it is taken in split doses during the day (actually the way that the patient information recommends it should be used, although this was designed for its original and now redundant use of dissolving gallstones). The other approach, if you are struggling with it, is to start with a very low dose and build up. In fact, UDCA takes a while to build up in the system (it needs to displace other bile acids in the bile pool) so takes a while to have its full effect. Slowing this a little further by phasing the commencement does not, therefore, make any meaningful difference to the long-term effectiveness. Other issues reported by some patients include slight hair loss and weight gain. These are not normally, however, significant enough to act as a barrier to the use of UDCA in practice.

One dosing issue that people do need to be aware of is an interaction with cholestyramine (Questran) which is a standard therapy widely used for itch. Cholestyramine works by binding to bile acids in the bowel and transporting them out into the stool. As UDCA is a bile acid this binds to cholestyramine as well, meaning that if the two are taken together you lose the effectiveness of both of them. The interaction isn't harmful; it's just that you lose the benefit of both.

A major advance in understanding UDCA treatment, and the answer to many of the questions raised in the early days of its use, was the observation by the Paris and Barcelona teams that the response to it was variable in terms of its adequacy. In simple terms, some patients got a sufficient response to it to return their risk of death to that seen in the normal healthy population, whilst some only got a partial response. These groups have been termed "UDCA responders" and "UDCA non-responders" respectively. This terminology isn't strictly correct as most people show some degree of response. The terms UDCA "full-responder" and "partial-responder" would probably be more accurate. The terms responder and non-responder have, however, entered widespread clinical use.

The existence of UDCA response and non-response have now been confirmed in very large populations, and assessment of UDCA response has entered into normal clinical practice. It is essential for all PBC patients on UDCA to know their response status. If you don't know ask your doctor! The identification of UDCA non-responders is really important because it is now standard practice to move to additional treatment; second-line therapy.

The Newcastle protocol for using UDCA in practice is outlined in Appendix 3.

The concept of second-line treatment: The concept of UDCA response and non-response is easy to understand. Its application into practice has been more complex and the source of much confusion! The reason why UDCA is incompletely effective in some people is not fully understood. It does not appear to be that the drug is changed in any way in non-responders. Similarly, it doesn't appear to be a resistance process as such. My suspicion is that it all relates to the aggression of the disease process in some people, and an imbalance between the severity of the disease process and the capacity of UDCA to modify it. The analogy I use in the clinic is one of trying to put out a fire with a bucket of water. If it is a waste-paper bin fire, it works fine. If it is a house fire, it does not. This idea is supported by the mode of action of almost all effective second-line therapies of PBC identified to date, which is to give an active cholestatic (bile acid production reducing) effect, complementing the more passive, bile-acid displacing role of UDCA. In terms of second-line therapy in practice there is currently one drug, **Obeticholic Acid (*Ocaliva*)** which is licensed for use in PBC. A second drug, **Bezafibrate** (generic so no trade name) has been shown, in a high quality trial, to be effective in PBC and is licensed for use, but its license does not include PBC. A number of other drugs are under clinical evaluation at present. In all instances it is current practice to continue with UDCA therapy when starting second-line therapy (i.e. we move to a combination of treatments rather than changing treatment).

What does licensing mean and does it matter to patients? A licence for a drug means that it has been assessed by a regulatory body (the Food and Drug Administration (FDA) in the USA and the European Medicines Agency (EMA) in Europe) as being both safe for use in a disease and effective. In many ways, safety is the primary concern as the licensing process in its current form arose in response to drug injury scandals, such as that linked to Thalidomide, where unsafe drugs were made available to vulnerable patients. Effectiveness is clearly important as well, as a safe but ineffective drug would indirectly harm you by not treating the disease. Drug licensing implies that a high bar has been cleared for both safety and effectiveness;

something which should give patients confidence. A licence per se does not mean that a drug will be available to all patients though. Depending on the health care system there will typically be a second stage of assessment of a drug by the body that will pay for it if the patient isn't paying directly (the NHS through NICE in the UK and the insurance companies in the USA). In this second stage the licensed drug will be assessed as to whether it is effective enough to justify the cost.

In order for a drug to be licenced it will need to have been shown to be effective and safe in clinical trials. The process of evaluating drug effectiveness and safety in clinical trials involves several stages or phases. In Phase 1 trials the drug is given to healthy volunteers to assess blood levels for given doses (starting with very low doses), and to ensure that there is no toxicity (in cancer Phase 1 trials are sometimes done in patients). Phase 2 trials are where the drug moves to patients. These are small trials with a short duration, principally to show that the drug is safe in patients who might be very different in their age and physical status to healthy volunteers. We are also looking in Phase 2 for evidence that the drug is effective for the disease, typically through improvement of an aspect of the disease which is meaningful and measureable (such as blood tests). If a drug is safe, and there is evidence to suggest that it is effective, then it moves to Phase 3. These are the larger and longer clinical trials with an end-point, or trial question, that is highly relevant to patients (ideally survival or avoidance of a major and meaningful endpoint such as, in the case of liver disease, liver transplantation). A typical phase 3 trial might still only involve the patients getting the drug for a couple of years so it is common to have what is called a long-term safety extension where the drug is, if participants in the trial want it, available for, typically, another 5 years during which the longer term effects are monitored.

In all good quality trials the effect of the new drug needs to be compared directly with either a dummy or placebo (if there is no currently available treatment in the space) or with the current most effective treatment ("standard of care") if such a treatment is available. Trials include a high level of monitoring of participants. This is partly to ensure safety but also to ensure that all the possible evidence to support the drug being licensed is collected (it would be a disaster if a drug clearly works but the tests collected don't manage to show it because they are the wrong ones; it happens!). To license a drug the FDA or EMA will typically want to see that the drug is safe and that it is effective in a minimum of 2 Phase 3 trials. In the case of rare diseases (ones, such as PBC, where there are fewer than 500 patients per million of the population) trials are more difficult to carry out. In such rare disease states, and where there is real unmet need, licensing may come on the back of one Phase 3 trial and one Phase 2, provided both support the drug. There typically, however, then needs to be another trial, this time after licensing, to confirm that the drug truly is effective.

Once a drug is licensed it will be provided with a "label". This is a description of the situations in which it is approved for use (the disease area, the types of that disease and, importantly, the situations when it shouldn't be used). This is all important in practice in a disease such as PBC where there are only limited numbers of licensed and labelled drugs (i.e. drugs licensed for use specifically in PBC). If a drug is licensed and labelled for use in a disease, and the patient meets all the conditions for use (typically around kidney function being normal/acceptable, pregnancy, breast feeding etc) then a doctor can prescribe it with full legal protection (the issue of whether the health authorities or insurance companies in their country will pay for it and thus "allow" it to be prescribed is a slightly different question). At the other end of the spectrum, an un-licensed drug can only ever be used as part of a clinical trial that has gone through all the approvals to check for safety and which is being monitored closely (the route to the drug becoming licensed). The grey area is where a drug is licensed for use in another disease area but not PBC (i.e. licensed but not labelled for use in PBC). This is important because a number of the drugs widely used in PBC fall into this category, most notably bezafibrate which is increasingly being used as second-line therapy, and rifampicin which is a key drug for the management of itch, and which will be discussed in **Chapter 7.**

Obeticholic Acid: Obeticholic Acid (*Ocaliva*, typically abbreviated to OCA*)*, and previously known by its development code-name INT-747, is the only currently licensed drug with a label for second-line use in PBC. It also has a label for use as alternative first line therapy in patients unable to tolerate UDCA (UDCA is obviously the other drug which is licensed and has a label for first line use in PBC). The criteria for use is in patients "showing an inadequate response to UDCA". As I will discuss later, this sounds a more straightforward thing to identify in theory than is the case in practice because of the different test sets that people use. It is important to note, however, that the label to use OCA doesn't specify any numerical criteria. It is typically used as an add-on to UDCA (i.e. patients taking OCA typically continue on UDCA as well), although an additional Phase 2 trial has shown that OCA is highly effective on its own. Unlike UDCA, the dose is not adjusted for patient weight; instead, patients are started on a low dose (5mg daily) and, if they are tolerating it well and have not responded fully, the dose is increased to 10mg/day.

One critically important issue with OCA is that it must be used either very cautiously, or in some cases avoided completely in people with cirrhosis. This is because the body can struggle to handle the drug if advanced cirrhosis is present. What does this mean in practice? The first thing to say is that for the vast majority of PBC patients who might benefit from OCA it has no implications at all as most such people don't have cirrhosis. Indeed, the whole "point" of using OCA is to stop them getting cirrhosis. Where people do have cirrhosis it is critical to assess the severity before deciding if OCA is suitable. Guidance in the USA says that OCA shouldn't be used at all in people with "decompensated cirrhosis". Technically this is defined as Childs B or C cirrhosis or Childs A cirrhosis with evidence of portal hypertension (I said it was technical!). Your doctor will be able to advise you as to whether this apples to you or not. In essence it means that the drug should not be used in people with varices, and may not be suitable for people with jaundice, ascites or hepatic encephalopathy. People with early, uncomplicated cirrhosis can take OCA but the dose must be adjusted. We take a very cautious approach in all patients and start at 5mg once a week with a very cautious increase to an absolute maximum of 10mg twice per week.

The trials of OCA in PBC have given a very consistent message. They have all been conducted in patients who are UDCA non-responders (there is currently no reason to use OCA in patients who are able to tolerate UDCA and have responded to it, although, as we will discuss later in the book, there are now trials going on to explore its use in different settings in PBC) and show a response rate of around 50% (compared with 10% in the placebo group). As is the case with UDCA, patients not meeting the response criteria for OCA almost always show some level of improvement, just one that falls short of the pre-defined response cut-offs. The trials suggest that, with the exception of two issues discussed in the next two paragraphs, OCA is very safe in PBC. The more our experience of its use grows (and it has now been used in thousands of PBC patients around the world) the more confident we become with regard to its safety.

OCA appears to work through very specific actions on key processes that contribute to PBC liver injury. Firstly, it reduces the production of bile acids in recipients. This is in keeping with its predicted mode of action as an activator of the Farnesoid X Receptor (FXR), the body's natural sensing system for bile acids. When activated, FXR switches off bile acid production (both directly and through the release of another molecule called FGF-19 which is released by the bowel in response to FXR, travels in the portal venous blood to the liver and has the switching off effect). Given the pivotal role for hydrophobic bile acids in PBC, this mechanism is likely to be directly beneficial. Secondly it appears to reduce both inflammation and fibrosis in the liver.

What OCA doesn't appear to have (at least in the ways we currently use it) is any beneficial effect on PBC symptoms. In fact, the only clear symptom effect of OCA is to worsen itch in some patients. The reasons why OCA worsens itch are not at present clear, but it does appear to be typical PBC itch. Importantly, it responds to the same approaches as non-OCA itch, in particular rifampicin (**Chapter 7**). In our clinic we take the approach of "dealing with the problem before it arises" by assessing potential OCA candidates for itch prior to beginning the drug and aggressively treating it. If, after OCA has been started, itch arises or worsens despite treatment then dose reduction in OCA is tried. This is ideally short-term, before it is built back up again to full dose. As experience of OCA use in normal clinical practice grows, so the issues with itch seem to have lessened and we are now at the point, I think, where the concerns are a little over-stated. Why is itch less of a problem than it initially seemed to be? I think there are a number of factors at play. Firstly, we use lower doses than was the case in the original trials where the problem was first seen (these used up to 50mg a day in comparison to the 5mg a day we start people on today). Secondly, we are now aware of the problem and can both warn patients in advance and control the symptom before we start OCA. This makes a big difference. Finally, if itch does develop we now understand how to treat it effectively (including through the use of a combination of OCA and bezafibrate). If OCA is the right treatment for your liver disease then the risk of itch is a perfectly manageable consideration.

There is a final, really important, consideration which is how far do the benefits of OCA go in terms of actually changing the course of PBC? We know with confidence that it significantly improves liver function test values. We also know that the worse the liver function test values the greater the risk of dying from PBC or needing a liver transplant. Therefore OCA must be reducing the risk of death or need for transplant, mustn't it? That is a reasonable extrapolation but it is an extrapolation all the same. There is always the potential for a drug to improve liver function test numbers independently of any improvement in the underlying disease (breaking the connection between the blood values and the actual risk). The only way to truly answer this is to do a long-term clinical trial of OCA, compared to placebo, with death or transplant as the disease outcome. The problem is that this is simply impossible in the real world in 2023 when the drug is already available. Would you want to go into a 10 year clinical trial involving a placebo arm, having been told that you are high risk, when you could just get the treatment on the NHS? Thought not.

How, then, do we know whether drugs such as OCA are actually benefitting people (in which case they are a good thing) or are just making some numbers better without real benefit (in which case you are potentially missing the opportunity to get better treatment whilst wasting a lot of money). This is where a very interesting concept of "virtual trials" incorporating "real world data" come in. This has been a major area of progress in PBC since the first edition of this book and one that points the way to progress in other disease areas which are "stuck" in terms of progress. At the heart of this approach is the data that have been collected as part of the very big PBC studies run by UK-PBC and the Global PBC Study Group. Between them they have over 20,000 records of test results for PBC patients together with outcome information (essentially what happened to people). In an actual trial a group of people would be identified who met the criteria for disease severity and they would randomly be given OCA or a placebo. We would then look at what happened to them over a length of time. Amongst the 20,000 people in the UK-PBC and Global PBC databases there are people who met the study criteria and had been treated with OCA by their clinicians as part of normal practice. There are also people who have similar disease but who didn't get OCA (mainly because they had disease before the OCA era). Can we compare what happens to these two groups of people as if they were in a trial? A virtual trial if you like. The short answer is that you can and it is a very powerful tool indeed. This has been done in PBC and shows, to a very high degree of certainty, that people who were UDCA non-responders who took OCA lived longer, and were more likely to avoid transplant, than equivalent people who didn't take OCA. This provides the best evidence to date to suggest that OCA really does improve outcomes in PBC and not just improve blood tests. Is this approach as accurate as a clinical trial? No, it is subject to potential biases such as the reason why people didn't get OCA (if there disease event was in the OCA era). The data derived using this approach are, however, infinitely more helpful than even the world's most perfect trial if that trial can't actually be done!

Bezafibrate: The second drug which is widely used as second-line therapy in PBC is bezafibrate (its cousin fenofibrate is also used but to a lesser extent). It is a drug that originally entered use to treat high cholesterol levels, although its use in that setting largely died out with the advent of the statins (probably more effective and have a cardiac protecting effect not seen with fibrates). It, as is the case with OCA, acts on the pathways regulating bile acid synthesis, although it doesn't work through FXR. Instead it works on another nuclear receptor called PPAR (peroxisome proliferator-activated receptor). Although it is increasingly widely used, the evidence to support its use is more limited than for OCA (a single formal trial and a number of earlier case series in which the effect of the drug was observed in groups of patients but a placebo group was not included). The key bezafibrate trial had a similar design to the OCA trials (the drug was compared to the effect of placebo in a group of patients who were non-responders to UDCA (although, as with the OCA trial participants, continued UDCA)) and a seemingly similar response profile. One important difference was that the bezafibrate trial used a lower level of abnormality of alkaline phosphatase as an entry criterion meaning that the treated group had less severe disease. This means that the effects of the 2 drugs are not directly comparable, and it raises a slight question as to how effective bezafibrate will prove to be in patients with the most aggressive disease; the group where it is most important to see a benefit. Unlike OCA, there are no data to suggest whether it is effective in patients not also taking UDCA. There was no real evidence from the trial to suggest an effect on fatigue. In marked contrast to OCA, though, there was no worsening of itch and subsequent studies have suggested that, in fact, the drug has a useful anti-itch action. There is some evidence from real world studies to suggest that bezafibrate improves survival in PBC. The approach taken was, however, less sophisticated than for the equivalent OCA study and the findings must therefore be regarded as less robust

Bezafibrate can have some side effects in PBC patients, including kidney impairment (usually reversible) and, on occasions, worsening of liver biochemistry. One issue is that, unlike itch with OCA which typically comes on early after the drug is started, renal and liver issues with bezafibrate can develop years down the line, often at a time when an "eye has been take off the ball" in terms of blood test monitoring. If people take bezafibrate long-term in PPBC they really do need their blood tests to be checked AND THE RESULTS LOOKED AT regularly. As is the case with OCA, bezafibrate should only be used with real caution in cirrhotic patients, especially if the bilirubin is elevated. The potential toxicity issues draw attention to the main issue with bezafibrate therapy in PBC. Although it is a licensed drug (and has been for many years) its label is for lowering cholesterol. It has no label for use in PBC. One aspect of this is that it has not been evaluated for durability of its actions and long-term safety in PBC to the same degree as OCA. This means that the question of its suitability for long-term use in PBC (the normal situation in PBC where we are looking for effective and stable regimes for long-term use) has a question mark against it.

In some countries, notably the USA, bezafibrate is not licensed at all meaning that it is not available to PBC patients other than in the setting in the trial. Other similar drugs are available and the most widely used is fenofibrate. The data in relation to fenofibrate use in PBC are, if anything, even more limited than they are for bezafibrate and there are no direct comparisons to guide us.

Other Drugs: All other drugs being used for second-line therapy in PBC at the time of writing are still experimental and are undergoing clinical trials. They really split into two groups, anti-cholestatics and others. The anti-cholestatics (in other words the drugs that actively suppress toxic bile acid production) really build on the actions of OCA and bezafibrate with the hope of identifying increased effectiveness or better tolerability. Although non-OCA FXR agonists have been explored in PBC (for example **Tropifexor**) none appear to offer any advantage over OCA (all still cause itch in a small number of people) and none are currently heading towards licensing and clinical use. The drug category where there has been most activity is the

PPAR agonists (i.e. drugs working on the same receptor type as bezafibrate). One of the reasons why there appears to be potential for improved action (compared to the original version bezafibrate) is that unlike FXR, PPAR comes in a number of different forms with different actions. The PPAR agonist drugs all work in slightly different ways with a differing "mix" of activation of the different receptor sub-types (think of it as being like a musical chord; one sound made up of different notes). The two key PPAR subtypes in PBC are alpha (α) and delta (δ). Bezafibrate, the archetype drug in the class mainly works on α with a small amount of action on δ. In contrast, fenofibrate (often thought of as having equivalent action to bezafibrate but to be slightly less effective) works entirely on α (i.e. it is actually a little different in action). This observation hinted at the possibility that PPAR agonists with more δ activity may be an interesting option in PBC (there are also some more specific rationales for why PPARδ agonists may be more effective related to receptor distribution and cell expression pattern). Is this the case? This is where the two emerging novel PPAR agonists come in, both of which are now in phase 3 trial and showing promising results. **Elafibranor** is a mixed α and δ agonists but with a greater level of δ than α (i.e. a little bit like bezafibrate but with the proportion of activity reversed). **Seladelpar** is a pure δ agonist. What do we know about these two drugs from the phase 2 trials? Both appear very effective at improving liver biochemistry (more so than bezafibrate) and both also appear to significantly improve itch. There are some signals around fatigue improvement, largely, I suspect, as a result of their anti-itch effect improving sleep. What we don't as yet know is whether safety is an issue long term (i.e. do they have the same potential safety issues as bezafibrate) and, of course, whether they improve actual survival. The important thing to say is that both are undergoing proper long term trial evaluation (which is what hasn't happened for bezafibrate) meaning that we will be able to answer the safety issues and then use a virtual trial/synthetic control model as was used for OCA in order to get some information about disease efficacy.

What about the other, non-cholestatic drugs? Are there options for other drugs that don't work through modulating bile acid biology? One such drug which has trial evidence to suggest benefit in PBC is **budesonide**. This is a drug which probably has a number of different modes of action. One is a steroid-like effect but without side-effects. Budesonide acts like prednisolone but, unlike prednisolone, is broken down in the liver and does not reach the general circulation. It thus has an effect on the liver but no side-effects beyond the liver (in theory at least). The whole issue of steroids and PBC is a complex one. We don't ever use them (other than in overlap), however there is trial evidence from many years ago to suggest that they are actually beneficial in PBC (albeit not sufficiently beneficial to outweigh the side effects). A drug which had the benefits of prednisolone without its downsides would thus be, in theory, useful. Budesonide may, however, have an additional action in the liver which is to increase the protective bicarbonate umbrella which reduces the injury to the bile duct cells caused by toxic bile. Does it work in PBC? The answer is yes and no. The primary endpoint of the recent trial of use in UDCA non-responders (the main question if you like) was around improvement in liver biopsy. This wasn't met so technically budesonide was shown "not to work". However, and it is an important however, liver function tests (the primary end point in all other recent PBC trials) did improve significantly. If biopsy hadn't been included (as it isn't in other trials) we would be saying that budesonide was an effective drug. A reasonable conclusion would be that budesonide has interesting potential applications in PBC and warrants further investigation.

A second different mode of action drug is **setanaxib**. A completely different approach to PBC treatment. It is an inhibitor of an enzyme called NADPH oxidase (and the only such drug in trial use at the moment). NADPH oxidase plays a major role in inflammation, contributing to free radical production and oxidative stress in diseases such as PBC. Given the importance of these mechanisms of tissue injury in the bile duct it is a logical therapy. The trials to date, again in UDCA non-responders, suggest that it has some LFT improving action but a more marked effect on Fibroscan. At face value this suggests that it may control or even reverse scarring or fibrosis in PBC. If so it is the only drug yet shown to have this effect. This is currently being explored in further trials. Setanaxib also appears to have a significant impact on fatigue, something which I will expand on in the next section. I strongly suspect that both budesonide and setanaxib will turn out to be beneficial in PBC. I also suspect that they may have their greatest use in combination with conventional anti-cholestatic therapy such as UDCA and OCA. How we will navigate the pathway to developing these combination therapies will be a key question in PBC.

The final group of drugs for discussion in this section is the one that is missing. These are the new and powerful immuno-modulating drugs; drugs that we might imagine would be useful in PBC given its autoimmune component. All drugs which have targeted the autoimmune response in PBC to date have been found to be ineffective (perhaps with the exception of budesonide although even that might be to do with non-immune actions. This seemingly paradoxical lack of activity is especially the case for a group of powerful immune system modifiers known as biologicals. Highly effective in a number of other autoimmune diseases, they seemed a logical choice in PBC. Why were they so ineffective? It seems likely that the time-point chosen to use them, after UDCA failure, was one where the features of cholestasis were predominating. In simple terms they were probably used too late in the disease. It may be that to be effective they either need to be used much earlier in the disease when the immune features are predominating, or alternatively in combination with one of the potent second-line anti-cholestasis drugs to ensure that all aspects of PBC pathogenesis are being addressed.

When to Use Second-Line Therapy and Which to Choose: In current practice, second-line therapy is used once first line therapy with UDCA has been proven to be ineffective. This is, conventionally, after a year of therapy at the appropriate dose (13-15mg/Kg). What constitutes proof that UDCA has not been effective is more complex than it perhaps needs to be, with multiple different criteria having been defined, all of which are variations on the theme of ongoing elevation of alkaline phosphatase, bilirubin and, less frequently, alanine transaminase. If these tests all return to normal with UDCA then a patient has responded fully and no further treatment for disease risk needs to be considered (although this may change over time if control of the disease slips meaning that long-term monitoring of test results is needed). Where the blood tests are slightly abnormal after UDCA the risk appears to be limited, and watching and seeing how things develop is the correct path. Where the blood tests remain significantly abnormal, risk is increased, and second-line therapy is appropriate. All the different criteria proposed give a slightly different answer to the question "what constitutes significant abnormality of tests" in the above approach and this is where confusion can arise. All were developed in a specific patient group, and shown to be valid in that population, and all remain accurate in other populations (although the level of accuracy varies from population to population and is typically lower in the second population than the one in which they were specifically developed). Each has its advocates, usually the people who derive them! The net result is, however, confusion for patients and frustration for clinicians who want a binary answer (yes or no for using second-line therapy) but can get a different answer from different criteria.

It is my view that the biggest risk to patients with severe PBC is that they do not get second-line therapy when they need it because of this confusion, and that this risk far outweighs the risk that you end up using the wrong criteria. Simple is good. In our clinic, the cut-offs we use are an alkaline phosphatase of 1.67 times the upper limit of normal (a value of 217 for our laboratory) and a bilirubin of greater than the upper limit of normal (a value of 20). These are the criteria used for the licensing of OCA, meaning that they are the ones with the most direct link to therapy decisions (they are called the "POISE" criteria after the Phase 3 OCA trial of that name). As I will discuss in **Chapter 9** it is really important for patients to push for the right treatment. Knowing the targets for blood tests is a really good way to do that. As I will discuss later, it is likely that we will see, over the next few years, a tightening up of what we see as acceptable results as out treatment options improve and we become more ambitious about the quality of care in PBC

Which second-line therapy to use is also quite a contentious issue. OCA is the licensed therapy with the best understood safety profile and probably should be first choice. My exception to this rule is in patients with milder PBC (UDCA non-responders but only just if you like) but severe itch. In this situation, where the gain from OCA may be relatively minor and the downside from itch potentially significant (although remember that the issues with OCA aren't quite the problem that people originally thought they were, bezafibrate can be a more logical choice. Many clinicians are using bezafibrate rather than OCA for reasons of costs. They should be cautious. Appropriate practice is to use licensed and labelled therapy where available and there are no good reasons not to use it. If labelled therapy is not available for the indication then it is appropriate to use the unlabelled drug (if licensed, remember unlicensed drugs should only ever be used in clinical trials). An example of this being acceptable is rifampicin for significant itch. When doing this patients should be advised that the drug is not labelled for PBC use, and the reasons for choosing it explained. Using this logic, it is appropriate to use bezafibrate in a UDCA non-responder with significant itch or who had not responded to OCA (in each case there is a specific and reasonable justification for using it). Choosing bezafibrate over OCA simply for reasons of price would probably not be seen as reasonable were the patient to not get good disease control or to get side effects. In this situation the patient (or their lawyers!) might reasonably ask whether they had had the recognised treatment.

If you are taking bezafibrate ask your doctor why. There may be a good reason that relates to benefit to you. There does, however, have to be a good reason and you need to understand what it is!

The Newcastle protocol for using second-line therapy in practice is outlined in Appendix 3.

Overlap and its implications for management: PBC-AIH overlap is one of the most controversial areas of PBC therapy and one of the biggest challenges for clinicians. The proposed process is a combination of both PBC and AIH occurring in the same patient at the same time. The questions are 4-fold. Does it actually really exist, if so how common is it, what else could it be and if it is present how do you manage it?

My view is that overlap definitely exists, but that it is rare. Many of the people said to have it in the past probably did not and do not have it, although many are still being treated incorrectly for it. The issue revolves around the liver biopsy appearance of interface hepatitis and the presence of anti-nuclear antibodies (**Chapter 4**). Until recently, both were thought to be features only of autoimmune hepatitis, meaning that patients with either or both of them were diagnosed as having an AIH component to their disease. If they also had AMA, or biopsy features of PBC, this meant they had both conditions and the label of overlap was given. Interface hepatitis is now known, however, to occur in aggressive PBC. Furthermore, PBC-specific ANA are just that, ANA which suggest PBC not AIH. The conclusion is that the "cardinal features of AIH", which underpin the diagnosis of the AIH component of overlap are no such thing. They can both equally be features of high risk PBC. The net result of conflation of these findings with a diagnosis of overlap has been rather too many PBC patients being treated with prednisolone and azathioprine (the standard treatments for AIH), often for long periods of time, and with little or no improvement in their liver biochemistry. This should have alerted their doctor that this is not an AIH-related process, as this condition typically improves very rapidly indeed with prednisolone. If you have been told you have PBC-AIH overlap and have taken prednisolone or azathioprine (or 6-MP or MMF variants of azathioprine) for a long time do discuss with your doctor whether the diagnosis needs to be reviewed in the light of current knowledge. It may be that you need second-line PBC therapy instead. It is critically important, however, that **you do not stop or reduce prednisolone or azathioprine without getting your doctors approval**. Suddenly stopping these drugs can be very dangerous. You need to be weaned off them. The reality is that I probably see one patient a month who has been on long-term prednisolone for "PBC-AIH overlap" with blood tests that remain abnormal, who has then normalised when switched to second-line PBC therapy.

One of the real challenges about overlap, however, is that it actually really does exist (it's just that many of the people thought to have it don't). To formally diagnose it you need to have, in addition to a diagnosis of PBC, 2 out of

- ALT above 5 times the upper limit of normal (above 200 typically)
- An IgG of above 30 (a test used in AIH where the upper limit of normal is 15) OR one of the autoantibodies associated with AIH (AIH-type ANA (the diffuse staining patters) or anti-smooth muscle antibody)
- Biopsy suggestive of AIH (the challenging one for the reasons outlined above although there are detailed features beyond interface hepatitis that help distinguish overlap from bad PBC.

If these criteria are met, then people do need to be treated with a combination of PBC and AIH therapy. The PBC therapy is as for PBC alone. The AIH element will normally be treated with high dose prednisolone which will be weaned down to lower levels reasonably rapidly (30 mg to 10mg over 1-2 months). The aim will be to stop the prednisolone and replace it with azathioprine for the long-term. If it is true overlap the blood tests will improve rapidly. If they do not then the diagnosis needs to be reconsidered, even if the patient met the formal criteria for the diagnosis.

How do I approach the specific challenge of patients coming to the clinic who have been diagnosed in the past with overlap? I suggest the following

1) In everyone with a diagnosis of overlap, whether that is correct or not in the light of current understanding needs to be thought about

2) In people in whom the interface hepatitis is, or was, accompanied by either an *IgG* of over 30 or an *ALT* over 5 times the *upper limit of normal* the diagnosis is likely to be correct and immunosuppression appropriate

3) In all patients with a diagnosis of overlap, the pattern of *liver function tests* after the introduction of immunosuppression needs to be reviewed critically. Was there a significant and rapid improvement? If so, the diagnosis of overlap is likely to be correct. If not it is likely that this is high risk PBC rather than overlap

4) In all patients with PBC and immunosuppression, as is the case with patients with autoimmune hepatitis itself, it is appropriate to try to wean down the immunosuppression to see whether it is still needed at the current dose (or in fact at all). THIS SHOULD ONLY BE DONE UNDER MEDICAL SUPERVISION. If the liver function tests deteriorate then, again, the diagnosis of overlap is probably correct. If the liver function tests don't deteriorate then it is likely that this is high risk PBC.

5) In all patients with a diagnosis of overlap, the possibility of high risk PBC should be considered and, therefore, whether second-line PBC treatment is appropriate. We would use our standard second-line PBC therapy criteria of an alkaline phosphatase of more than 1.67 times the upper limit of normal OR a bilirubin above the upper limit of normal.

MANAGING CIRRHOSIS (STAGE 4 DISEASE)

The classical description of the liver changes in PBC divides the disease into 4 stages (**Chapter 3**). In this classification, stage 4 represents the development of cirrhosis, the state of networked fibrosis accompanied by liver cell regeneration forming liver nodules introduced in **Chapter 1**. It is likely that, over time, this focus on disease stage will decrease as assessment of disease progression will be entirely by Fibroscan. This approach gives rise to a numerical value on a continuous scale (in essence 1 to 40KPa), although it is possible to convert this into the equivalent values for stages. In my experience, PBC patients put great store by their disease stage, and particularly worried about the onset of stage 4 disease, fearing the implications for their health.

The reality is somewhat different, however, for two linked reasons. The first is, as discussed in the section on liver biopsy in diagnosis in **Chapter**

4, PBC is frequently a very patchy disease, meaning that even if there is stage 4 disease in part of the liver other regions may be non-cirrhotic, taking the pressure off the liver. The second is that PBC patients appear to tolerate cirrhosis very well indeed (potentially, of course, because of the presence of non-cirrhotic areas of their liver). All PBC clinicians will be familiar with PBC patients who have reached stage 4 in the disease but remain well, with normal liver function for many years afterwards. The important point is that although cirrhosis/stage 4 disease has the risks described in **Chapter 1**, and the rest of this chapter will explain our approach to mitigating them in the clinic, it is not the presence of stage 4 disease per se that is the issue, but the state of function of the remaining liver tissue. A patient with a bilirubin of 50 in stage 3 is at much greater risk than a patient with stage 4 disease but a bilirubin of 10. The message with stage 4 disease is **don't panic**, but work as hard as you can in getting really good control of the disease.

Put simply, the goal of all management in PBC in the future should be to stop progression to stage 4 disease. The goal of management of the PBC patient who has already progressed to stage 4 disease is two-fold. The first is to ensure that everything possible is done to maintain the remaining liver function. The second is to manage the additional risks that can be associated with each of the complications. Management of the underlying disease remains largely the same in patients with stage 4 disease as it is in early disease. It could be argued that effective disease control is even more important in stage 4 disease than in earlier disease because, in the case of varices for example, it can literally make the difference between having a bleed and not having a bleed. UDCA doses do not need to be adjusted in stage 4 disease. Both OCA and bezafibrate should be used carefully (and in the case of OCA at lower dose) in stage 4 disease because the liver can sometimes struggle to handle them. This is especially the case if the patient has an elevated bilirubin. Patients with definite or likely stage 4 disease (and the approach to determining this is outlined in **Chapter 4**) should be screened for the complications of cirrhosis on a regular basis.

Before I describe the individual complications of cirrhosis/stage 4 disease there is one really important, over-arching point to make. Even where cirrhosis complications develop in PBC they are tolerated much better than is the case in almost all other liver diseases (because of the cholestatic nature of the disease). Thus, most people with PBC never develop cirrhosis (and the number is falling all the time with ever-better disease treatment), where people develop cirrhosis most of them don't develop complications and in the small group who do develop complications they are very well tolerated. Almost all the patients we see with cirrhosis complications have presented very late with the disease meaning that there has been no opportunity to treat it and prevent progression.

Porto-systemic varices: Rather as stage 4 disease, in general, is feared by patients this is the complication that worries patients the most. This is because of the risk of bleeding. The reality is that in our clinic we have not had a PBC patient experience a bleed from varices for several years. Why not? The answer is the same one that will be repeated throughout this chapter, a combination of good management of the underlying disease and good management of the complication risk is really effective in practice.

There are two aspects to varices management. Bleeding prevention and managing a bleed if it happens. Prevention is, unsurprisingly, much preferable to managing an actual bleed. Screening for varices is done through endoscopy (typically known to patients as a "telescope test") which is a quick and well-tolerated procedure to visualise the common sites for varices. This should be done in all patients with proven or suspected stage 4 disease on an annual basis. If significant varices are found then the standard approach is to start treatment with a beta-blocker (especially propranolol or carvedilol), tablet medicines normally used to manage conventional hypertension, but which also reduce portal venous pressure in portal hypertension. Very rarely, if the varices are big, thought to be at high risk of bleeding, or if the patient can't tolerate beta-blocker, we may use some of the invasive management approaches, such as banding, which are normally reserved for managing a bleed, in a preventative way.

A patient with stage 4 PBC who vomits blood or passes black tar-like stools containing blood which has been digested as it passes down through the bowel (melaena) should be treated as if they have had a variceal bleed. This is an emergency. In a newly presenting patient in whom assessment for stage 4 disease hasn't taken place yet bleeding should be assumed to be variceal until proved otherwise. If there is a possibility of variceal bleed then it is essential to get urgent medical attention. This is one of the times when it is correct to call for an emergency ambulance. Variceal bleeding can sometimes occur without any overt signs of blood loss (vomiting blood or passing blood in the stools). In these situations the bleeding is typically in the upper bowel and the blood is in the process of passing down the bowel, but hasn't yet emerged in the stool. In these situations, the signs of bleeding can be more subtle and include light-headedness, palpitations or a fast heart rate.

When a variceal bleed is suspected the absolutely critical first step to treatment is, irrespective of the type of bleeding seen, to put a cannula or tube into a vein to allow the patient to be given fluid to replace the blood loss. This needs to happen quickly and can only be done in the hospital setting or by a paramedic. If bleeding continues it can become more difficult to insert a cannula because the veins collapse, so early attention is key. Initially, the fluid will be clear fluid (a saline drip). In hospital, once blood has been cross-matched it may be blood and plasma. Once fluid is being given it is usual to give an intravenous drug called glypressin. This causes the bleeding vessels to clamp down on themselves applying pressure to stop the bleeding. This allows the situation to stabilise.

The mainstay of treatment is through an endoscopy, this time done to treat rather than look for varices. The current state of the art is to apply small rubber bands onto the bleeding vessel which pinch it off. This is highly effective. Once varices have been banded the bleeding should stop and things can be allowed to settle down. It is then normal to repeat the endoscopy and banding every couple of weeks until the varices have been completely obliterated.

Rarely, banding and glypressin don't control the bleeding. In this case, most liver units would use a procedure called TIPSS (trans-jugular intra-hepatic porto-systemic shunting). In this procedure a cannula is put into the jugular vein in the neck and navigated down into the liver where it is used to make a connection between the hepatic vein (the vein running out of the liver taking blood back to the heart) and the portal vein. This connection is then widened, and a plastic tube or stent is inserted to keep it open. The effect of this connection is to relieve the pressure in the portal vein, taking away the driving force for the bleeding. This is a more invasive and risky procedure than endoscopy, so tends to be reserved for situations where the bleeding can't be controlled in any other way. It is, however, literally life-saving in those situations.

If bleeding recurs despite the use of these treatments then, once the patient is stable, the possibility of transplantation should be considered. Transplant would never be considered acutely in the context of an active bleed, however.

Ascites: Ascites is another manifestation of portal hypertension and is, again, uncommon in PBC. The mainstay of treatment is with diuretics ("water tablets"). Typically, this is with either spironolactone alone (a useful drug as it has a specific action on the fluid accumulation mechanism in ascites) or spironolactone in combination with frusemide. If the volume of the ascites is very large, and in particular if it is causing problems with breathing, then it is sometimes necessary to drain it through the abdominal wall using a temporary tube. This makes patients more comfortable very quickly but, of course, increases the risk of infection getting into the ascites (peritonitis). Sometimes bacteria can get from the bowel into the ascites and cause a low-grade infection; a process known as spontaneous bacterial peritonitis (SBP). If SBP is thought to have arisen, a small sample of ascites is taken through the abdominal wall (a small syringe-full with a small needle) for examination in the laboratory. If SBP is found then the treatment is with antibiotics. SBP development does, however, indicate a higher risk liver disease state and is one of the events that would make us think actively about transplantation.

TIPSS can also be effective for the control of ascites where diuretics are no longer working, although not if SBP has been present because of the risk of the stent becoming infected.

Hepatocellular carcinoma: HCC is probably seen less frequently in PBC than in any other form of liver disease. This is partly because of the cholestatic nature of the disease protecting the hepatocytes until very late in the disease, and partly because male sex is a risk factor for HCC (through the actions of testosterone). Women with PBC do get HCC occasionally, but the risk is very low. Male patients do have a higher risk and particular attention should be paid to screening all male PBC patients with stage 4 disease.

The art with HCC is early diagnosis through screening. If identified when small (as a result of the recommended 6 monthly screening with ultrasound and a blood test called alpha-fetoprotein which often, but not always, rises when an HCC is developing, followed by further imaging with CT or MRI if a suspicious lesion is seen) there are a number of treatment approaches. If it presents late when large, or when the liver function has started to deteriorate it rapidly becomes untreatable. Approaches used for small cancers include

- TACE (trans-arterial chemoembolization). This is a procedure in which the artery supplying the cancer is identified and chemotherapy is injected into it, followed by a plug to block off the artery to lock the chemotherapy in and take away the tumour blood supply
- RFA (radiofrequency ablation). In this procedure a microwave probe is inserted through skin into the tumour and the tumour is killed in situ by a pulse of radio-waves
- Transplant. An effective approach in small cancers and should be considered because once one cancer has developed the rest of the liver is at risk
- Surgical resection. In practice only rarely possible because of the presence of cirrhosis.

Chemotherapy options are relatively limited at present and the effectiveness low. Drugs like sorafenib are mainly used where the physical approaches outlined above cannot be used because the cancer is too large.

Liver failure: The function of the liver is, initially, maintained very well in stage 4 PBC. Over time, however, it can deteriorate to the point at which the patient enters liver failure (insufficient functioning liver for their needs). There can be acute deteriorations in liver function with other complications such as variceal bleeding or SBP, as well as with inter-current illnesses unrelated to the liver. Largely eliminated as a problem by the combined benefits of UDCA and transplantation, it represented the end-stage of the disease in the "bad old days" of PBC.

The critical step in managing PBC liver failure is to look for, and manage, the event or complication that has triggered the acute worsening of liver function. This is normally bleeding from varices or an infection. If there is a trigger such as this for deterioration then it is usually the case that we can return people to the level of liver function they had prior to the deterioration. If liver failure becomes established, and does not reverse with supportive care, then liver transplantation should be actively explored.

Hepatic encephalopathy: Encephalopathy is very uncommon indeed in PBC (I haven't seen anyone with it for several years). It is really important that it is distinguished from the cognitive symptoms of PBC which can occur at any stage of the disease, but which can mimic encephalopathy in its earliest stages. If hepatic encephalopathy occurs as part of an acute liver failure deterioration then it will typically improve as the event is treated. In my experience, the complication to be certain you look for is variceal bleeding as most sudden onset encephalopathy occurs as the result of a bleed. If it becomes chronic then we treat encephalopathy with lactulose or rifaximin, both drugs that reduce the bacterial and protein load in the bowel. In practice, however, we would always consider a PBC patient who had had an encephalopathy episode for transplantation.

WHEN TO CONSIDER LIVER TRANSPLANTATION
Liver transplantation is an effective treatment for end-stage PBC. The practicalities of transplantation will be discussed in **Chapter 6**, however its use should be considered as a normal part of the management pathway for the disease. In other words, it is a completely normal treatment that should be thought about in all PBC patients, even if it is dismissed very quickly because the disease is too mild or is well controlled with first or second-line therapy. We always set out to "de-mythologise" transplantation in PBC for our patients.

There are actually two reasons (or indications in medical terminology) for considering liver transplantation in PBC. Overwhelmingly the commonest is when the disease has advanced to its very end stages and the likely risk of the complications of advanced disease that would be seen if you did not have a transplant have become greater than the risk of the operation. The development of cirrhosis/stage 4 disease is not, in and of itself, a reason to consider transplantation. Most patients with PBC cirrhosis in fact remain well with it (although they need to be watched very carefully). This is because the liver has a lot of reserve capacity. Although cirrhosis reduces the functional capacity of the liver, for many people all that does is reduce the reserve. It is only once the reserve has run out that problems arise and transplant becomes more relevant. In practice, loss of reserve in PBC is best indicated by a rising bilirubin level. The vast majority of PBC patients, including most patients with cirrhosis, have a normal bilirubin level. It is only once it starts to rise that transplant needs to be thought about. A value of around 3 times the upper limit of normal (50-60 in UK units, 3-4 in USA units) is conventionally the point at which transplant is first thought about and 6 times (100 and 6 in the UK and USA respectively) is when it should be actively pursued. As outlined in the section on monitoring below, however, the disease can deteriorate rapidly once the bilirubin has started rising and it is critically important that the opportunity to consider transplant is not missed. I would much rather know of all patients in the catchment area for our transplant programme with an abnormal bilirubin so that follow-up can be taken in our clinic that links directly to transplantation. "Fore-warned is fore-armed" is an expression I use frequently. Patients with cirrhosis will occasionally develop difficult to manage complications (such as variceal bleeding, ascites not manageable using diuretics or hepatocellular carcinoma) without a rising bilirubin. Transplant should be considered in these situations because we know that each of these complications suggests that the patient is, either directly or indirectly, at significantly increased risk. Rarely, the albumin can begin to fall without either complications developing, or a bilirubin rise. If this is definitely related to PBC then it is an adverse finding. In most cases, however, there is another explanation related to bowel dysfunction or nutritional problems.

The other, very occasional, indication for transplantation in PBC is for the management of symptoms other than those of cirrhosis complications. The only such symptom indication for transplantation in PBC is itch. Transplant is a highly effective treatment for itch if needs be. It is important to be clear, however, that it is only a very small number of people indeed who have truly uncontrollable itch. In most cases, it is just that all the treatment options for itch (outlined in **Chapter 7**) haven't been explored. Over 90% of the patients referred to our clinic for transplantation for uncontrollable itch end up with effective medical treatment and no transplant!

A number of years ago fatigue was regarded as an indication for transplantation. Whereas there is no question as to the potential impact of fatigue on patients, our experience is that patients transplanted mainly or purely for fatigue have only a limited symptom improvement. The reasons why this is the case aren't clear, but probably include the negative effects of immuno-suppressive drugs on functional status, and the possibility that the process underpinning fatigue in PBC has a chronic and irreversible element to it so that by the time patients were reaching transplant the process could no longer be reversed. This possibility has helped shape current thinking about the need to treat fatigue early in the disease course moving forward.

MANAGING PBC IN PRACTICE

PBC disease management is a life-long process. It consists of two elements; **monitoring** the disease to ensure that no changes to treatment or additional treatments are needed and **supporting** you as a patient.

Monitoring PBC: PBC should be thought of as a condition which is almost always controllable with current treatments. Although the direction of travel for research in the future must be towards cure this is not currently achievable. PBC also only very rarely resolves itself. The result is that PBC should be thought of a life-long condition that should therefore be managed life-long. Even when treatments are seemingly working well it is usually the case that this represents effective control of the disease by the treatment being used rather than any fundamental change to the underlying disease process. As this situation can, and does, change it is important that someone monitors disease and acts on changes. Patients themselves can make a huge contribution to effective monitoring by being aware of their test status, and the test values at which a change in treatment may be needed. This allows them to work with the doctor to agree and effect any changes that are needed.

In clinic follow-up, the team are (or should be) asking themselves three important and largely independent questions.

a) Is the treatment to control PBC as outlined in the previous sections working as effectively as we would like?

This represents the main question for follow-up and itself has a numbers of elements to it. We structure our thinking, and look at this in terms of

- **Is the patient on UDCA and is the dose correct?** Remember that body weight changes with time meaning that the dose of UDCA may need to be adjusted. It needs to be within the 13-15mg/Kg range and if your weight changes the dose also needs to change. If someone is not taking UDCA, why not? If it is difficulty in tolerating it, can we try introducing it very slowly. Can we split the dose? If tablet size is an issue what about the liquid suspension version?

- **Is second line therapy necessary?** At the heart of this is the question of UDCA response status. Is the patient a UDCA responder? If not, are there reasons to not use second-line therapy (it should be this way around; in the same way as everyone with PBC should be on UDCA unless there is a specific reason not to so second line therapy should be actively considered in everyone who is a UDCA non-responder). If a patient is truly unable to tolerate UDCA then should we be considering second-line therapy in its place? All approaches to monitoring UDCA response (and, indeed, response to second-line therapy) are based on liver blood biochemistry (liver function tests).

- **Is there any evidence to suggest that the patient has PBC/AIH overlap syndrome?** Given that this has probably been over-diagnosed in the past it is sensible to always review a past diagnosis of overlap. It is also worth remembering that unlike the central process of PBC, which does not tend to fluctuate, the AIH component in overlap can "come and go" over time. Again, liver biochemistry plays an important part, with immunoglobin levels (especially IgG) being very useful. The presence of AIH-specific autoantibodies, such as a diffuse nuclear pattern anti-nuclear antibody (but not, as we have seen, the more focal PBC-specific anti-nuclear antibody; the 2 are different and have different significance) and anti-smooth muscle antibody, is very suggestive. Looking for overlap, and guiding its management, is one of the situations where liver biopsy is still appropriate in PBC.

- **Has the patient progressed to the point at which liver transplant should be considered?** For the vast majority of patients the answer will be no. Transplantation is, however, an important and effective treatment for a small group of patients with aggressive disease. The topic of transplantation is covered in detail in **Chapter 6**. The important message for this section is that this should be thought about in all patients, and at every review in the clinic. If the bilirubin is normal, there are no features of cirrhosis and symptoms are not very severe then the thought need go no further. In people with a rising bilirubin, however, the disease can progress fast and there is a constant danger that the opportunity for transplantation is missed. In my career I have looked after too many people who were referred in to our centre too late to be transplantable because the potential for the disease to deteriorate rapidly had been ignored.

b) Does the patient have cirrhosis, or sufficiently suggestive features of cirrhosis, to warrant the risk screening programme to look for (so we can manage) varices or hepatocellular carcinoma?

This can be more tricky than people think for the simple reason that the historic way of looking for progression of PBC, as with any liver disease, was through follow-up liver biopsy where the characteristic features would be obvious. We, correctly, no longer follow-up PBC using biopsy, meaning that this information is rarely available. How, then, do we look for cirrhosis? The following are commonly used approaches. Which are used in different centres is down to local experience and availability of the necessary tests.

- **Transient elastography** (most often referred to by the trade name of the most widely used approach "Fibroscan") is a non-invasive method of assessing fibrosis severity in the liver. It works on the same principle as sonar, with an ultrasonic "pulse" being fired from the probe. The amount of that pulse that is reflected back is counted. The more solid the liver is, the more of the pulse will be returned, as solids transmit sounds better than fluids and fibrosis makes the liver more solid. It is widely available in Europe but less so, at the time of writing, in North America. Limitations are the upfront cost of the machine and the need for trained technicians who do enough tests to maintain skills. Once the technology is in place, however, it rapidly becomes an indispensable tool. The costs per scan once the equipment is in place are minimal and it is a very acceptable test to patients (it feels very much like having a conventional ultrasound scan). Fibroscan was originally shown in studies to be highly predictive of the degree of fibrosis in the liver on a biopsy that was done at the same time as the Fibroscan and, on this basis, Fibroscan started to be used as an alternative to biopsy to get "stage" information. More recently it has been shown that Fibroscan is directly predictive of risk of death and complication development in PBC. This suggests it is perhaps an even more useful clinical tool than originally anticipated. This work identified three Fibroscan values as being important in understanding risk. The first is 7.8KPa. This value is a little higher than the one that would be seen in someone with a completely normal liver (where it would be 4-5), however a value below 7.8 is associated with a very low risk indeed of complication development. Between 7.8 and 15.1 the risk was elevated, but not dramatically so. However, values of above 15.1 were associated with significant risk of complication development. The third value is a slightly older one of 17.9 KPa. This was the value in the biopsy studies that was suggestive of cirrhosis or stage 4 disease development. The reason why the 15.1 cut off for high risk is lower than the 17.9 cut-off for cirrhosis is probably that once the value has gone above 15.1 progression to 17.9 and cirrhosis is almost inevitable.

- **Enlarged spleen on ultrasound**. Cirrhosis leads to an increase in the pressure in the portal vein that drains blood from the bowel to the liver leading, in turn, to the spleen increasing in size. This does not typically cause any problems, but can be measured on ultrasound and is a useful suggestion of portal hypertension and thus, by extrapolation, cirrhosis. Given that the risk of varices is down to portal hypertension specifically, rather than cirrhosis in general, it could be argued that this is actually a very useful specific risk marker. The limitations are the possibility that an enlarged spleen has been caused by a different process (a blood problem for example), and the fact that some people don't have a spleen because they didn't develop one (something that is not infrequent), they have had it removed after trauma or it has died back naturally (splenic infarction, particularly common in sickle-cell disease).

- **Suggestive blood tests**. A low platelet count (one of the standard blood count measures in the universal "full blood count" test set) is suggestive of portal hypertension. It is a result of splenomegaly and is, therefore, an alternative to ultrasound detection of an enlarged spleen. If the platelet count is normal this is a cheap way of knowing that portal hypertension almost certainly isn't there. There are, however, a number of non-liver reasons why the platelet count can be lowered.

- **Blood-based fibrosis tests**. When the body forms scar tissue in fibrosis and cirrhosis it is not a uni-directional process. The scar is, in fact, dynamic, being broken down and re-formed on a continual basis. The breakdown of fibrotic tissue leads to breakdown products from it being released into the blood. There are a number of, largely commercial, tests that can measure these breakdown products and, accordingly, suggest the level of fibrosis. These can be costly and are not in widespread use in the clinical setting. A limitation is also that fibrosis and its remodelling can occur in most tissues in the body, and a number of other fibrotic conditions such as systemic sclerosis (see **Chapter 8**) are associated with PBC. A fibrosis remodelling signal may, therefore, not result from PBC.

- **Complications**. Perhaps self-evidently, if any of the complications of cirrhosis, such as ascites development, hepatocellular carcinoma or varices arise then the patient should thereafter be assumed to have cirrhosis.

c) Are there PBC symptoms that warrant treatment or a change of treatment.
The symptoms of PBC and their practical management are explored in detail in **Chapter 7**. Symptoms can only be treated if clinicians ask about them and patients talk about them. It is worth noting that the presence of a symptom does not automatically mean it needs treatment. Many people with PBC itch experience the symptom at a level that does not actually trouble them (it is there if you ask about it but when people are not being asked about it they can forget about it). All symptom treatments have side-effects, sometimes making other symptom domains worse. Anti-histamines used for itch can make fatigue worse, for example. It can therefore be counter-productive to treat a symptom which is not causing a problem. When screening for symptoms it is therefore important for the clinician to gauge the degree of impact. I always ask whether it is "bad enough for us to think about adding or changing treatment?" The recent UK audit of PBC care (carried out in 2021) suggests that only half of all PBC patients are being asked about their

symptoms. This is despite the importance of those symptoms, their treatability (mainly in the case of itch) and the fact that the guidelines that doctors follow to manage PBC all state that symptoms must be assessed. We must improve this. Patients can absolutely help with this by ensuring that they talk about their symptoms every time they see the doctor or nurse.

How does this all translate into practice in the clinic? There are, in fact, no established rules for how, how frequently and by whom PBC patients should be followed-up. Treatment guidelines only suggest that follow-up should take place. The following represents our approach. We are, however, flexible in this approach, adjusting it according to the needs of the individual. We aim to find a follow-up model that is, on the one hand, frequent enough to allow change in the disease to be responded to in a timely fashion whilst, on the other, not being so burdensome to the patient that they slip into a state where the disease rules their life. It is also important to remember that the more clinicians there are who are involved in managing a patient, the more different versions and interpretations of information will be imparted. Inconsistency in information given, even if seemingly innocuous, can be very unsettling for patients and can breed a lack of confidence in their clinicians. Simple, readily understandable and consistent messaging is a really important part of follow-up

ANNUAL FOLLOW-UP: Everyone with PBC should be followed up at least annually, with assessment of the diseases status and action taken if there has been important change. The following would represent a key follow up information set

- **Clinical Review**: What has changed in the last year in terms of the disease and its impact? What changes in medication for PBC and for other conditions have taken place and why? Are you tolerating your PBC treatment or are there side-effects which are getting in the way of the treatment?
- **Blood Test Review**: Liver function tests should be checked, and compared against previous values. The key values to look for are the bilirubin level (has this changed and is the value still within the normal range for the laboratory that did the test?) and the alkaline phosphatase. The key information with regard to alkaline phosphatase is what is the value as a multiple of the upper limit of normal (often referred to as uln) for the local laboratory (for example if your value is 390 and the upper limit of normal is 130 your value is 3 times the upper limit of normal (3x uln). The key value to watch out for in the UK is an alkaline phosphatase of over 1.67x uln. This equates, for most laboratories, to a value of around 200. As long as bilirubin is <1x uln **and** alkaline phosphatase is <1.67x uln) you are deemed to be responding well

to treatment. It is very likely that over the next few years the target for alkaline phosphatase levels with treatment will fall. The analogy is with blood cholesterol where the target number doctors aim for now is much lower than it was originally because it is now clear that there was still elevated risk in some of the people who reached the old target value.

- **Fibroscan Assessment:** The emerging data on the capacity of Fibroscan to predict complication risk means that Fibroscan will increasingly become part of normal follow-up. This may not need to be annual for people with low risk base-line values.

- **Symptom Severity Assessments:** Current treatment guidelines emphasise, correctly, the need to formally assess symptoms and suggest that this take place annually. Not asking about symptoms and their impact on quality of life is a sure fire way for doctors to ignore them and their impact. The standard tool used for PBC symptom assessment, the PBC-40, is too long to be useful in the clinic on an annual basis (it is a research tool that has its main use in trials of new treatments). A shortened version with 10 questions (the PBC-10) has recently been developed and is suitable for annual use. An alternative approach is to ask about severity of the symptom (at a minimum itch and fatigue) on a scale of zero to 10 where zero is no symptom and 10 is the worst symptom you can imagine.

Where people are tolerating and have a good response to the treatment they are on (alkaline phosphatase <1.67x uln and bilirubin <1xuln at the moment, although this may change), have no symptoms (or symptoms which are stable and at a level that don't need an increase in treatment) do not have clinical features of cirrhosis and are not in the high risk group on Fibroscan, then annual follow-up is appropriate. This can be in a hospital clinic or with your GP (provided they are aware about PBC and interested in it).

ENHANCED FOLLOW-UP: A significant proportion of patients end up on a follow-up programme that is more frequent. This is usually individualised to the needs of the patients. Reasons for more frequent follow-up can include, in our clinic

- Treatment change with follow-up to ensure it effective and being tolerated
- Changing clinical picture (deteriorating liver biochemistry or worsening symptoms)
- Second-line therapy being used (we follow all second-line therapy patients up closely)

- Cirrhosis (we follow up all patients with cirrhosis or suspected cirrhosis at a minimum every 6 months)
- Ongoing discussion about a treatment change (most obviously the process of thinking about transplantation which we introduce over several visits)
- Patient support. Some patients struggle with the diagnosis of PBC and support is a key part of their management.

SUPPORTING PBC PATIENTS

We put a lot of time and effort into supporting PBC patients to live normal lives. Management of PBC absolutely shouldn't start and finish with UDCA and LFTs! We will discuss in much more detail in **Chapter 9** what patients can do themselves to help ensure that they get the best possible treatment for PBC.

CHAPTER 6: **LIVER TRANSPLANT**

The 2-Minute Version

- Liver transplantation is an effective treatment for advanced PBC. The aim of our approach to treatment in PBC these days is, however, to avoid it ever being needed if possible. The effectiveness of current and emerging treatments means that, hopefully, the need for it will gradually disappear over time.

- Most patients who end up needing a liver transplant are either diagnosed very late (typically when advanced cirrhosis is already present) or have not been treated adequately. The risk of needing transplant in patients presenting with early PBC, and who are treated to the full extent of our current abilities, is probably vanishingly small.

- In the majority of cases, liver transplant in PBC is carried out because of the risks to life of very advanced disease. This could be through the complications of cirrhosis (difficult to control variceal bleeding, ascites with complications, liver cancer etc) or through liver failure (rapidly rising bilirubin is the usual sign).

- A small proportion of liver transplants are carried out for very severe itch (for which it is very effective). Transplant is not an appropriate treatment for fatigue (for which it is not effective).

- Before transplant patients go through an assessment process to explore the likely benefits and risks to them as an individual. PBC patients tend to be low risk compared to patients with other types of liver disease. The only matching between donors and recipients is for blood group and for organ size (to ensure the new liver will physically "fit").

- Early complications can include non-function and thrombosis of the hepatic artery. Both are rare but potentially significant. Advances in technique have reduced their frequency and impact.

- Rejection (the attempt by the immune system to "fight" a liver it sees as being foreign) typically first arises as an issue at around 7 days after the transplant, but can occur at any point after that. Patients typically take life-long immuno-suppression (usually a drug called tacrolimus combined with azathioprine or MMF) to prevent this. Rejection only rarely causes problems.

- Recurrence of PBC can occur. The latest data suggest that PBC patients should continue to take UDCA post-transplant as it is highly effective at preventing recurrence.

For all types of liver disease, the ultimate treatment option is to replace the damaged liver with a new one. This is liver transplantation. The good news about liver transplantation for PBC patients is that it exists as a treatment option. It is a great safety net to have. The even better news for PBC patients is that it is only very rarely needed! For most of the readers of the book, this chapter is for information and interest only as it hopefully will never be directly relevant to you. For the small group who are maybe heading towards, and the larger group of people who have already had, a transplant this is meant to inform and guide you and, hopefully, give you confidence. Transplantation policy and practice is one of the areas that can differ from country to country and, inevitably given the authorship, this chapter mainly focuses on policy and practice in the UK. For patients with more advanced disease understanding the opportunities around transplantation in your own health care system are important and you should discuss these with your clinical team.

THE BASICS OF LIVER TRANSPLANTATION

The term liver transplantation is short for "orthotopic liver transplantation". In this title orthotopic means that the old liver is removed and replaced, in the same place in the body, with a new organ (this contrasts with kidney transplants which are often heterotopic (i.e. the new organ is placed in a different location in the body to the old kidney; usually in the pelvis). There are four aspects to transplantation for all liver diseases. These are the donor organ, the operation itself, the assessment process before transplant and the follow-up after the operation. I will discuss these in general terms first and then, in the next section, discuss the specific issues in relation to transplantation for PBC.

Donor livers: In simple terms, there are two sources of a donor liver. Cadaveric donation (meaning from a person who has died) and living-related donation (a family member giving a portion of their liver). The vast majority of liver transplantation historically has used cadaveric donors. This was, until, recently, using what are termed donors by brain death (DBD). This is where the donor has suffered some form of significant brain injury (usually a bleed or head trauma) which means that they cannot survive, and will not recover. In lay terms they are "brain dead". They are on a ventilator (without brain function you don't breathe) but the heart continues to beat normally and the other organs of the body are getting their blood supply. Many countries in the world (but not all) have a legal framework by which the organs that are functioning well can be taken in an operation for use in transplantation. In the UK, historically, we used an "opt in" system, meaning that people carried a donor card, or put their name on a registry to indicate that in the event of brain death they would become a donor (provided their next of kin at the time also agreed). The UK is now moving to an "opt out" system where consent is presumed unless the person has indicated otherwise. DBD livers tend to be good quality because the events around their collection are controlled (the operation to remove them is planned and the body had a good blood pressure). People can sometimes worry about the imagery of an operation with surgeons and an anaesthetist removing organs. Doesn't this mean the donor is still alive? **The answer is absolutely not**. There are strict laws about ensuring that a person is brain dead before they become a DBD donor, and that the situation is completely non-recoverable. The anaesthetist is there to control the blood pressure in the organ removal operation, not to anaesthetise the donor. Even after brain death, the body still has reflexes and blood pressure can often soar in response to a cut being made at operation. This is not brain function, just a reflex. People often confuse brain death and persistent vegetative state (one from which very occasional people have recovered). A persistent vegetative state is a state of grossly affected brain function, but which falls short of complete brain death (i.e. there is some small neurological function). People in a persistent vegetative state are often breathing spontaneously. It is the existence of some ongoing brain function that makes all the difference.

The issue all transplant programmes face with DBD organs is that fewer and fewer are being donated. This is largely not because of reluctance to donate (although we can always do more on education and awareness), but because the causes of catastrophic brain trauma that lead to the brain death state are getting rarer (fewer intra-cranial bleeds because of better blood pressure control, fewer massive head traumas in road traffic accidents because of safety legislation etc.). These improvements in population health are, of course, to be applauded. In order to maintain the numbers of organs available for donation there has been a move towards the second type of cadaveric donor; the donor by cardiac death (DCD). Death in the conventional sense has always been recognised as the point at which the heart has stopped beating (which is why someone who has had a cardiac arrest is technically dead). DCD donors are donors who are dying for reasons that are not recoverable, and from whom the organs are removed immediately after the heart has stopped beating. The use of this approach has increased the number of potential donors significantly. It has, however, significant limitations. The obvious one is that the whole process is less controlled, and is more rushed, meaning that the condition of the organ is often less good. The cause of death can have a much greater impact on organ quality as well.

For all cadaveric donor organs, a detailed assessment of the donor is made in advance of the organ being retrieved. The organ is also assessed at the time of retrieval. Concern at either of these stages means the organ is not used. The pre-donation assessment is around underlying health state and cause of death. Contra-indications to donation include disseminated cancer and chronic infection such as hepatitis B or C, HIV or TB. Significant pre-existing liver disease would also be an obvious contra-indication. The assessment at the time of retrieval is largely around how much fat is in the liver. The liver naturally stores fat (it is one of its normal functions). As the levels of obesity in the population rise, so the levels of fat in the average liver have grown. In many people, this is harmless (although not ideal). In a growing number of people, this contributes to active liver disease in the form of non-alcoholic fatty liver disease (NAFLD). If a donor liver is too fatty it will not cope with the whole process of removal, transport and re-implantation and runs an increased risk of not functioning after re-implantation in the recipient. After removal from the donor, the liver is perfused with a special fluid that is designed to lessen the potential injury that might occur with the organ outside the body. Conventionally, the organ was then stored on ice until the operation to implant it into the recipient. More recently, a new technique of organ perfusion has been developed in which, prior to implantation, the liver is re-perfused on a machine, warming it and providing oxygen and nutrients. This approach is becoming routine and may make a significant contribution to increasing the health of organs for transplant in the future.

Living donation is a much newer approach and one that is growing in its scope. In some countries, the law does not allow cadaveric donation and this is the only route to organ donation. Predictably, these countries are the ones that have led the way in the surgical approach to living-related transplantation. In simple terms, a donor (usually a family member or spouse) volunteers to donate a section of their liver that is then removed at operation and implanted into the recipient. The technique was originally developed for children, where a parent would donate to a child. In this situation, the approach has proved highly successful. Living-related transplantation has key advantages, but also important challenges. The obvious advantage is that both donation and transplant operations can be planned and co-ordinated. This allows the health of the recipient to be optimised to reduce the risk of the operation, and for the time between removal of the donor organ and its re-implantation in the recipient to be minimised, reducing the impact on the liver. There are, however, two major challenges. The first is the need for, and impact on, the donor. Clearly, a donor cannot have any of the health issues which would preclude cadaveric donation and can't have liver disease (more of a challenge than you might think given how common fatty liver is in the community). They must also be emotionally able to donate, and to be doing so without any element of obligation or coercion. The whole issue of consent is critically important because the donor faces some degree of risk (resection of a lobe of liver, which is the operation they undergo, is a significant procedure). There have been instances (thankfully very occasional) where the donor has died after the operation but the recipient has survived. One of the reasons why the approach is so successful for child recipients is that most parents would regard risk to their own life to save the life of their child as being completely acceptable. The ties might not be so strong for a friend or a distant adult relative….. The other major challenge is organ size. Again, adult to child transplant works well as most of the child recipients are under 5 and only need a small amount of liver. This leaves plenty behind in the donor. At the other extreme, if a small wife is to donate liver to a large husband her liver may not be large enough to provide sufficient tissue for both. The challenges mean that, outside adult to child donation, living-related transplantation is something that tends to be considered as an option far more frequently than actually being performed.

One thing that often surprises people about liver transplantation is that there is no need to match the donor and recipient by tissue type, as would be the case for all other types of organ transplantation. The only matching done between recipient and donor is by blood group and body mass. Body-mass matching is important as a donor liver that is too large for the recipient can become compressed, pressurising it and making closure of the wound difficult. Too small a liver has the potential to twist around its blood supply putting it, in theory at least, at risk of blocking it off. In non-liver transplant settings, if tissue type matching isn't carried out the organ is at a much greater risk of rejection. This is not the case for livers for reasons that aren't entirely clear. It may be that the liver is just so large that the immune system does not attempt to reject it. Alternatively, the complex mechanisms that exist in the liver to allow us to tolerate protein from the diet without mounting an immune response may come into play.

Liver transplant surgery: The transplant operation itself is a significant one, taking between 4 and 12 hours. It has two symmetrical elements to it, the removal of the old liver and the implantation of the new. Removal of the old liver may, of course, be complicated by its diseased state and, in particular, by the presence of portal hypertension which can increase the risk of bleeding significantly. Previous sub-acute bacterial peritonitis (SBP) can also make the removal of the old liver difficult. It is now standard practice to use bypass to maintain the blood drainage from the bowel and lower half of the body. The portal vein and the inferior vena cava (the large vein carrying blood from the lower half of the body back to the heart (the counterpoint to the aorta) and which passes through the liver) are both removed as part of the transplant operation and therefore have to be clamped off. Without bypass, venous blood would not be able to drain from the lower body and the gut, potentially causing damage to the more delicate tissues such as the kidney and the gut. Implantation and anastomosis (the re-connection of the hepatic artery, vena cava, portal vein and bile duct) are normally technically straightforward, although there can be issues with size disparity between the donor and recipient blood vessels. This is particularly the case for the portal vein, which contributes a different proportion of the total liver blood flow in different people (ranging from 50 to 80%). Where there are likely to be issues with anastomoses these are avoided by changes in the operation. The details of the surgical technique are, however, beyond the scope of this book. The time of the greatest potential risk in the operation is when the new liver is perfused for the first time (the bypass is switched off and the arterial and portal venous blood flow allowed into the new liver). This is a time of great potential stress for the body as it washes out any remnants of the preservation fluid used for the liver in transport from the donor site, as well as any toxins that have built up in the liver during its storage. Blood pressure can fall and may need to be supported by the anaesthetist. This stress point is the main reason for the detailed assessment of cardiac function undertaken as part of the assessment process pre-transplant.

Liver transplant assessment: Before a patient ever comes to the transplant operation they need to have gone through the process of transplant assessment. There are two settings in which liver transplantation is performed; acute liver failure when it is an emergency procedure and for the complications of chronic liver disease where it is a planned procedure. Only the latter setting is relevant in PBC, a condition which never gives rise to acute liver failure (unlike, interestingly, the other autoimmune liver disease autoimmune hepatitis which can have a highly acute presentation). Although the exact timing of liver transplantation for chronic disease depends on when an appropriate organ becomes available, there is a formal process of assessment that takes place before someone can be placed on the transplant waiting list. Note that the terminology "waiting list" is in common usage but in reality there is no such thing; a patient will be transplanted at the time an organ best suited to them becomes available, which means there is no strict ordering of recipients. The format of assessment will vary from centre to centre but the aim is the same. The goal is to understand the benefit that someone might get from transplantation (the risk posed to them by their liver disease which might be reduced by transplantation), counter-balanced by the risk of the procedure to them in relation, in particular, to their cardiac and lung status. Most centres also use the assessment process as an opportunity for potential recipients to get to know the transplant team, and to understand more about the procedure. In my unit we admit people for a few days (other centres do assessment as an outpatient), undertake imaging of the liver to map the blood vessels and assess heart and lung function in dynamic tests. Once the risk and benefit data are collected together, all the potential transplant recipients are discussed in a formal assessment meeting with all the team members present (including the transplant co-ordinator, one of whose roles is to express the views of the patient). Our assessment process is very successful at avoiding "getting it wrong" (i.e. transplanting someone who goes on to have avoidable complications during the operation or who struggles to cope with the emotional side of the procedure). Once someone is accepted onto the list they continue to undergo close follow up to make sure there is no material deterioration of their condition that might impact upon successful transplantation.

Post-transplant management: Whereas patients often think of liver transplantation as being the end of the part of their life with liver disease, the reality is that it is the beginning of a new life as a post-transplant patient. Transplantation should not, therefore, be thought of as a cure, rather a procedure that avoids the complications of liver disease but is subject to its own long-term problems. An integral part of post-transplant management is to use drugs to reduce the risk of organ rejection. Organ rejection is the process by which the immune system recognises the new organ as being "foreign" and mounts an immune response against it. Think of this as a potentially much more aggressive form of an autoimmune disease process. The good news is that, unlike autoimmune disease, the point of first "recognition" of the new organ by the immune system is known in advance, meaning that treatment can be given to prevent the onset of the immune response. This is what is known as "immuno-suppression", a blanket term for a number of different drugs, several of which are typically used at the same time in liver transplant recipients.

Immuno-suppression will be started the day after theatre, and will essentially continue for life thereafter. Different units have different approaches to drug combinations, which will also be tailored according to the health of the recipient (do they have kidney problems for example) and the underlying liver disease. In most centres, a drug called tacrolimus (previously known as FK506) is the mainstay of treatment, usually accompanied by steroids (initially hydrocortisone injections replaced by prednisolone tablets when patients can eat and drink) and azathioprine or mycophenolate mofetil (MMF). The tacrolimus dose is adjusted up or down according to blood levels whilst the other drugs are given either at fixed doses or adjusted for dose according to patient body weight.

Post-transplant management begins immediately after surgery when patients are managed on the critical care unit. In the first 24 to 48 hours after a transplant operation the potential complications and problems are largely related to the operation itself (anaesthetic issues and bleeding from vessels around the operation site). The two specific complications that can happen in liver transplantation are hepatic artery thrombosis and primary non-function. The hepatic artery is, despite supplying a large organ, often a very small vessel (remember that a significant proportion of the blood coming into the liver comes via the portal vein), with a difficult anastomosis (the joining up of the donor and recipient arteries). For this reason, it is at risk of clotting off, typically in the first 24-48 hours after the operation when there is swelling in the artery wall that narrows it further. If the surgeons are concerned about the risk to the artery they will fashion what is called an arterial conduit, which is a linker between the donor and recipient arteries and which significantly reduces the hepatic artery thrombosis risk (but does slightly lengthen the transplant operation and make it more complex). Blood flow will typically always be assessed in the hepatic artery on the day after surgery using ultrasound, with a more detailed CT or angiogram study carried out if there are any doubts about the flow. If the hepatic artery does thrombose the effect is much less dramatic (in the short term at least) than people think it will be. Because of the portal vein blood supply, the liver will only lose a relatively small percentage of its total blood flow. The slight blood supply shortage will show up as a deterioration in liver function tests. Hepatic artery thrombosis is not, however, a benign process. The artery may only supply a fraction of the blood needed by the liver but it supplies the vast majority of the blood needed by the bile duct. Thrombosis of the artery can, therefore, cause ischaemia of the bile duct, which can lead to it necrosing and beginning to leak bile into the abdominal cavity (where it is highly irritant). Longer term, ischaemia of the bile duct can lead to stricturing or narrowing in the duct, which reduces bile flow and can, ironically, replicate many of the clinical features of PBC! The other complication of hepatic artery thrombosis is that it can leave areas of the liver with relative ischaemia. The loss of arterial flow is not enough to cause the liver to infarct (die) but it can become isolated from the immune system. The ischaemic zones can thus become areas where bacteria in the circulation can lodge and thrive, protected from the immune system. This leads the formation of liver abscesses that can be very difficult indeed to manage. The risks associated with hepatic artery thrombosis mean that it is an emergency, and there is only a relatively short time-period to restore flow before damage becomes permanent. In the first instance, the approach is radiological (insertion of a tube or catheter into an artery which is manoeuvred to the hepatic artery (a very skilled procedure!) where the artery is opened and a stent (a liner tube left in place to keep the artery open) is inserted). If this is not possible technically then an operation to replace the thrombosed artery with a conduit is likely to be needed. Occasionally, none of these approaches work, or it is not possible to restore blood flow and in these situations re-transplant may be needed

The other early complication is primary non-function (a state in which the liver simply does not start working in the recipient) or delayed function (a milder process where function is impaired for a while). Both of these processes are thought to be a consequence of preservation injury (damage caused to the liver in the removal and transport process). A major contributor to this is fat in the donor liver (an increasingly common problem in society as a whole and therefore in organ donors as well). In simple terms, livers with a lot of fat in them do not cope well with being ischaemic (losing their blood supply). The fat in the liver exacerbates the ischaemic injury. High fat level in the donor liver is the commonest reason for a liver to be deemed non-transplantable. Improvements in the science of organ retrieval and preservation, including with the preservation of fluid, have reduced the risks. It is likely that the new organ perfusion techniques, which are now entering into routine practice, will make a further major difference in the future.

The aspect of post-transplant management that everyone thinks about is, of course, rejection and its prevention by the use of immuno-suppression. As introduced above, rejection is the process by which the immune system recognises a transplanted organ as being foreign and attempts to mount an immune response against it. This injury can cause damage to the liver and, over time and without treatment, its loss. The term rejection is not helpful, however, as it conjures up images of dying organs. In reality, rejection is a process which, if it happens at all, is identified early when the changes in the liver are minor, and which is reversed, in most cases, by short burst of additional treatment followed by a slight increase in the long–term immuno-suppression. The net result is that rejection, once feared, is now more of an inconvenience for most people. It could be completely prevented by using higher levels of immuno-suppression, but that would open patients to significant risk of drug side effects. The optimal approach is to find, for each patient, their "sweet spot" where rejection risk is minimised whilst maintaining immuno-suppression at an acceptable dose. The typical pattern of rejection, where it occurs (at least 50% of patients never get an episode), is a slight worsening of liver blood tests at around 7 to 10 days after transplant. This is sometimes, but not usually, accompanied by a fever and aches and pains which can make the unwary think it is an infection. Rejection should always be confirmed using a liver biopsy, which reveals a typical pattern of immune-mediated injury to the bile ducts (the same bile ducts that are the disease target in PBC....). If significant rejection is seen on liver biopsy (determined by the nature of the injury and the extent of involvement) then standard therapy is pulsed intra-venous methyl-prednisolone (a very powerful form of steroids given as 2 doses a day for 3 days via a drip). After this, it is normal to go on to a reducing dose of oral prednisolone. At the same time, it is appropriate to review all the immuno-suppression being used to try and identify a treatable reason for rejection (there usually isn't one). For most people, getting rejection is a case of a single episode that responds well to treatment and does not recur. Occasionally, a first pulse of immuno-suppression is not sufficient and the 3 day course has to be repeated. On the rare occasions when this does not work then an alternative therapy, usually with one of the biological agents such as anti-thymocyte globulin (ATG), is appropriate.

There are 2 further forms of rejection which bring their own issues. The first is antibody-mediated rejection that typically arises very early and is driven by antibodies in the recipient that are specific for donor proteins (it can also be one of the explanations for a later episode of acute rejection that fails to settle with methylprednisolone). This doesn't mean that the recipient has previously been exposed to the donor, rather it is sometimes a consequence of a previous blood transfusion where the blood donor was coincidentally a partial match to the liver donor. Alternatively, it can be just bad luck (remember that the immune system works on the basis of making any immune response possible unless it is negatively selected because it is too close in sequence to one of the body's own proteins). Antibody-mediated rejection can be a very severe form of rejection (although thankfully it is rare) and typically needs action to be taken to remove the antibodies (antibodies are long-lasting in the blood and aren't removed by steroids or other conventional forms of immuno-suppression). Approaches can include the use of plasmapheresis (a form of dialysis that removes antibodies from the circulation) and of rituximab, a biological drug that removes B-cells (the cells that will go on to produce antibody) from the circulation, often in combination.

The second additional form of rejection used to be called chronic rejection to contrast it with the acute cellular rejection (i.e. mediated by the T-lymphocytes in the circulation) which is the typical early form of rejection. The term now used is ductopenic rejection. This is partly because it more accurately describes the process, and partly because the terms acute and chronic imply a sequencing that isn't in fact the case (ductopenic rejection can occur early and in patients who have not had acute rejection). Ductopenic rejection is a rare but very difficult complication of liver transplantation that is very hard to treat. The first step in management is normally to optimise standard immuno-suppression in case the process has been driven by under-treated acute rejection. The issue is probably, however, that the injured bile ducts enter into a cycle of ongoing damage where an initial rejection injury has given rise to bile acid retention which causes further injury. If this concept of a first "hit" followed by a cycle of chronic damage sounds familiar it is because it is exactly the model I discussed earlier for PBC itself. Perhaps the message is that there is something about the bile ducts that makes them particularly vulnerable to chronic injury. Where ductopenic rejection occurs it is troubling for PBC patients as, perhaps unsurprisingly, the clinical features are very similar to those of PBC, with cholestatic itch being particularly prominent. The approach to treating ductopenic rejection is, first and foremost, to try and avoid the cycle ever starting by getting really effective long term immuno-suppression regimes in place. One established, there is no recognised treatment, however we use, again unsurprisingly, UDCA and bezafibrate (although we have to be very careful about watching kidney function).

Immuno-suppression "does what it says on the tin" which can bring its own long-term problems. In fact, in many ways the complications or immuno-suppression are, these days, more of an issue for patients than rejection. This is the reason why we always try and find the treatment "sweet spot" of just enough but not too much immuno-suppression. The first obvious potential problem is infection. Given that the immune system evolved to protect us against infection, limiting the function of the immune system naturally increases infection risk. A bit like rejection, however, this is a manageable risk, and not quite the problem people think it is. There are certain very specific infections transplant patients can be at risk of. These include fungal infections such as pneumocystis and aspergillus. Both of these are important and dangerous infections which are avoided by prophylactic drugs (typically a weekly dose of specific antibiotic) and risk avoidance respectively. Aspergillus tends to hide in spore form in dust in old buildings so we always recommend transplant patients stay well away when building work is being carried out! There is also an increased risk of certain viruses such as cytomegalovirus (CMV) and human papilloma virus (HPV). We make sure people's vaccinations are up to date before the transplant to reduce risk and recommend normal vaccinations after the transplant BUT ONLY IF THE VACCINE IS NOT A LIVE ONE. In my experience, however, patients are not troubled by increased numbers of "ordinary infections". Sometimes, people worry about infection and avoid crowded places such as cinemas. My advice is to use common sense. Avoid people with known active infection if you are not immune to it, otherwise live your life! Other than the specific infection types outlined above (and then only very rarely), I have never seen a post-transplant PBC patient die of an infection.

The second immuno-suppression risk is of cancer. In large part, this is in relation to those cancers that are driven by viral infection such as cervical carcinoma and squamous cell carcinoma of the skin, both of which can be driven by HPV infection. It is important that all transplant patients (and indeed anyone on long-term immuno-suppressive therapy) gets all relevant cancer screening (especially cervical) and is aware of the potential skin cancer risk checking for unusual skin lesions and getting them checked quickly if they arise. The other main cancer risk is for lymphoma, a cancer of the lymph glands. This can be a particular issue if people have had one of the powerful biological drugs such as ATG, which, by their very nature, disrupt the immune systems checks and balances (that's how they work!). The commonest version of this is a condition called post-transplant lymphoproliferative disease (PTLD). This starts out as overgrowth of the B-cells that is not cancerous, but has the potential to turn rapidly into a lymphoma. It appears to be, as with the other transplant-associated cancers, driven by a virus; in this case Epstein-Barr virus (the glandular fever virus). Treatment is, in the early stages, to reduce or stop immuno-suppression to allow the immune system to be able to clear the virally infected B-cells. If necessary, rituximab can be used effectively to clear the B-cells. If PTLD evolves into an active lymphoma then the treatment is chemotherapy. The message that PTLD sends is to be cautious about the immuno-suppression you use. Hitting the immune system hard to avoid any chance of rejection may feel like a good idea as a clinician when you are focusing on rejection as an issue. Be careful, however, to ensure that the treatment is really needed as it can store up major problems down the line

The final major complication of immuno-suppression is one that people often don't think of. It is the metabolic effects of the drugs. The issues with prednisolone (weight gain and risk of type 2 diabetes) are well known and are one of the reasons why these drugs are weaned down and stopped whenever possible. What is less well known is that tacrolimus and cyclosporine, the mainstays of immune-suppression, have their own metabolic impacts. Tacrolimus can, itself, cause type 2 diabetes mellitus and an increased risk of ischaemic heart disease. Both tacrolimus and cyclosporine can cause renal damage if their levels are too high, and can, over time, lead to renal failure. Finally, both can cause neurological symptoms. These include a fine tremor (I once met a watchmaker taking tacrolimus who knew his blood level by the degree of hand tremor he had, and who would stop the drug when he was working on a very expensive watch!). Other problems can include headaches, confusion and even fitting on occasions. It is very important when taking tacrolimus or cyclosporine that the blood levels of the drug are monitored carefully, and the drug dose adjusted accordingly.

LIVER TRANSPLANTATION IN PBC
There is no doubt that liver transplant is a significant undertaking with challenges and risks. It is also, however, frequently life changing. The good news for PBC patients is that they are the group of liver patients who have perhaps the best results from the procedure. The even better news is that the numbers of PBC patients needing liver transplantation are going down year on year because of earlier diagnosis and better treatment. My personal goal as a PBC doctor is to consign transplantation for my patients to the history books because diagnosis and treatment will have improved to the point where it is no longer ever needed! In this section I will look again at the 4 aspects to liver transplantation but this time specifically in relation to PBC.

Donor Livers: This is the aspect of transplantation that has fewest PBC-specific features as the nature of the donor organ is beyond the control of patients (other than, of course, if living-related transplantation is being considered). PBC is perhaps the setting (other than the special case of paediatric liver disease) where living related donation may be most relevant. This is for two reasons. The first is that PBC patients, in my experience (and forgive the generalisation), have strong and supportive family structures with spouses and family members frequently asking about volunteering as donors. This is not the case for all types of liver disease! The second reason is that the majority of PBC patients are women. This means that their liver size is smaller, and it is therefore much easier and safer for a brother or a husband to act as a donor than it would be the other way around (in simple terms a smaller fragment of the donor liver needs to be removed). As yet, the opportunities potentially offered by living related donation in PBC haven't really been realised because the systems, in the UK at least, are not well developed.

Liver transplant surgery: Liver transplantation surgery is typically straightforward in PBC. There are two reasons for this. The first is that all the complications of cirrhosis are less of an issue in PBC than they are in cirrhosis of most other aetiologies (largely because it is a cholestatic liver disease). Portal hypertension leading to large vessels on the abdominal wall is not a particular issue, nor is ascites and, in particular, spontaneous bacterial peritonitis which can cause a lot of scarring within the abdominal cavity making removal of the original liver very difficult indeed. The second reason why the transplant operation is relatively straightforward in PBC is because the patients are, other than for their PBC, typically in reasonable physical shape with less in the way of the heart and lung problems than can be common in patients with other types of liver disease. This all makes the anaesthetist's job much easier! The one issue that can sometimes arise is pulmonary hypertension; elevation of the pressure in the artery taking blood from the right side of the heart into the lungs to be re-oxygenated. Pulmonary hypertension can cause serious cardiac issues in general, and in particular in the transplant operation. It appears to be slightly commoner in PBC patients than in other people for reasons that are not well understood. Even in PBC, however, it remains rare.

Liver transplant assessment: As discussed in the previous section, PBC patients tend to have fewer other disease processes that might complicate liver transplantation than patients with other forms of chronic liver disease. In that sense, transplantation assessment is relatively straightforward. The challenge in terms of transplant decision making is, paradoxically, in the other direction with patients sometimes being perceived to be "too well" to need transplantation. In my experience such patients can sometimes go on to deteriorate quickly and sometimes miss out on transplantation. What is going on? As outlined earlier in the book PBC, as a cholestatic as opposed to hepatocellular disease (the injury is primarily to the biliary epithelial cells rather than the hepatocytes), behaves very differently to the way that many less experienced clinicians believe it will. Rather than a long, usually slow and, crucially, predictable decline, which gives time to recognise the risk and plan for transplant assessment, PBC patients can decline very rapidly once the end-stage of disease is reached. Crucially, the onset of this decline can be very difficult indeed to predict unless you are aware of the nuances of PBC. Danger signs include varices or ascites development, a rise in the bilirubin (even within the normal range) or a fall in the blood albumin level. All these things can happen in people who end up not being at significant risk so they should not worry people, it is just that these are the first signs in people who do go on to deteriorate. In other words, if you don't have varices or ascites, have a stable bilirubin within the normal range and a normal albumin then it is incredibly unlikely that you will deteriorate at any point in the near future. As I will discuss in **Chapter 9** it is really key for patients to "own" their disease and be aware of all the potential issues. Do not rely on your doctor to be aware of risk, know whether you have any of these risk factors, and if you have, discuss them with your doctor and ask about transplantation. DON'T DIE OF BEING TOO POLITE!

Post-transplant management: The early post-transplant management of PBC is usually very straightforward, with no specific risks. Indeed, given the dramatic impact of transplantation on itch, PBC patients can get a really good early "bounce" from transplantation. None of the early surgical complications are seen at an increased rate in PBC, and rejection does not seem to be a particular issue compared to transplant for other aetiologies (this is not the case with autoimmune hepatitis where acute cellular rejection appears to be common). PBC does, however, have a particular post-transplant issue that is disease recurrence. It is now clear that PBC can recur post-transplant, with about a third of patients having some features by around 5 years after the operation. It is important to be clear that in most people this will either be a change in blood tests or mild biopsy findings (many centres do routine liver biopsy after transplantation to monitor the organ and, unsurprisingly, they are the ones that see recurrent PBC most frequently). Occasional patients can, however, develop clinically significant recurrent PBC, with some people getting itch, and very occasional people getting recurrent cirrhosis. This possibility naturally worries people and it is important to be clear that the risk of getting a form of recurrent disease that causes harm is very low. For this reason, the risk of recurrent PBC should not deter anyone from being assessed for transplantation if they need it. It does, however, emphasise again the importance of doing everything we possibly can to avoid the need for transplantation by diagnosing the disease earlier and treating it better.

What can we do to reduce the risk of post-transplant recurrence (other than, of course, from avoiding the need for transplantation in the first place!)? An obvious question is what about UDCA? Given that we know that in "normal" PBC it works best when given early in the disease, what about the earliest point imaginable which is in a brand new liver? The logic is clear and for that reason many centres routinely give post-transplant PBC patients UDCA (and if I had had a transplant for PBC I would, without question, take it). What was lacking, until recently, was any evidence, as it would be almost impossible to carry out a conventional clinical trial to answer the question. The real world evidence approach which has helped our understanding of the effectiveness of OCA has, however, come to our assistance. Data from the Global PBC Study Group (a group that curate data from many thousands of PBC patients from across the world going back decades, including large numbers of post-transplant patients, some of whom got UDCA after transplant and some of whom didn't) strongly suggest that UDCA given from the point of transplant for PBC onwards significantly reduces risk of recurrent disease and, crucially, harm from recurrence. For this reason, I think preventative UDCA will rapidly become standard practice.

The other potential approach is an intriguing one. Several studies have suggested, and the Global PBC Study Group have confirmed, that recurrence is significantly more likely if tacrolimus is used as the main immuno-suppression drug rather than cyclosporine, its older and now less widely used counterpart. Cyclosporine is a crucial drug in the history of all organ transplantation as it was the first drug that really effectively prevented acute rejection. It has, however, significant side effects including, in particular, renal failure if dosing is too high. Tacrolimus is a drug of the same type that emerged after cyclosporine, and has fewer (or, probably more accurately, different) side-effects with, in particular, a lower rate of renal issues. A major UK trial showed that it was more effective at preventing rejection and led to better organ survival in liver transplant. This finding led to pretty much universal use. We therefore have a paradox. Tacrolimus is probably better than cyclosporine for preventing rejection, but definitely worse for permitting/facilitating disease recurrence. At this point in time, this information does not influence immuno-suppression decisions in PBC and it isn't clear whether it should. If, however, you are a post-transplant patient with no history of rejection but significant recurrence of your PBC then a change from tacrolimus to cyclosporine is definitely something you should consider.

CHAPTER 7: **SYMPTOMS IN PBC**

The 2-Minute Version

- Symptoms are much more frequently a problem in PBC patients than is progression of the disease to cirrhosis. Treating symptoms is, therefore, just as important as slowing disease progression and should be just as high a priority for doctors and nurses.

- The two main symptoms are itch and fatigue. Fatigue is commoner but itch is easier to treat.

- PBC itch is typically deep under the skin, often feeling like "creepy-crawlies". It can often affect the palms of the hand and the soles of the feet; areas of the body rarely affected by other types of itch. It is never accompanied by a rash; any skin changes seen arise as a result of scratching.

- There is a well-established "ladder" of treatments for PBC itch if patients need them. Just having itch isn't, however, a reason to treat it. You should treat it if it is causing problems (for example difficulty in sleeping). UDCA should already have been started, but will typically not particularly help.

- The first-line treatment is cholestyramine (Questran). This can taste unpleasant and adding fruit juice or chilling (it is a drink) can help. If this does not work, or you can't tolerate it, the next choice in most centres is rifampicin. This is effective, but can make the liver worse, so liver function tests need to be measured after 4 weeks on it. Anti-histamines don't work. A recent trial has suggested that bezafibrate is highly effective for the treatment of itch (although issues with renal dysfunction need to be remembered). It may well replace rifampicin as second-line treatment for PBC itch.

- Fatigue can have peripheral ("it feels like my batteries are running down") and central ("it feels like I have brain fog") components. Central fatigue is often accompanied by memory and concentration problems. There is no specific therapy, although a supportive approach is effective.

- The first step is to look for and treat other conditions that can also cause fatigue (such as thyroid disease or anaemia; this is discussed more in **Chapter 8**). The second is to look for and treat associated features such as depression (not a cause of fatigue in PBC but it can make it worse), sleep disturbance and blood pressure regulation. The third, and really key step is to develop a coping strategy to minimise the impact. This is discussed in detail in **Chapter 9**. Exercise seems to be really helpful for reducing fatigue severity.

- Abdominal pain can occur in PBC. It is usually over the right side of the upper abdomen (i.e. over the liver). People think it is caused by gallstones, although this is rarely the case. It appears to improve with UDCA and may be caused by cholestasis causing swelling of the liver capsule.

- Audit of clinical practice suggests that assessment of the impact of symptoms on PBC patients is frequently not included in clinic follow-up, despite guidelines recommending that patients are asked about fatigue and itch on every clinic visit. This needs to change!

One of the major steps forward in the management of PBC, in recent years, has been the appreciation, by most clinicians at least, of the extent to which symptoms can occur and can impact on peoples quality of life, and the importance of treating them (patients, of course, have always known about them!). Traditional thinking held that PBC was initially asymptomatic and, as it progressed towards cirrhosis, so symptoms developed. The implication was that symptoms were, therefore, a feature of advanced disease and, indeed, a bad prognostic feature. It is now recognised that this is completely incorrect. The fallacy arose because of the inclusion of jaundice and abdominal swelling from ascites as disease symptoms. Given that they are exclusively features of cirrhosis/stage 4 disease it is unsurprising that they are seen in advanced disease!! The advent of tools to allow us to measure symptoms and their impact on people have allowed us to fully explore the clinical picture of PBC. The most widely used of these is the PBC-40, a 40 question questionnaire that was derived in the UK entirely in PBC patients and which uses patients own words to form the questions. This patient-derived and disease-specific approach to its development makes the PBC-40 highly relevant to patients, and allows their experiences to be captured (to the extent that a questionnaire can ever accurately capture what are, in practice very complex, problems). The PBC-40 has been applied very widely in PBC and can allow us to make some broad conclusions about symptoms in PBC.

- There are a number of symptom sets in PBC that can occur at any point in the disease course (i.e. they are NOT features of advanced disease) and contribute to quality of life impairment.
- Of these symptom sets the commonest is fatigue, followed by cognitive symptoms (issues relating to short-term memory and concentration) and itch. Symptoms suggestive of social isolation are also common, as are emotional issues. There are also a series of additional symptoms including abdominal pain and bone pain.
- Additional symptoms can arise as a result of associated conditions. These include dry eyes and dry mouth from associated Sjogren's syndrome.
- Symptom sets are inter-connected (for example, sleep disturbance resulting from itch at night can have knock on effects on fatigue and cognitive symptoms the following day).
- Social isolation symptoms can, in particular, complicate all other symptom sets (fatigue can cause social isolation because people haven't got the energy to work or to socialise, itch can cause social isolation because people are self-conscious about scratching in public).
- The severity of each of these symptom sets is unrelated to disease severity or degree of liver function test abnormality, and none

appear to respond to either first line or second-line therapy (at least as currently used). This lack of a disease severity association is one of the reasons why clinicians have, in the past, questioned the link to PBC (a link that in my experience patients never had any difficulty in making!)

- Patients with complications of cirrhosis have additional symptom sets (outlined in **Chapter 2**). These are in addition to the non-stage-related PBC symptoms and mean that quality of life in PBC is typically at its very worst in patients with very advanced disease with complications.

- There are, undoubtedly, PBC patients who are completely asymptomatic (and often wonder what I am talking about when I ask about fatigue and itch). This group, who definitely have PBC and definitely don't have symptoms, are both fortunate and very helpful in helping to understand why PBC symptoms develop,

One of the important conclusions of our work is that symptoms in PBC are a problem in their own right, and should be assessed and treated on their own merit as part of normal PBC management. Assessing and treating symptoms is one of the steps we need to take to manage the disease, in just the same way that assessing severity and treating to prevent progression is an end in its own right. In fact, given that symptoms impact on more patients than disease progression they are actually a priority for many patients. The unfortunate reality, however, is that symptoms are, all too often, not thought about or asked about in many clinic visits. Data from the audit of UK practice (reported in 2022 with data for the calendar year 2021) suggests that 50% of PBC patients are not being asked about their symptoms when they go to the clinic. This is despite assessment of symptoms at every clinic visit being a clear recommendation in all PBC treatment guidelines. It is a simple, if obvious, truth that you can't treat symptoms unless you know that they are there and you won't know they are there if you don't ask about them! We all need to work together to increase awareness of PBC symptoms and "enshrine" their assessment in everyday PBC clinical practice.

In the rest of this chapter I will consider each of the symptoms in turn, looking at current thinking as to causes and impacts before looking at treatment options. This is an area which is developing very rapidly and where I anticipate real progress being made in the near future.

ITCH

Itch is, in many ways, the archetypal PBC symptom although, given that it is the symptom with the greatest range of treatment options, its impact is substantially less across the population than it was in the past. The itch described by PBC patients is not actually unique to them as it can occur in a number of cholestatic conditions (conditions characterised by abnormality in bile flow). This strongly suggests that it is caused by some aspect of the deranged bile production pathway rather than a PBC process per se. It is often described by patients as being "deep under the skin" with "creepy crawlies" there and is often made worse by a hot bath. Its characteristics are, therefore, very different to an allergic type of itch which tends to affect the surface of the skin. The body distribution is also characteristic with affected areas including the soles of the feet and the palms of the hands, as well as the scalp. Perhaps inevitably, the first thought of clinicians is that itch has a skin cause rather than being a feature of a distant disease process. PBC (and other cholestatic itch) patients do not, however, have any rash or skin abnormality (other than where they cause skin damage through scratching) and the absence of rash should always make clinicians think of another cause. The severity of PBC itch ranges from a mild sensation which is present, but which doesn't warrant treatment, all the way through to a life-altering, very severe symptom. Fortunately, the former is far commoner than the latter.

The actual cause of itch in PBC remains unclear. The response to treatment, however, gives us some clues. The most striking response to treatment of PBC itch is that seen following liver transplantation. Itch disappears immediately (patients tell me it has gone by the time that they wake up after the operation) and, in my experience, rarely if ever comes back. This suggests that a fully functioning liver clears whatever it is that causes itch (or at least sets off the chain of events that leads to itch) very quickly. We also know that an approach called naso-biliary drainage, in which a tube is used to drain the bile from the bile duct out of the body, is also highly effective. These two observations point to something which is present in the bile contributing directly to itch. Furthermore, the first-line treatment for itch is a drug called cholestyramine which acts, within the bowel, to bind bile acids and prevent them from being taken back up at the end of the small bowel (the ileum) and recycled to the liver. To take the bile link further, one of the new classes of itch treatment which has been successful in trials is an iBAT inhibitor which specifically blocks the uptake of bile acids within the ileum. These observations all point to bile acids either being directly responsible for itch, or acting as triggers for the itch pathway. Whatever the underlying cause of the stimulation, the actual sensation of itch is mediated by activation of nerve receptors in the skin which then signal to the brain. Interestingly, drugs that block the actions of opiates (the morphine family of pain killers which are also present in the natural state in the body to act as an internal pain control system) are effective for PBC itch suggesting that the activation of nerve sensors in the skin may be via natural opiates.

The current "state of the art" thinking for itch in PBC and other cholestatic diseases is that there is a bile-acid driven activation of an enzyme called autotaxin which may itself be produced by stressed biliary epithelial cells. Autotaxin promotes the generation of another chemical called lysophosphatidic acid which may well be the direct stimulating factor for nerve sensors that then signal irritation to the nerves that communicate to the brain through natural opiates. If this model is correct then it has important implications for potential treatment approaches, including drugs that can block the action of autotaxin, which are currently under development.

Treating itch in PBC: Treatment of itch in PBC can be very effective and can make a huge difference to quality of life. We take a stepwise approach. The first step in managing itch is to understand whether treatment is actually needed at all! For many people, understanding that itch is part of the disease, and is treatable if needs be, is enough. The art with controlling itch is to be able to forget about it or block it out. The brain has highly developed pathways to prevent sensory overload by information coming from the skin; none of us normally thinks about being able to feel our clothes on our skin, yet once you do think about it you can indeed feel them. This continues for a few minutes until you "forget" about the sensation again. The art with itch treatment is, therefore, to help people to get to the point where they can forget about the sensation. Awareness of itch during normal activities, the need to scratch and, in particular, significant itch at night are the features that suggest treatment may be necessary. Sleep disturbance from itch can be a particular issue as it can have knock-on effects in terms of fatigue and cognitive symptoms. The issue of night itch is partly a result of the symptom being worse at night, and partly the lack of other daytime distractions at night meaning that the brain has less in the way of other stimuli to focus on.

The first stage of itch treatment is to ensure that patients are on an effective dose of UDCA. This is partly for all the other good reasons for using UDCA, and partly because a number of patients report that it is effective at controlling itch (although, paradoxically, about 5% of patients report that it can make their itch worse and can actually be a reason for UDCA dose reduction). Before moving to drug-based therapy many patients try moisturising creams and, in particular, vitamin E cream. These have never been formally tested in clinical trials but they are very safe and as this is a purely symptom issue (the only goal is symptom control as disease risk is managed via different routes) if they work for a patient then they are effective. One preventative step that patients can take is to avoid opiate painkillers (e.g. codeine phosphate, dihydrocodeine etc). These can add to the level of activation of the body's own opiate signalling system, which, as we have discussed, probably signals itch in the skin.

First-line treatment for itch, once a decision has been taken to go down the medicine route, is cholestyramine. This is the only licensed drug for itch in PBC and has the advantage of being very safe (it stays in the bowel and has its actions there). It is, however, limited in its actions and can be unpleasant to take (it has a bitter taste and an odd texture). We suggest to people to try adding fruit juice to it (it comes as sachets that are mixed into a drink) or chill it in the fridge before use; both of which patients describe as making it more palatable. Cholestyramine should always be spaced away from UDCA or OCA therapy as both of these drugs are themselves bile acids which will obviously also bind to cholestyramine and lose their activity. We recommend that cholestyramine is taken three times a day, with UDCA and OCA being taken 4 hours after the last sachet later in the evening. The use of cholestyramine as first line treatment for PBC itch often comes as a surprise to GPs, whose first thought with itch management is always to use anti-histamines. In fact, anti-histamines are to be avoided in PBC for two reasons. The first is that they do not particularly work for cholestatic itch. The second is that they are even more sedating in PBC patients than is normally the case (and sedation is their commonest side effect).The one time I use anti-histamines in PBC patients with itch is in people with real difficulty in getting to sleep because of the itch. In this situation the sedating property is actually quite useful! When they are used, people need to be really careful about hang-over effects. They can be slow to clear from the circulation in people with cholestasis meaning that if they are taken late at night they can still be acting in the morning. Something to be very cautious about if you are driving to work…..

If cholestyramine is not effective, or people simply can't tolerate it, and itch is severe enough, then consideration should be given to second-line itch therapy. It is important for patients to understand, though, that although none of the second-line drugs are particularly risky as such, they do have more in the way of side-effects than cholestyramine. Using them definitely means that the stakes are rising. It is also important to remember that none of the second-line therapies are labelled for use in PBC itch. There are a number of licensed, unlabelled drugs that are widely used, as well as new drugs that are, as yet, unlicensed and undergoing evaluation in clinical trials. Practice differs from centre to centre but our preferred second-line therapy is still (in 2023) a drug called rifampicin. This is an old antibiotic, originally used for the treatment of TB and still used for preventing disease in the contacts of people with bacterial meningitis. Its actions in PBC are unrelated to its antibiotic actions. Instead, it probably works by promoting the breakdown of autotaxin. In a sense, the mechanism of action doesn't matter; it is used because clinical trials, backed up by long clinical experience, suggest that it is effective. Rifampicin, however, represents a clear step up in both potency and potential side effects compared to cholestyramine. It is therefore really important to be certain that cholestyramine is not effective before moving on. All too often, we see patients with "intractable itch" who, in practice, have only had a couple of days or weeks here and there with treatments. In almost all these cases, going back to the beginning and using the earlier therapies again but properly this time results in good itch control. The issue with rifampicin is that it can (thankfully rarely) cause liver injury. This is not particularly worse in PBC patients than it is in patients getting the drug for other reasons, but the concern about additive injury is obvious. The good news is that the injury, if it happens, settles down very quickly if rifampicin is stopped. We start people on a low dose (150mg (1 tablet) daily and check liver blood tests at 2-4 weeks). If there has been a deterioration, in particular a rise in ALT or bilirubin, the rifampicin should be stopped and the blood tests watched until they return to the levels they were before it was started. If the blood tests are fine (as they usually are) then we monitor the effect on itch. If it isn't controlled completely we slowly increase the dose as far as 600mg daily (4 tablets). If we get good control of the itch at a lower dose then there is no need to keep increasing the dose. In my experience, about half of patients get good control just on the lowest "test" dose of 150mg. One thing we always warn people about with rifampicin is that it can colour urine, sweat and even tears pinky-orange; a real surprise to people who are not expecting it. Although this discussion of side effects might give the impression that rifampicin is a problem drug this would not be correct. For most people it is a safe and very effective treatment for itch and it is our "go to" treatment once cholestyramine has failed. The other good news with rifampicin is that, unlike some drugs such as naltrexone which will be discussed in the next section, the effect does not appear to "wear off" over time. I have patients who have been on the same dose of rifampicin, with complete control of their itch, for more than 20 years. In fact, the one thing I always tell people is, if the drug is working and there are no problems with it DON'T FIDDLE WITH THE DOSE. I have seen a number of people who, after a long time on rifampicin with good itch control wondered if the itch had in fact gone away and tried stopping the drug. The itch then comes back and appears to no longer respond as well to rifampicin……..

In my experience, the majority of PBC patients get good itch control on UDCA with either cholestyramine, rifampicin or a combination of both. There are, however, a small number of patients who do not get good control. We run a specialised service for itch so see patients from all over the country, meaning that we have more experience of this than most. The important first thing to say is do not panic. There is always a treatment for everyone. We just need to find what the right one for you is! After rifampicin, the drug we used to use most commonly was naltrexone, an oral blocker of opiates. This is, however, an area where practice is changing and increasingly, we are using bezafibrate early in the itch treatment "escalator". We have discussed bezafibrate in some detail in **Chapter 5** as one of the therapy options for patients who do not respond to UDCA. In addition to this blood test improving effect (and, potentially impact on disease progression) it also seems to significantly reduce itch severity and has trial data to support its use.

The caution, of course, is, as is the case for its use in treating underlying disease, the risk of renal impairment. One scenario we encounter not infrequently is the patient with significant itch as well as UDCA-non-response level bloods. In this setting bezafibrate makes a more logical agent than rifampicin that has little if any effect on the disease process. In people with well-controlled liver blood tests rifampicin is still my preferred second-line itch therapy simply because of the long experience that we have of long-term use.

If neither rifampicin nor bezafibrate proved effective we would then consider the opiate-blocking drug naltrexone. As outlined above, natural opiates produced by the body appear to be elevated in PBC (they may be produced by the sick biliary epithelial cells) and act as transmitters, signalling from the itch sensors in the skin to the nervous system. Blocking this transmission is a logical way of interrupting the signals so that the brain gets less of an itch signal. Naltrexone was developed to help people with opiate drug addiction stop their drug habit and has also been used to help people with alcohol addiction. It can therefore feel like an odd drug to use in PBC. It does, however, work well and has clear trial evidence to support its use. Why, given the evidence as to how well it works, and the logic behind it, do we use it only after rifampicin and bezafibrate has failed? There are three very practical reasons. The first is that if patients have had high levels of opiates for a long time (remember these are not opiates taken as tablets or injections but ones produced naturally by the body in PBC, probably over long periods of time) then blocking them can lead to a withdrawal-type reaction (like going "cold turkey"). This can involve shivers, cramps and nightmares. We mitigate this by either starting on the lowest tablet dose possible (realistically 12.5mg which is a quarter of a tablet) or, if starting the drug is still problematic, bringing people into hospital to give intravenous naloxone (the injectable version of naltrexone) which can be started at very low doses indeed. Although most people get through any cold turkey quickly (a couple of days is normal) there are some people who never manage to take naltrexone because of this issue. The second problem with naltrexone is, in my experience, the predictable one of pain. The body produces its own opiates to be able to control pain. If that benefit is blocked, aches and pains seem to be worse in people. I have come across people with real problems from toothache and shingles for example. The third reason is a wearing-off of the beneficial effect over time. The effects of opiates on pain can reduce over time, leading to a need for ever-higher doses to get the same effect. The same is true of the action of naltrexone as an itch treatment. It is possible to "reset" the effect by discontinuing the treatment for a period of time. This gives rise, however, to the obvious problem of the itch returning until the treatment can be re-started. The end-result of these issues is that, although naltrexone clearly "works", it is a drug that in practice doesn't end up helping that many people.

If we are still struggling to control itch at this point there are a number of further options and it is often a case of trial and error. Clinical guidelines suggest that a good drug to try is sertraline (the anti-depressant drug) with a clinical trial showing benefit. Our experience, however, has been unimpressive, with few, if any, patients responding. Paradoxically, we do use a drug which a trial has suggested does not benefit, but which in our experience works well. This is gabapentin, an anti-epileptic drug which is widely used for pain control. It slows transmission of pain signals to the brain. The similarity in the signalling paths between pain and itch gives a logic as to how it might work. In our experience low doses (as low as 150mg or 300mg daily but increasable well beyond that if needed) work well, and don't have too many in the way of sedation-related side-effects (something that can happen when higher doses are used).

There are a very small number of people (and it is a very small number) where drugs fail to control itch. At this point it is very important to take a step back and just be certain that this really is PBC itch, rather than itch for another reason that happens to be in a PBC patient (the treatments outlined above will only work for cholestatic itch). If this really is PBC itch, and all the treatments outlined above have not worked, then there are two broad options. The first is trial medication and the second is a broad category of what I call "physical approaches". Improved treatment of itch for PBC and other cholestatic liver diseases is an area of real research activity at the time of writing, with drug trials both ongoing and planned. Approaches with potential include iBAT inhibitors (drugs that block the re-uptake of bile acids in the small bowel and thus, in theory at least, acting as "super-cholestyramine"). Another approach is around improved opiate antagonists (in essence naltrexone equivalents but engineered to not have the "cold turkey" withdrawal effect). A little further in the future there may be drugs that block the action of autotaxin. Clinical trials have been very successful in PBC and have undoubtedly led to rapid progress in how we treat the disease, so considering taking part in one is an important option. Not everyone will meet the study criteria, or want to take part, of course, so discuss the opportunities with your doctor. My personal observation is that people typically find taking part in trials in PBC a very rewarding experience and never regret it.

The physical approaches represent the last option set for treatment of severe or otherwise untreatable itch. The ultimate physical approach is liver transplantation. As outlined in **Chapter 6** transplantation is performed (rarely) for intractable itch. Before considering this it is really important to be clear it is indeed PBC itch, and to think through the ramifications of going for transplant to manage it (particularly if you are otherwise low risk with regard to your PBC). As discussed previously, transplantation is a balance of risks between the risk of having the operation (the complications of the surgery, rejection and medication side effects) versus, normally, the risk of not having it (risk of death from the complications of PBC). The challenge in considering transplant for itch is that the risks of the operation remain the same but the risks of not having the operation are very different (a risk of poor quality of life rather than a risk of death). This needs careful consideration and long discussion. Transplant is very effective for itch if there really is no alternative, but the risks of transplant need to be weighed against the nature and degree of likely benefit.

The two other physical approaches are best thought of as emergency interventions. These are MARS (a version of dialysis that removes the itch-causing toxins from the blood) and the previously introduced approach of naso-biliary drainage (drainage of bile from the bile duct via a tube that removes the toxins in bile). Both are effective, but are very invasive, require a hospital stay and are not without risk. They also only have a short-term benefit (one to 2 weeks of itch control at most). The capacity to offer them, however, gives a crucial benefit. The mere existence of a "big-gun" approach that will definitely work, and work quickly, is incredibly valuable to patients who are really struggling with their itch. The sense of loss of control is, in my experience, a major factor for patients ("I am at the mercy of the disease"). The existence of an intervention that is available rapidly if they need it allows people to regain control. My centre offers naso-biliary drainage as an intervention. This has benefitted far more people than have actually received the treatment! The others benefit from the knowledge that it is there if they ever need it. Because of the challenges and risks of these interventions they really should only be provided in very specialised centres with experience of the approach.

There is one final, and important, aspect to itch in PBC which is the challenge of itch in the context of OCA therapy. Itch was a significant side-effect in the early OCA trials, which typically used far higher drug doses than are used in practice now. At the typical doses used in the clinic the issue is much less and should not get in the way of using OCA if that is the right drug for disease management. In my clinic's OCA programme we have not had any patients who have needed to stop OCA because of itch. In our experience there are two aspects to the effective avoidance of itch issues with OCA. The first is to look for any evidence of itch before starting OCA and treat it. The other is to be aggressive with itch developing on OCA. It is the one situation when we would advocate early treatment for itch rather than waiting to see the impact. Where we are managing itch in the context of OCA we tend to go to rifampicin as the first line treatment because cholestyramine is rarely effective and it can bind to OCA meaning that both drugs lose their effect. A slow introduction of OCA over a few weeks can also sometimes be a useful approach.

The Newcastle approach to itch management is outlined in the Appendix 3

FATIGUE

In my experience, the most challenging symptom in PBC is fatigue. It is challenging for several reasons. The first and most obvious reason is that, unlike itch, we currently have no effective drug treatments. This means that our management approach in the clinic is purely supportive. This can make an important difference to people, but falls some way short of a solution. The second reason is the "normality" of fatigue. What do I mean? Itch is something abnormal. We never normally have itch other than perhaps as a fleeting sensation. It is, therefore, easy to compartmentalise as something that is abnormal as part of the disease. This does not, of course, reduce its impact but it does make it easier for patients to understand it as part of their disease. Fatigue is very different. It is something that many of us feel as part of ordinary life (working too hard, too many late nights etc). This leads many patients to struggle with understanding whether their fatigue is part of the disease or not. Is what they perceive real? It is no coincidence that one of the important steps in managing fatigue in the clinic is to explain it in the context of PBC, and to describe the experiences of other patients. Patient groups facilitating meeting with other patients with similar experiences are also very helpful in this regard. This, again, does not reduce the fatigue but it does make it easier for patients to accept it. The third reason is the attitude of the medical and nursing professions to fatigue. This is, unfortunately, often very negative. Far too many patients describe doctors tutting, rolling their eyes, saying that they "only treat proper problems" and saying how tired they are because they were "on-call" last night. One of the things I find most puzzling in PBC is why doctors find it so easy to accept that itch is "real", whilst at the same time believing adamantly that fatigue is not. I suspect the fact that the former is easy to treat whilst the latter is not has a lot to do with it.

One of the main challenges with fatigue is that the concept itself is difficult to explain. Whereas pain or itch are quite easy to explain and understand, and the terms largely mean the same thing to different people, the term fatigue is challenging. I once met a patient after a lecture who told me that some days it was her fatigue that was bad and some days her tiredness. I had used the terms inter-changeably in the lecture, but to her each had a distinctive meaning. The problem is that the same words may well have meant different things to another patient. When using patient descriptions of their own experience, fatigue appears to be present in approximately 60% of patients, with around 25% of all patients having significant fatigue. Tools such as the PBC-40 are, as with itch, very useful for allowing us to quantify fatigue; something which is an important step if we are going to understand it and treat it. As with itch, one of the important groups of patients is that of people who are clearly not affected. It is the comparison of these people with patients with fatigue that has been most informative in understanding the problem.

There appear to be two main variants of fatigue in PBC, neither of which is associated with disease severity (it is as likely to be seen in people with mild disease as severe). Patients can have one, both or neither. The first type is a very peripheral form, which patients often describe as feeling like their "batteries running down". This type of fatigue is associated with real struggles doing day-to- day things (people often describe planning shopping trips to shopping centres where they know they can sit down half way round). There can often be a sense of a finite amount of energy that, once used up, means that the rest of the day is a struggle (mornings are often much better than afternoons for this reason which is an important part of the approach to coping with fatigue that we work with patients on). Resting re-stocks energy to a degree, but it is normally only the next day that people can get going again. Another common phenomenon is that of "good days and bad days". A number of years ago a patient who, earlier in life, had been a keen runner said to me that her fatigue felt just like she had "finished a half marathon" with her legs turning to jelly. Based on this, we did a study looking at the extent to which people could repeat a physical task (squeezing a hand grip-strength meter). Healthy controls and PBC patients without fatigue showed a drop off in the strength of repeat squeezes of about 25%, but after that could continue without any problems. The fatigued PBC patents were very different, showing a rapid drop off that continued to the point at which they could not carry on. Their batteries appeared to have, indeed, run out of power. A number of years later the advent of new scanning technology allowed us to explore what was actually happening in people's muscles when they had fatigue. We used an MRI scanner to "look inside" leg muscles during repeat exercise to see what was happening to energy levels. What we found was that PBC patients, as a whole, had very abnormal patterns of muscle function. Whereas in healthy controls the pH in muscle (the degree of acidity) was very stable with exercise, PBC patients showed a significant build-up of acid. This was lactic acid, which is a breakdown product of inefficient, anaerobic exercise. Given that this is what happens at the end of a bout of exercise when people are exhausted our former runner patient was exactly right (something I learned a very long time ago was to always listen to patients! The exact words they use are very telling). Interestingly, although the degree of acid build up in muscle did not associate with how fatigued people were, their ability to recover from it did, with people able to recover fast having much less fatigue that those recovering slowly. Given that ability to recover from exercise is built up by exercise training this is an important reason for PBC patients to exercise, even if their level of fatigue mean that they feel at first that they can't. It will improve! This is another part of the coping strategy for PBC fatigue and a key aspect of "self-ownership" of the disease and its problems.

The second type of fatigue is what we call central fatigue. As its name suggests this is more about brain function than peripheral muscle capacity. Patients typically describe this as "brain fog". Concentrating can be hard and short-term memory can be a real problem. People feel like they have to make a huge effort to concentrate enough to do things. In its purest form this is very distinct from the peripheral type of fatigue although, of course, the two can co-exist in the same person. One potential mechanism for the co-existence is that in some people central fatigue is the initial problem. This leads to people wanting to, and being able to, do less. This means that they lose physical fitness, which means that their muscles work less well and are more inefficient, reverting to anaerobic metabolism too quickly. This results in lactic acid build up and the increased acid levels that we see in our MR studies. This in turn results in a signal being sent back to the brain to say that the muscles are stressed which gives rise to the sensation of fatigue. This cycle is known as de-conditioning. There are parallels with other situations. An unfit person trying to run a half-marathon at the same speed as a fit person will soon have to stop because of lactic acid build up in their muscles. If that person trained, then next year they could run further and faster before the acid build up stopped them. The other analogy is the fit person who breaks their leg and has it put in plaster. They very rapidly lose muscle bulk and function on the immobilised side. If you did the MRI muscle studies described earlier on them just after the plaster came off, then the previously immobilised side would show greater acidosis (i.e. look more like a PBC patient) than the non-immobilised side. This is of much more than academic interest. The impact of de-conditioning is such that even if we found a "cure" for central fatigue it, on its own, would not really help people because although the motivation and capacity to initiate activity will be increased the muscles will need to re-adjust to be able to do that. This will take time and rehabilitation. The athlete with the broken leg needs to rehabilitate and so, I suspect, will PBC patients recovering from central fatigue.

The study of the brain in PBC is an area of real interest and activity. It is also an area of real progress that offers much promise for better treatments. Perhaps the most striking finding is that there are measureable, visible changes in the brains of people with PBC with central fatigue when we use state of the art MRI imaging techniques. These are largely about the effectiveness of pathways of the brain that link from the lower to the higher parts. The higher brain (the cortex) is where information processing and activity initiation happen. If you see an apple and want to pick it up and eat it the sensors in the eye signal to the brain that there is something there. The occipital cortex (the area at the very back of the brain) processes that information and, accessing memory areas, converts the sensation of a green sphere into awareness that it is an apple. The information is fed into the connection network which leads to the motor cortex which controls the arm and leg muscles and which initiates the activity of picking up the apple and eating it. The sensors for smell and taste then function to send signals about the taste which the higher brain again interprets. If the decision is that the apple is good the motor action for eating is continued. If it is rotten the taste and smell sensations are interpreted in the context of memory of rotten food, the motor signal is to throw the apple away. Much of the function of the brain occurs, however, at a more automatic level. There is an "engine room" that controls many functions in a way that means we don't have to think about them. Take breathing. If you want to you can breathe as fast as you want. This shows that breathing can be controlled by the cortex. If, however, you stop actively thinking about it you still carry on breathing normally. This is the automatic side of the brain function. It itself can be reactive to situations. If you encounter a threat (you see a tiger in front of you) then as well as the visual stimulus leading to a motor effect (running away!) your breathing will also increase in frequency to help you run away by increasing the blood oxygen supply. You do not, however have to think about it. Other body functions are controlled by the brain in an (almost) entirely automatic function. Think about heart rate and blood pressure. Your heart rate is controlled by brain function through specialist nerves that supply the natural pacemaker in the heart, but at a completely automatic level. Blood pressure is partly controlled by heart rate and partly by how narrow or constricted the blood vessels are in your legs. If they tighten up the blood return to your heart goes up along with your blood pressure. If they relax, blood pools in your legs and blood pressure falls. This is all controlled by the nervous system, but this time originating in the lower areas of the brain. Some of these automatic functions can be over-ridden by cortical control. The most obvious one is potty training a small child. Bowels and bladder will both empty automatically when they are full, but we can learn, at an early age, to control it. Although heart rate cannot normally be controlled, some people can teach their body to do it by intense concentration. Examples include professional violin and snooker players (!) where a high heart rate can lead to tremor which affects performance. Breathing control is a trick of free divers (who dive to great depths without an air supply). There are other "deep" brain functions that are crucial but typically happen automatically. These include the initiation and maintenance of sleep and memory creation and recovery. Trying to go to sleep or remember something rarely works, but, typically, just after you have stopped trying they happen spontaneously!

Central fatigue rarely exists on its own. It appears to be linked to two other processes which are important in terms of its clinical impact. The link to a third is very controversial. The first clear link is with dysfunction of the autonomic nervous system, the part of the brain and nervous system that controls the most fundamental automatic functions such as heart-beat and blood pressure, sweating and the function of the bowel. One of the key roles of the autonomic nervous system is to adjust the blood pressure up and down in response to changes in the body position and function. A simple example is standing up in the middle of the night. Blood pressure falls at night in general as the blood vessels dilate up. On top of that, if you suddenly stand up the blood literally rushes to your feet as gravity takes over. If there were to be no response to this you would feel dizzy and then black out as the blood supply to the brain was compromised. This is actually a protective mechanism as blacking out makes you lie down again, removing the gravity problem! Normally, of course, this doesn't happen. The instant the blood pressure begins to fall the drop is sensed by receptors in the veins in the neck (the baroreceptors). They signal to the brain and the brain activates the autonomic nervous system to tighten the blood vessels in the leg returning the blood pressure to normal. This all normally happens in an instant without you ever being aware of it. In PBC patients with fatigue this "reflex" is either poorly functioning or fails completely. This means that the blood pressure continues to fall when you stand up. A fail safe then kicks in which is the release of adrenaline to speed up the heart. This is not the most effective way of increasing blood pressure if the problem is dilation of the blood vessels in the leg (it is a bit like stamping on the brake pedal very hard when the fault is a leak of brake fluid) but it is enough to stop blacking out. The adrenaline release can lead to sweating and palpitations (fast heart rate). Ultimately, if this fail safe doesn't work you will get dizzy and eventually black out. This is fortunately rare in PBC patients (although it does happen). What is common is a sense of dizziness when standing up accompanied by palpitations. All of this is particularly common in patients with fatigue. What is the link to fatigue? We do know that autonomic dysfunction is a feature of many chronic conditions with fatigue as part of their clinical picture, suggesting that the link is real. It may be that it is at the level of blood pressure regulation in the muscle with poor blood flow in to the limbs (necessary to supply nutrients and oxygen). Perhaps more likely is a dysfunction of the muscle draining blood flow. Pooling of venous blood may lead to poor run-off of lactic acid contributing to the muscle acidosis and dysfunction discussed previously. Given that increasing venous drainage of lactic acid is part of how we adapt in exercise training this would fit with the finding that exercise training helps in PBC fatigue.

The second key association is with sleep disturbance. Fatigued PBC patients very frequently have abnormal sleep patterns. The commonest pattern is daytime sleepiness. This can sometimes be severe enough to get in the way of work or family life. People tend not to have the extreme sleep patterns seen in the condition narcolepsy (where people can even fall asleep driving a car) but on occasion it can fall not far short. Obviously, disturbed sleep can occur in lots of conditions (and, of course, can be just the way people are). It can be very difficult to "unravel" abnormal sleep because we are not good at sensing our own sleep patterns. Many of our patients, therefore, go to the sleep clinic to have a formal sleep study where the stages of sleep are assessed. This can be done in a hospital sleep lab during an overnight stay or, more commonly these days, at home using portable equipment. One of the recent revolutions in healthcare has been the rapid development of digital health monitoring technology. These days a "Fitbit" or "i-watch" can give really quite accurate sleep data at relatively low cost. It may be, therefore, be that we will be able, in the near future, to introduce sleep assessment into everyday practice. One simple step which may help with sleep is ensuring that vitamin D levels are normal.

The controversial question is around depression. Fatigue is a common feature of depression. It is also, however, a common feature seen in people with a number of chronic illnesses who are not depressed. To put PBC fatigue down to depression is, therefore, a rather casual, lazy assumption. In my experience (and the scientific literature supports this view) actual depression is not at all common in PBC. Some people do get down, and occasional people get depressed, but this seems to be more a response to the frustration they feel about their fatigue than a primary problem. Treating fatigue with anti-depressant drugs such as sertraline is not effective in my experience (other than in people with secondary depression in whom the drugs treat the secondary depression but not the fatigue!).

Treating fatigue in PBC: Our approach to managing fatigue in PBC is, in many ways, a complete contrast to itch. Whereas there are a number of effective drug treatments for itch, and the issue is finding the right agent for an individual, there are, regrettably at present, no drugs effective for treating fatigue in PBC. There are, however, clinical trials now ongoing or about to start targeting fatigue in PBC meaning that this currently rather bleak picture may improve. In the absence of drug therapies our approach at present is to minimise the effects of fatigue on people and to help them to find a way to live with the symptom. We have developed a 4-step approach which we teach to many other doctors and nurses. It will only work, however, if the doctors and nurses start from the point of view that fatigue is an important problem that needs a solution. Negative attitudes are highly counter-productive. We have a saying when training people in the approach which is "don't fail before you start". We have christened our approach TrACE after the 4 steps.

STEP 1: TREAT THE TREATABLE

As I will explore in **Chapter 8**, PBC rarely exists in isolation. Patients typically have one, and frequently more, other conditions which themselves might be linked to fatigue, and where the fatigue may be easier to treat than it is in PBC. These conditions can either be ones that are directly linked to PBC or ones that are co-incidental, but may be commoner in people of the typical age and gender as PBC patients. The linked conditions are typically the autoimmune conditions which associate with PBC because of the shared genetic risk factors linked to control of the immune response. The two most relevant associations are with thyroid disease and with autoimmune conditions that cause anaemia. An underactive thyroid is very common in PBC patients and is caused by autoimmune injury to the gland. Its classic symptom is fatigue, often accompanied by weight gain and constipation. These effects are all caused by a "slowing down" of the metabolism because of the reduced levels of thyroxine being released by the damaged gland. It is really easy to test for using blood tests and really easy to treat using thyroxine tablets. Anyone with PBC and fatigue should have their thyroid function tested.

Anaemia is the second common issue. There are 3 causes for it that are linked to PBC. The first linked condition in this setting is celiac disease. This is an immune disease in which a dietary protein (gluten from wheat) triggers an immune response, which then also targets the lining of the small bowel. This is seen in one form or another in around 2-5% of PBC patients. Clinically, it presents either with diarrhoea (nutrients in the diet cannot be absorbed by the damaged small bowel so carry on through the bowel and out) or with shortage of particular nutrients. These include iron, hence the anaemia link. This form of the disease can be much more subtle, and is only diagnosed if people think about it. Again, diagnosis is easy with a blood test (an antibody test akin to the AMA test in PBC) which is usually followed by an endoscopy to take a piece of the small bowel for examination under a microscope. Treatment is not, as you might imagine, with iron supplements as in patients with celiac disease the issue is not the amount of iron in the diet (typically normal) but the ability of the body to absorb it. Treatment is with a gluten-free diet to take away the immune irritant. Gluten-free foods are now easily available (most supermarkets have gluten-free sections) making this easier to manage in practice than has been the case in the past. One really important thing is that if celiac disease is there it needs to be diagnosed formally. Gluten sensitivity has become something of a popular meme (possibly because of the easy availability of gluten-free food) and we come across quite a lot of incorrect self-diagnosis.

The second autoimmune anaemia is pernicious anaemia. This is, as is the case with celiac disease, an immune response against the bowel wall. In this case it is directed against the stomach and, in particular, the cells that produce a protein called intrinsic factor which is essential for absorbing vitamin B12 from the diet. Intrinsic factor shortage, therefore, leads to deficiency of the vitamin B12 which is essential for normal red blood cell production, hence anaemia. In practice, pernicious anaemia is the commonest cause for vitamin B12 deficiency, although it can also be seen in people following a strict vegan diet or, possibly, who are taking long term proton pump inhibitor drugs for acid-related gastric problems. Treatment is with B12 supplementation which has to be by injection (typically every 3 months) because, of course, the abnormality in pernicious anaemia is not in the level of B12 in the diet but the capacity to absorb it from the diet. This means that tablet B12 would go the same way as dietary B12, which is straight through the bowel and out again. Although endoscopic examination of the stomach is not needed to diagnose pernicious anaemia the condition is one of chronic damage to the stomach lining which can, very occasionally, turn cancerous so checking of the stomach lining for pre-cancerous cells is a sensible precaution.

The third autoimmune anaemia is haemolytic anaemia where the immune response is directed at the red blood cells themselves leading to their breakdown. This is a very rare association in PBC. It is diagnosed using blood tests which look for the presence of the antibodies that cause the injury. Treatment is aimed at suppressing or removing the antibodies.

The other treatable causes of fatigue are the age-related associations. Conditions such as Type 2 diabetes, mild renal failure and heart failure can all cause fatigue and occur in the same age-group as PBC. None of these are associated with PBC, other than through age, and are thus no more common in PBC than in the age-matched general population. They do, however, need to considered, looked for and where present treated before treatment for PBC fatigue specifically is considered. It is also really important to consider the possibility of menopausal symptoms where relevant. PBC as a condition is seen significantly more frequently in women than men, and the peak age for disease development is in peoples' 50s. Menopausal symptoms include fatigue and "brain fog", and these can clearly be additive to PBC symptoms. What makes the association particularly important is the fact that menopausal symptoms can be treated using hormone replacement therapy (HRT). The menopause does not completely explain fatigue and brain fog in PBC (male patients also get symptoms (albeit less frequently than women) and the most symptomatic groups seem to be pre-menopausal women), however to not use HRT in relevant patients may represent an important missed opportunity to reduce overall symptom burden. One reason for under use of HRT has been past concern about the safety of the approach both in general (because of blood clot and cancer risk) and specifically PBC. It is likely, however, that these concerns have been a little overstated, and we have many patients who have now been treated with HRT both safely and effectively for a number of years. One precautionary step that a number of PBC clinicians recommend is to use patch-based medication rather than tablet to reduce the high levels of liver exposure to the drug if it is taken up from the gut after being ingested in tablet form.

One condition that cannot co-exist with PBC is chronic fatigue syndrome (CFS). CFS is a diagnosis of exclusion, meaning that it is a diagnosis that is only reached by excluding all other potential conditions that could be causing fatigue. As PBC is a condition that causes fatigue its presence alone prevents a diagnosis of CFS from being possible.

The last element of "treating the treatable" is to make sure that all the other aspects of PBC management have been addressed. Effective treatment of the disease itself is really important not because it will improve fatigue directly but because if cirrhosis develops it typically reduces quality of life further. This is avoidable by proper treatment. A second aspect of effective PBC treatment is to look for and treat AIH overlap. As outlined in **Chapter 5** this co-existence of PBC and autoimmune hepatitis has historically been over-diagnosed. It does, however, exist and the presence of the autoimmune hepatitis element typically adds to the fatigue levels. This component of the fatigue is relatively easy to treat with immuno-suppression. The third aspect is itch. Night-time itch in particular causes fatigue through sleep disturbance and is therefore something that can be effectively targeted to improve fatigue.

STEP 2: AMELIORATE THE AMELIORATABLE

This step is about addressing those problems that are clearly part of the fatigue process and which make it worse. These include, as we have discussed, sleep disturbance, autonomic dysfunction and depression.

The potential for sleep disturbance to make fatigue worse is obvious. We therefore explore to see if there is significant sleep disturbance and then look for ways to reduce it. The first and obvious question in the clinic is about night-time itch because of the clear link. Assuming that there isn't significant night-time itch, what do we do next? The first step is to understand the type of sleep disturbance (is it difficulty in getting to sleep, a tendency to wake during the night, early morning waking or a tendency to fall asleep (or want to sleep) during the daytime). Each has its own causes and treatments. Difficulty in getting to sleep can be a result of taking stimulants (tea, coffee, energy drinks etc) too late in the day (I have always wondered why people who cannot sleep go downstairs to make a cup of tea........that is the last thing they should do!). Waking during the night is often a consequence of sleep apnoea (a process of airway collapse that leads to a temporary cessation of breathing which results in the patient waking up). A useful suggestion that this might be the case is snoring, something we ask partners about in the clinic. Sleep apnoea is an important diagnosis to make as there are effective treatments that can be delivered by sleep clinics. Waking early is a classic feature of depression, although this phenomenon seems uncommon in PBC. The commonest manifestation of sleep disturbance in PBC is daytime sleepiness, which can often be very prominent. Its impact depends on the lifestyle, and obligations, of the individual. For people who are retired it can be an irritation (perhaps having to cancel a social event at short notice), but people adapt to "go with the flow". At the other end of the spectrum are people who have tight and inflexible timetables in their work (teachers are the classic example) where worry about being overcome by sleepiness can be as big a problem as the sleep itself. In our experience, the sleep pattern is rarely dangerous (people do not fall asleep when the car has stopped at traffic lights as, as we have discussed, people with narcolepsy do), but it is difficult to address. Our approach is to explore all aspects of sleep with the sleep clinic in order to attempt to "push-back" sleep into the night-time. There is often an element of poor night-time sleep that contributes. Very occasionally we use stimulant drugs such as modafinil. Developed as sleep suppressants they have got a bad name through their abuse as "cognitive enhancers", and even study aids to help students stay awake to revise for exams. They are also misunderstood in PBC. They are not a treatment for fatigue in PBC as has been suggested by some people. They are a way to control daytime sleepiness if that is having an impact on peoples' lives. In such people, they will improve fatigue as well as the sleep pattern, but it is the sleep abnormality that we are treating. They are particularly effective when we use them to address a specific problem. An example was someone who was in danger of losing their job because they were falling asleep on their computer at work. This approach can be very short term and targeted. Another patient was terrified that she would fall asleep at her daughter's wedding. A couple of days of modafinil were enough to both remove the threat and the anxiety. Taken to its extreme this approach can involve just giving people a small supply to take if problems arise. Many of our patients who have benefitted from modafinil have never actually taken it! If you are going to use it, blood pressure needs to be really carefully monitored and some experimentation is useful to work out the optimal time in the day to take it.

The second modifiable process is autonomic dysfunction and, in particular, the problems with dynamic control of blood pressure. This is really common in PBC and the tell-tale feature is dizziness or light-headedness on standing up. Most hospitals now have a clinical service dedicated to autonomic function (usually called a falls clinic or something similar because autonomic dysfunction is a common cause of falls and fracturing). Their testing approach can be very helpful in PBC, however. If autonomic dysfunction is present (and it is seen to some degree in most fatigued patients) then the treatment approach is to try and restore effective muscle perfusion and venous flow control. There are several ways to do this. The simplest, and most effective, approach is to reduce blood pressure lowering treatments that many PBC patients are on, and which may no longer be needed. As PBC develops, blood pressure tends to naturally fall. If blood pressure treatment isn't adjusted to take account of this natural drop then people can end up "overshooting" with low blood pressure. The "lower the better" mindset for blood pressure that many doctors have doesn't help (very low blood pressure can be as risky as high; blacking out because of low blood pressure as you are crossing the road in front of a bus is not good for you!). PBC patients with fatigue, blood pressure treatment and features of autonomic dysfunction should have their blood pressure reviewed by their doctor. It goes without saying, however, that you **must not adjust blood pressure treatment without discussing it with your doctor**. If blood pressure treatment is not the culprit then there are some simple steps you can take. The first is to increase your fluid intake (our saying is 2 litres before lunch). This will increase the intravascular volume. Make sure this isn't sugary drinks (diabetes risk) or tea or coffee (they will add to sleep disturbance and are actually fluid depleting as they have a mild diuretic or water tablet effect). Another simple measure is graded pressure stockings that squeeze the lower limb and increase venous return (these are available in pharmacies). Beyond these simple measures, there are drugs such as fludrocortisone and midodrine which directly increase blood pressure. Given the risks for very high blood pressure these are, as you might expect, very specialised drugs that should only be used in specialised clinics.

The final associated problem is the challenging one of depression. In my experience, the role of depression in PBC fatigue tends to be over stated, with true depressions being uncommon. Clearly, if present it needs to be managed through talking therapy and anti-depressant treatments as appropriate. Lower levels of depression can be seen and can contribute to the overall perception of reduced well-being. This tends to be a consequence of the problems that people perceive; the limitations to life that people perceive accompanied by worry about the future. This is one of the reasons why self-management is so important. Taking as much control as you can is a natural way to reverse these feelings. Sometimes drugs (in particular the SSRI drug such as sertraline) can help and counselling and psychological support are often needed. Patient groups have an important role to play to bring people with similar problems together and to offer mutual support.

STEP 3: COPE

Coping strategies are really fundamental to living well with PBC fatigue. These are explained in detail in **Chapter 9**. The really key issue is owning the problem so that you can own the solution. Understand what is going on and why, and how you can plan and live your life to minimise the impacts. This can improve symptoms and absolutely improve well-being.

STEP 4: EMPATHISE and EXERCISE

The "E" in step 4 of the TrACE model was originally "empathise". This step was mainly for doctors and other clinicians but is a useful thing to think about for partners and family members. It is about understanding and caring for your patients/loved ones. In my experience, PBC patients with fatigue don't want their doctors to sympathise; to feel sorry for them. They want them to understand and appreciate how horrible it can be. They want someone who will help them to come to terms with it and make it as good as it can be. If you as a doctor do not think fatigue is "real" or a "proper problem" than you will be unable to work effectively with your patients and you shouldn't be managing PBC patients.

In this second edition of the book I am adding another "E". This is for exercise. We have known for a while that de-conditioning (a loss of "physical fitness" is part of peripheral fatigue in PBC) and that exercise is a good way to reverse this effect. We had specifically shown in a small study carried out a number of years ago in Newcastle that exercise was helpful in reducing fatigue. Recently, however, a larger study led from Birmingham has shown very clearly that exercise really does reduce fatigue severity and improves quality of life. The goal is 30 minutes of exercise three times a week with a level of intensity sufficient to make you mildly short of breath. A more accurate way of determining the right level of exercise is to look at heart rate. As we exercise our heart rate naturally goes up. We can calculate the maximum possible heart rate using the formula 220 minus your age in years (i.e. a 60 year old has a maximum possible heart rate of 160). In order to reduce fatigue in PBC you should be aiming for a heart rate of 60-80% of this maximum heart rate (i.e. 96-128). It is really easy to track your heartrate using a "Fitbit" or other type of heart rate tracker. PBC patients frequently struggle to get going with an exercise programme, often worrying that it will harm them or make their fatigue worse. It won't! If you struggle to get started with an exercise programme then drop the frequency and the intensity. If you can't do 30 minutes three times a week then do 15 minutes once a week and build it up from there. Try it. It really will make a difference.

The Newcastle approach to managing fatigue is outlined in Appendix 3

COGNITIVE SYMPTOMS

These are the symptoms of poor memory and concentration which are experienced by a number of PBC patients. The distinction between these and the symptoms of central fatigue (fatigue with "brain fog") is probably arbitrary, and these are best thought of as part of the same central fatigue process. It is likely that treatments in the future that benefit central fatigue will also benefit these symptoms. They can, in practice, be really troublesome for people, particularly if they have jobs that require a lot of concentration or information processing. They can also be a real concern to people who worry that they are developing dementia. It is interesting that in the clinic people will often talk about fatigue but rarely about memory problems (unless we ask them). I suspect that this is because of the deep down worry about dementia. The important thing for patients to realise is that dementia is no more common in PBC than in the non-PBC population, and that although these symptoms can be a real nuisance they do not progress to dementia. In the absence of a specific treatment, the approach is to find ways to cope with the problem. Writing lists and trying to finish one thing before starting another are the sorts of things that patients do which help.

I think it is likely that there will be real progress in our understanding of cognitive symptoms in PBC over the next few years, and that this will lead to real improvements in treatment. There are emerging data to suggest that the process of cholestasis leads to changes in the blood brain barrier (the "lining" of the brain that under normal circumstances shields it from exposure to toxins in the blood), making it leaky. This then allows toxins into the brain which can cause similar cell damage processes to those seen in the liver in PBC. Potentially crucially, OCA, if used early in the cholestasis process, can reverse these changes (and the accompanying memory loss) in animal models of cholestasis. This raises the fascinating question as to whether OCA might also reverse "brain fog" in PBC patients if given early in the disease (as opposed to our current practice of using it relatively late after UDCA failure).

DRY EYES AND MOUTH

Dry eyes and mouth are not really PBC features. They are problems resulting from Sjogren's syndrome, an autoimmune condition which causes problems with tear and saliva production that is very commonly associated with PBC. Sjogren's syndrome is, like PBC, an autoimmune condition. In this case one where the targets of injury are the salivary and tear glands. It does not cause risk to life, but can be associated with problematic symptoms. Poor tear production leads to dry and gritty eyes which can be irritating and which can cause knock-on symptoms through disturbed sleep and thus fatigue. Profound loss of tear production can lead to corneal ulceration and, conceivably, threat to vison through corneal damage. Treatment is, in the first instance, through the use of artificial tear preparations of which a number are on the market. They lubricate the eye and reduce irritation, as well as protecting the cornea from injury. Their limitations come with the number of times they need to be applied per day in the most severe cases. A really innovative approach of plugging of the tear ducts is, in my experience, really effective (and isn't nearly as bad as it sounds!). The logic is simple. Put small plugs in the tear ducts and this stops the tears draining away. This means they are retained in the eye. Do the procedure in someone with normal tear production and they would end up with profuse tears. In someone with limited tear production it can mean that the tears that are still produced are much more effective. It is an outpatient procedure and once the correct size plugs have been established they can be replaced very easily (they last around 3 months typically).

Poor saliva production causes a number of problems. These split broadly into difficulty with swallowing (saliva is important for lubricating the oesophagus and helping food to pass down easily) and mouth problems (mouth infections, bad breath etc) which arise because saliva has a mild disinfectant role. Simple lack of saliva can also be quite uncomfortable. Dry mouth is more difficult to treat than dry eyes in my experience. Saliva stimulating treatments do not work particularly well because the problem is with the ability of the salivary glands to produce saliva. This means that stimulating them further doesn't really work. There are a number of artificial saliva preparations on the market which are designed to replace saliva. They often take the form of sprays. In my experience, they are not terribly effective and the taste/texture can sometimes be an issue. Simple steps are usually the most effective for helping with dry mouth. Drink plenty of fluid when eating, particularly if it is dry food, and make sure you chew well before swallowing. A lot of people find that fizzy water is more effective than still. For the mouth issues good basic oral hygiene is key with regular teeth cleaning and use of an antiseptic mouth wash.

ABDOMINAL PAIN

One of the symptoms in PBC that patients often talk about, but doctors seem to only rarely think about, is abdominal pain. This is often a dull ache in the upper right-hand side of the abdomen (tummy). This is, of course, where the liver is situated. One obvious possible cause of this pain is gall-stones which are known to be seen more frequently in PBC patients (because of the connection of the disease to altered bile flow patterns). Gallstones can cause pain in a number of ways. The commonest is through what is called biliary colic (which isn't actually a colic-type pain but the name has stuck). This is a constriction or squeezing of the gallbladder around a gallstone that can't get out. The pain pattern (patterns of pain are very important for the identification of the source of a pain) is typically one of a growing sense of a squeezing type discomfort that gets worse and worse over several hours and then eases off. These episodes can be repeated. The pain can be severe, and is sometimes associated with nausea and vomiting. Episodes can be more common after a fatty meal as fat stimulates the gallbladder to contract. A second, and really important, type of gallstone pain is a much sharper one (it can double people up) which worsens and eases much more frequently than biliary colic (ironically this is much more typical of a colic pain than biliary colic!). This type of pain is caused by a gallstone that has got out of the gallbladder into the bile duct and is being passed down the duct. If the stone gets stuck (typically at the bottom of the bile duct where it joins the duct draining the pancreas and enters the bowel) it can block the bile duct. This is a medical emergency because of the damage the blockage can do to the pancreas, and because of the risk that the bile which can no longer drain can become infected. This is the only gallstone problem that is characterised by jaundice (caused by the blockage). The presence of jaundice should, therefore, ring real alarm bells.

Gallstone problems have become much less frequent in PBC in recent years because of the widespread use of UDCA. It is a little known fact that UDCA was originally developed as a treatment to dissolve gallstones to reduce the need for surgery. It is not terribly effective at this (it takes too long to work) but its early use in PBC has been very effective at stopping gallstones from developing. Surgery for biliary colic should only be considered if the severity of the pain and, in particular, the frequency of the episodes warrants it (I say to patients if it is an episode a year forget it, if it is an episode a day have surgery and for most people it is somewhere in between). If a stone has got into the bile duct then the approach is to clear it using an endoscopic approach (called ERCP). This is usually done after the blockage has been confirmed using an MRI scan called an MRCP. If stones are getting out into the bile duct then it is almost always appropriate to have gall-bladder surgery.

Gallstone pain of the type described above is not, in practice, that common in PBC any longer because of the actions of UDCA (it slowly dissolves gallstones). What is much commoner, particularly before UDCA treatment has been started, is a dull ache over the area of the liver. It does not come in day long waves like biliary colic but is a sense of uncomfortable "fullness" that is always there. The liver can sometimes be a little uncomfortable if you push on it. In my experience this is a really common issue. It is not really understood, but my theory is that it is the liver capsule being stretched. The liver has no nerves within it so it can never be painful per se. It does, however, have a lining around it to hold it together (the liver tissue itself is really soft and floppy). This is the capsule and it does have nerves supplying it. If you have a liver biopsy the painful bit is going through the capsule. The other way that the capsule can cause pain is if it is stretched by the liver swelling. My theory is that when PBC first develops there is a build-up of bile in the liver, and inflammation resulting from it, all of which stretches the liver capsule causing pain. Again, in my experience, this also tends to settle with UDCA and, where needed second-line therapy. This is another good reason to treat the disease effectively!

BONE PAINS

Clinicians tend not to think of bone and joint pains in PBC but recent work done by UK-PBC to explore the impact of symptoms suggest that they are in fact a common issue. It is not entirely clear why it arises. It may be related to the metabolic bone problems that some people with PBC experience (**Chapter 8**) and appropriate management of bones is an obvious important step. Otherwise effective pain control is the correct step. As with most drugs, people with PBC, other than those with advanced cirrhosis, are able to take pain-killers to manage the pain.

CHAPTER 8: **ASSOCIATED CONDITIONS**

The 2-Minute Version

- PBC patients frequently have additional medical conditions. These are, typically, either conditions with a linked aetiology (i.e. other autoimmune diseases) or those that are common in people with the typical age and gender pattern of PBC patients. There are also conditions that occur as a consequence of PBC.

- Of the autoimmune conditions, the most frequently seen is Sjogren's syndrome. The tear and salivary glands are affected, leading to a lack of tears and a dry mouth in this condition. The former leads to painful, gritty eyes. The latter leads to difficulty in swallowing and/or issues with mouth hygiene.

- Other commonly seen conditions include autoimmune thyroid disease (usually an under-active thyroid) and celiac disease (a condition of the small bowel). Pernicious anaemia (a lack of vitamin B12) and other autoimmune anaemias are also common. All of these conditions can also cause fatigue, and should always be thought of when patients are symptomatic.

- Less common overall (because they are, unlike thyroid disease, very rare conditions), but with a stronger specific association, are features of systemic sclerosis and CREST syndrome, including Raynaud's (a problem with blood flow to the fingers that is worse in cold weather) and skin thinning and mild lupus.

- Age-related conditions such as Type 2 diabetes are common in PBC, but only because of the age profile of the condition and not because they are more frequent in PBC. Despite much concern (and internet mis-information), neither cancer (with the exception of liver cancer which can occur in people with cirrhosis of all causes, including PBC) nor heart disease are associated with PBC.

- Osteoporosis can arise as a complication of PBC, compounded by the fact that the majority of PBC patients are women; another risk factor. PBC patients are, perhaps surprisingly, more likely to smoke (another osteoporosis risk factor) than non-patients. Screening for osteoporosis, with prevention through calcium and vitamin D, and treatment using bisphosphonates mean that fractures of the hip and spine (the main concern with osteoporosis) are much rarer than they once were.

- Cholesterol levels are frequently elevated in PBC patients and the source of much concern. In fact, this is usually harmless high-density lipo-protein (HDL or "good" cholesterol) rather than the type that is associated with heart disease risk and, as pointed out above, there is no increase in cardiac risk in PBC.

As is the case with many, if not all, chronic conditions, PBC often occurs in the context of other conditions. Some are specifically associated with PBC and are, as a result, seen more commonly in PBC patients than would happen by chance. Some are common in PBC patients simply because of the age and gender distribution of the PBC population. All can, however, change the ways in which PBC affects people and is treated. There are also some important conditions that worry people but that are actually not associated with PBC. I will explore each of these groups in turn.

PBC-ASSOCIATED CONDITIONS

These divide into two important groups. Those that are associated with PBC because it is an autoimmune disease and those associated with PBC because of its mechanisms.

Autoimmune Diseases: Other autoimmune diseases are common both in PBC patients and in the family members of PBC patients. The reason is the genetic predisposition to PBC discussed in **Chapter 3**. The vast majority of the genetic influences in PBC are, as we discussed earlier, factors that regulate the immune response (controlling, in essence, its on and off "switches"). Because of their general mode of action a number of these risk genes are, perhaps predictably, shared with other autoimmune diseases.

The most challenging autoimmune disease association in PBC is with autoimmune hepatitis. As outlined in earlier chapters the nature and extent of this association is quite complex because many of the features of autoimmune hepatitis are also seen in the more aggressive forms of PBC. Interestingly, there appears to be no association between PBC and the other autoimmune liver/biliary disease primary sclerosing cholangitis (PSC).

The most frequently seen associated autoimmune condition in PBC is *Sjogren's syndrome*. This is an autoimmune condition affecting the salivary and tear glands, as well as causing fatigue and joint inflammation. Up to 70% of PBC patients experience Sjogren's syndrome symptoms to some degree. They tend not, however, to have the full clinical complex. This is a theme that will recur in this chapter, as many of the associated autoimmune diseases seen in PBC patients appear to be in a milder form than when they are seen as an isolated condition in someone without PBC (the joint problems in particular appear to be less of an issue). PBC patients with Sjogren's syndrome also do not tend to express the typical autoantibody patterns of isolated Sjogren's syndrome having, instead, a typical PBC pattern. This apparent difference in the disease type have led to the question as to whether this is truly two associated diseases, or whether it is in fact the case that PBC patients can have Sjogren's-like symptoms. In practice, it does not make much difference. The Sjogren's features are rarely significant enough to need anything beyond symptom reducing therapy. The approach to the management of the symptoms of Sjogren's is covered in **Chapter 7**.

In terms of other associated autoimmune conditions, some associations are more common than others (type 1 diabetes, a classical autoimmune disease is, for example, hardly ever seen in PBC patients). In terms of overall risk, the commonest other autoimmune disease in PBC is *autoimmune thyroid disease*. This level of thyroid disease isn't especially elevated in PBC, but the condition is common in the population in general meaning that even a small increase can lead to an appreciable number of patients with both PBC and thyroid disease. Autoimmune thyroid disease takes two forms, with underactive and over-active thyroid states. The underactive state (also known as Hashimoto's disease) is where an immune response damages the cells of the thyroid gland and reduces their capacity to produce thyroid hormone (thyroxine). The clinical features are entirely as a result of reduced thyroxine levels. These can include weight gain, constipation, slow heart rate, low mood and skin changes. They can also, importantly, include fatigue, meaning that an underactive thyroid as a consequence of autoimmune thyroid disease is an important condition to look for and treat as the first stage in managing PBC patients with fatigue (the "treat the treatable" stage outlined in **Chapter 7**). Diagnosis of an underactive thyroid is very simple using blood biochemistry tests. The thyroxine level is low and thyroid stimulating hormone (TSH; the hormone released by the brain which signals to the thyroid to produce thyroxine) level is high (because the brain is sensing that the thyroxine level is low and is signalling to the thyroid, unsuccessfully because the thyroid can't respond, to produce more thyroxine). Treatment is also normally simple, with thyroxine given in tablet form.

The over-active form of autoimmune thyroid disease (thyrotoxicosis, or Grave's disease, which is much less commonly associated with PBC than underactive thyroid) arises because an autoantibody stimulates the thyroid to release more thyroxine than it should, mimicking TSH. The symptoms revolve around a "speeding up" of body processes, with weight loss, diarrhoea, fast heart rate (including the development of atrial fibrillation) and anxiety. Again, diagnosis is easy with very high levels of thyroxine and a very low level of TSH (the body is trying hard to stop the production of thyroxine as it senses that the level is too high but, as a result of the antibody effect, has lost control). Treatment can be a little more complex than for hypothyroidism. There are three options. This first is drugs to control the production of thyroxine such as carbimazole. These are not without side-effects, and it can be a challenge to get the right level of blockade. The second option is radioactive iodine. Thyroid hormone includes iodine in its structure, which has to be taken up into the thyroid gland from the circulation. This concentrating effect for iodine means that a small dose of radioactive iodine will concentrate in the thyroid and, in essence, obliterate it with minimal risk to other tissues (almost a targeted form of radiotherapy). Radioiodine is passed out in the urine meaning that care has to be taken regarding other people in the house during the treatment phase (especially children). Long-term, the thyroid tends to be obliterated completely following radioiodine therapy, meaning that patients end up needing, paradoxically, to take thyroxine. This is, however, a much easier treatment to balance and get the dose right for than carbimazole. The third option is surgery, removing most of the thyroid gland. This is quite a delicate operation, which runs the risk of damaging one of the nerves that makes the voice box (the larynx) work (the recurrent laryngeal nerve). Removal of the thyroid can also mean removal of the parathyroid glands. These are associated physically with the thyroid gland, although they are not related to its function. They are essential for the balance of calcium in the body. It is important, in thyroid surgery, to try and identify these glands and leave them behind in the body. With all the treatments for thyrotoxicosis, it is often very helpful to control the heart rate using Beta-blockers as a first step. This makes people feel much better, reduces the risk of heart failure from a fast heart rate and makes surgery (if that is the chosen approach) much safer. Beyond the very short term, however, they can worsen fatigue.

Pernicious anaemia is an autoimmune anaemia. As outlined in **Chapter 7**, anaemia of any cause can make fatigue worse and is an important treatment target. In pernicious anaemia the target for autoimmune damage is, paradoxically, nothing to do with the actual process of red blood cell formation. The target is, in fact, the cells lining the stomach that produce a protein called intrinsic factor that is essential for the take up from the diet of vitamin B12, which is, in turn, essential for the production of red blood cells. The diagnosis is made from the blood count (the characteristic pattern is anaemia in the context of larger than normal red blood cells) followed by a vitamin B12 level (which is very low). The presence of autoantibodies directed against the cells of the stomach lining is a useful additional finding. Treatment is with vitamin B12 injections every 3 months (tablet supplements are not useful because the issue is not shortage of B12 in the diet but the capacity to absorb it). Endoscopic screening of the stomach is also important because the chronic inflammation resulting from the autoimmune process can result in a slightly increased risk of stomach cancer.

Amongst the strongest associations, in increased relative risk terms, are with the connective tissue disorders. The most important of these is with *systemic sclerosis/CREST syndrome*. This is an immune-mediated fibrosing or scarring condition. It has a number of manifestations, some of which are common in PBC patients and some of which are very rare. As with Sjogren's it is, once again, the more severe complications which are, fortunately, less frequently seen. The commonly seen features include

Raynaud's, a problem of vascular flow to the fingers and toes. Raynaud's is common in PBC although it is usually mild. It is characterised by sensitivity to cold, with the development of white, painful fingers in cold settings. There can then be a painful reddening of the fingers as blood flow is restored when they warm up. The process underpinning it is one of spasm in the blood vessels and it is a clinical diagnosis (i.e. there are no diagnostic tests). Treatment is, in the first instance, through avoiding cold triggers (avoiding putting your hands in the freezer, gloves, hand-warmers etc). The drug nifedipine, which dilates blood vessels, can be useful, especially taken in a preventative way. In extreme cases intra-venous treatments such as prostacyclin can be necessary to prevent damage to the fingertips. Other skin features of SS/CREST can be seen, including scarring of the finger tips and around the mouth (leading to a "pursed lip" appearance) and calcinosis (chalky lumps under the skin). Fortunately, the most significant complication of systemic sclerosis, such as scarring to the lungs, kidney and bowel are rare in PBC patients.

Clinical features of *systemic lupus erythematosus (SLE)* are also common in PBC although, again, the more significant complications of the disease such as kidney and brain injury are very rare indeed. Variants of the characteristic butterfly-shaped rash across the face are common. The milder *cutaneous lupus erythematosus (CLE)* characterised by skin rashes only is also seen.

The final immune disease process commonly encountered in PBC is *celiac disease* which can be seen in around 2-5% of the patients (although in most people it is very mild). It is best thought of as an autoimmune disease directed at the wall of the small bowel which is triggered by the gluten protein found in wheat and other cereals. In people reactive to gluten, exposure to even minute amounts can lead to a significant immune response to the small bowel lining. This, in particular, damages the villi which are the very small finger like extensions from the surface of the bowel wall cells that dramatically increase the surface area of the bowel wall to allow absorption of food. Loss of the villi leads to a failure of absorption. The clinical effects include loss of weight because of nutritional deficiency and loose bowel motions because of non-absorbed food passing through the bowel and out. There can also be specific nutritional deficiencies, most commonly iron deficiency which leads to anaemia, worsening fatigue. Diagnosis is through clinical suspicion confirmed by blood tests (a specific antibody test) and then endoscopy to take a biopsy from the upper part of the small bowel which confirms the loss of villi. Treatment is, in the first instance, through avoidance of gluten (complete avoidance because of the potential for even tiny amounts of gluten to activate the process). This is much easier than it used to be because of the easy availability of gluten free foods in most supermarkets. The celiac society is also a very useful source of information regarding which processed foods do and don't contain gluten (this is more complex than you might imagine because of the variable inclusion of gluten in different manufacturing processes). The response to a gluten free diet is the final diagnostic test for celiac disease as the improvement can be rapid and dramatic. Very occasionally, steroids are needed to control the disease. This is, however, rarely the case in PBC patients. There has been an increasing tendency in recent years for people to self-diagnose with gluten sensitivity (perhaps a by-product of increased awareness and the availability of gluten free foods). This is to be avoided at all costs. Celiac disease is an important condition which if present needs to be monitored properly. If not present, then there is no need to avoid gluten. There is no real evidence to suggest a food intolerance to gluten out with celiac disease.

Non-autoimmune diseases: The most important non-autoimmune associated condition in PBC is *osteoporosis*. This is a condition of bone thinning that can predispose to fractures (especially of the hip and spine). It is common in the population in general, with a number of risk factors including age (more common in older age), female gender, smoking, low body weight and reduced activity levels (rather like muscle, bone strengthens with exercise). Clearly, a number of these risk processes are common amongst the PBC population, putting them at risk before any additional disease-specific effects. Liver disease in general increases the risk of osteoporosis and, as a cholestatic disease, the risk is higher with PBC (probably through reduced absorption from the diet of calcium and vitamin D). Diagnosis and treatment of osteoporosis (or, even better, prevention) are important to reduce fracture risk. We screen for bone density using the radiological approach of bone mineral density assessment. This should be carried out at diagnosis of PBC, and thereafter every 1 to 5 years depending on the first value (more frequently the closer to being osteoporotic people are). The data from the bone density are added to an online scoring system (called FRAX) that also includes the other risk factors such as gender, age and smoking history which guides us as to the need for therapy. Where there is evidence of bone thinning that falls short of osteoporosis (this is called osteopenia) the advice is to optimise all risk factors (especially increasing activity and stopping smoking!) and then to take an oral calcium and vitamin D supplement. Where osteoporosis is present, and the risk of fracture is increased, specific treatment has made an important contribution to reducing fracture risk. It has been very noticeable, over the 30 years I have been looking after PBC patients, just how rare fractures have become. The mainstay of treatment is bisphosphonate drugs. These can be given as a tablet (typically given once a week) or as an injection. The tablet forms are most commonly used and can cause irritation to the gullet (meaning that people need to stand up after they take them!). It may also be that there is a limit as to how long people can safely take them because of the potential, paradoxically for bone injury as a side effect. The treatment of osteoporosis is a rapidly developing and specialised area and if problems continue despite bisphosphonates, or people are struggling to take them, then specialist review is appropriate. Historically HRT was widely used to prevent osteoporosis in women after the menopause. HRT can be useful in PBC patients to help treat menopausal symptoms (which can add to the overall quality of life burden) but there are better ways to address the osteoporosis risk.

Although the osteoporosis risk in PBC is, perhaps, lower than was previously thought to be the case (this may be because of the use of UDCA to reduce cholestasis levels) there is still an issue with bone fractures. Part of the reason for this apparent paradox is that there is an issue with PBC and *falls*. Clinicians tend to think of osteoporosis as the main driver for fractures but, in practice, falls are an important predisposing factor to the trauma that leads to fracture. The falls risk in PBC is largely related to the autonomic dysfunction outlined in **Chapter 7** which is common and which appears to be a major factor in fatigue. The potential falls risk (which increases dramatically if people are losing consciousness with their autonomic dysfunction) is another important reason, beyond treating fatigue, for taking an aggressive approach to addressing autonomic dysfunction. As a patient, there are two things that you can do to help yourself. The first is to be aware of the risk and mention to your doctor that you are getting dizzy or light-headed when you stand up (and certainly mention if you have had a fall!). The second is to minimise risk of black outs. In addition to drinking plenty of fluid, as mentioned previously, if you are getting light-headed when standing up (the commonest first feature that warns of future fall risk) then take care, when getting up from lying down, to pause in the sitting position to let the blood pressure stabilise before standing up. Ideally, have something you can hold on to and, if you do feel very light-headed, sit down again. One of the areas of real advance in medicine in recent years has been in pro-active prevention and management for falls so make sure you take advantage of the services that are now available.

A second important, and slightly complex, area is hyperlipidaemia and, in particular, *high cholesterol*. This is something that is very common indeed in PBC and causes a great deal of (misplaced) anxiety. Across the PBC population, total blood cholesterol levels are typically higher than in the non-PBC population (often substantially so). In an era when people tend to know their cholesterol number, and the need to reduce cholesterol levels is hard-wired into peoples' thinking, this can cause real worry. The important thing to be aware of, however, is that cholesterol elevation in PBC is part of the disease process, and that the elevation is almost always of the "good" HDL form of cholesterol that actually reduces the risk of vascular disease. The total cholesterol number is, therefore, of little use in PBC. PBC patients are, of course, not protected against getting heart disease (indeed smoking, the main risk factor for ischaemic heart disease, is commoner in PBC patients than in the general population) so due consideration does need to be given to "hidden" hypercholesterolemia. When assessing cholesterol in PBC it is essential that the differential cholesterol levels are measured (i.e. the LDL and VLDL cholesterol forms where elevation is associated with cardiac risk) not just total. If there is elevation of either, or both, then treatment is appropriate to reduce cardiac risk. Statins, the mainstay of drug treatment for elevated cholesterol, are safe in PBC and can be used. One slight complication with regard to cholesterol management in PBC is the use of bezafibrate for the treatment of the disease itself (**Chapter 5**). Bezafibrate is also a cholesterol lowering drug and was used reasonably widely before the advent of the statins. It fell out of use for hypercholesterolemia with the advent of statins, largely because statins are more effective and seem to have an additional cardio-protective effect over and above that resulting from their cholesterol-lowering action. It is very important that people do not take both a statin and a fibrate at the same time because of the risk of drug reaction, so if a patient needs a fibrate for management of their PBC then they should rely on this as well for cholesterol control. If this is not effective for cholesterol control then the combination of a statin and OCA should be considered. It is important to note that statins have, unlike bezafibrate and the other fibrates, no disease modifying action for PBC. Many GPs are not aware that bezafibrate and the other fibrates are used in PBC to treat the disease and suggests swapping them for statins. If this is suggested to you then explain why you have been prescribed a fibrate by your PBC doctor!

CONDITIONS NOT ASSOCIATED WITH PBC

This may seem like an unusual topic to cover but it is important in two ways. The first is to remember all of the many medical conditions that can affect people, and in particular people with the age profile of PBC, that are completely unrelated to PBC. There can be a tendency for doctors and other clinicians to ascribe all the problems that people have to their PBC. This is usually not correct, and can lead to missed opportunities for better treatment of those conditions (sometimes exacerbated by a fear of using medications because of the risk associated with liver disease). A common example is type 2 diabetes, which is common in PBC patients because it is common in the population in general, especially at the sorts of ages that people develop PBC. The presence of PBC should not alter the management of type 2 diabetes at all. In conditions such as hypertension (high blood pressure) the issues are a little more nuanced. High blood pressure is not a problem that is associated with PBC, but there can be some challenges around blood pressure regulation and autonomic dysfunction. Because people with PBC lack the normal "fine tuning" for their blood pressure because of autonomic dysfunction they can end up with a profile for their blood pressure that is "spiky". By this I mean that there are falls in blood pressure with standing, and sometimes an over-compensation. This can mean that one-off blood pressure values seem high. The important thing is to understand this possibility, and for doctors not to rely on one-off measurement. Twenty-four hour blood pressure monitoring is much more appropriate and readily available. The other issue around blood pressure is the potential for anti-hypertensive therapies to contribute to the expression of autonomic dysfunction in fatigue. This is explored in more detail in **Chapter 7**.

The second reason why the issue of conditions not associated with PBC is important is to challenge some fallacies that are out there, and that are busy being propagated by the internet. These are about rumoured associations between PBC and cancer and heart disease. The data regarding cancer are very clear indeed. Other than the specific association with hepatocellular carcinoma discussed earlier (and which is only relevant to the small group of people with advanced cirrhosis) there is **no additional cancer risk in PBC.** This is really important because a number of patients have been worried by reports of an association with breast cancer. It is essential to know that these were very early studies when people described cases of patients with both PBC and breast cancer. Breast cancer unfortunately affects one in 12 women in the UK and that includes 1 in 12 female PBC patients. We will therefore inevitably see people with both. This does not mean that they are linked! We very rarely see prostate cancer in PBC but that is not because PBC is protective against it, it just means that most patients with PBC do not have a prostate because they are women! When we do proper studies looking at thousands of patients no cancers other than hepatocellular carcinoma are seen more frequently in PBC than they should be based on the population risk. The same is also true of ischaemic heart disease (heart attacks). What PBC patients need to be aware of is that they run the same risks of these diseases as the non-PBC population. You should take steps to reduce your risks (stopping smoking, increasing exercise etc) but the need to do so is just the same as it would be for anyone else.

CHAPTER 9: **LIVING WITH PBC**

The 2-Minute Version

- At present, we do not have a cure for PBC (although we can control it). This means that patients need to learn to live with their disease and ensure that it does not take over their lives. We call this "owning the disease" and it can be really empowering for people. If you own the problem, you can also own the solution.

- There are two critical aspects to owning the disease. The first is to understand it, the reasons why issues arise and what the possible solutions are. You are reading this book so that's a great start! The second is to not be shy about asking your doctors about your treatment and making sure you get the best treatment possible. Do not die of not wanting to challenge your doctor.

- In terms of good disease control, if you are not on UDCA ask why not and ask to be started. Also, know your ALP and bilirubin levels on UDCA. If they are still elevated after UDCA has been used for at least a year ask whether additional treatment might be appropriate. OCA is the standard additional therapy. If you are offered something else ask why it is not OCA.

- If you have itch make your own decision about whether it is bad enough to warrant treatment. If you get it for half an hour every six months it isn't. If it is all day every day (or all night) it is. Most people are somewhere in between and it is your decision.

- The contribution you can make to fatigue control is enormous (much more so than any drug treatments). Steps you can take include learning to pace yourself (use energy wisely) and to arrange your days so that important things are scheduled for the morning when energy levels are normally at their highest.

- It is critically important that you maintain your social networks. This includes carrying on working wherever possible. Cutting yourself off from the world can save energy, but it usually makes quality of life worse, and is a false economy.

- Try and exercise as much as you can. It can often feel like a challenge but it is really good for fatigue (and, if you do it in a group, for social networks). Try and eat a healthy balanced diet.

- Many things that people think are problems in PBC are not at all. This includes pregnancy and taking most drugs for other diseases. There are a lot of myths out there so check these things with your doctor. The PBC Foundation is also a great source of accurate information.

- Men get PBC as well as women. The impact is slightly different, however. It tends to be diagnosed later, to be a little less likely to respond to UDCA and less likely to have bad symptoms. The treatment is exactly the same as in women.

- Across the world there are many patient support groups who do an excellent job supporting and advising PBC patients and supporting the research efforts aimed at better understanding of the disease and improved treatments.

- DON'T FORGET TO LIVE YOUR LIFE!!!

PBC is a condition that is not, currently at least, curable. It is also not a condition that resolves spontaneously. This means that, for the vast majority of people diagnosed with PBC, they will have the condition for the remainder of their lives. PBC is, however, a condition that can be controlled and with which people can and do live a completely normal life. Learning to live with PBC, and the approach that you take to living your life, is therefore, of the greatest imaginable importance. In my experience it is quite simple. The patients who want to do everything that they can to control the condition and its impact are the people who do best; the people who live the longest and have the best quality of life. Doctors and nurses can help, but ultimately you yourself determine what happens to you. As someone who attempts to understand the condition and its impact, and who has spoken to many, many people with PBC over the years, but at the end of the day can't know what it really feels like, I am not perhaps the best person to write this chapter. The many excellent groups who support people with PBC such as the PBC Foundation, LIVErNORTH and the PBCers to name but a few, are the people with most to contribute to this area. I did feel it was important to include this chapter to help people who are perhaps struggling to "get started". These are my purely personal views on the steps that I think people can take to make a difference for themselves.

OWN THE PROBLEM

One of the most common phrases I end up using in clinic with patients is "in life we have to play the hand we are dealt". What I mean by this is that if you have been diagnosed with PBC there is nothing you can do about it other than get on with living with it. There is nothing you could have done to prevent it. It is basically a random event. There is, therefore, no point in looking backwards. There are three ways of looking at it that I think are quite helpful. The first is that although no one wants to be diagnosed with an illness, if you have PBC and it is not diagnosed it doesn't mean that you don't have the condition. A tree that falls over in a forest with no one there does still make a noise. The good news about having the diagnosis is that it allows us to, collectively, get on with treating it, and we know that the earlier treatments are started the more effective they are. If you had PBC and it hadn't been diagnosed it would actually have made things worse for you! The second, hopefully helpful, way of looking at it is, that if you have the symptoms of PBC, and have been struggling to understand them, a diagnosis gives you an explanation. The symptoms are real and the diagnosis of PBC goes a long way to explaining them. Over the years, I have told many people that their symptoms are exactly like those of all the other people with PBC. All of sudden they realise that they are not alone, and not "going mad". The third helpful way of looking at it is that if you are going to be diagnosed with a condition then at least be diagnosed with one which is well understood, and is relatively straightforward to manage. There are far worse conditions to have than PBC, particularly in the current era with the rapid progress that we have made in relation to treatment. One of the best life coaches I have heard talk to people about managing challenges is Paul McGee (if you haven't heard him talk or read his book then you should). He is also called the SUMO guy. His mantra is Stop, Understand and Move-On. This is perfect advice to take after a diagnosis of PBC. Take a pause, understand what it is and what it means and take control of what you and your clinical team are going to do about it. Most of all. Don't feel sorry for yourself. That will achieve nothing.

To help you with "owning the problem" I have developed a summary of tests, and the values that you should be looking for in your clinic visits. This is in **Appendix 4**. Use it to know exactly how your disease is doing!

OWN THE SOLUTION

One area where you can make an enormous difference to your care is by understanding what the current state of the art approach to treatment of PBC is and **making sure you get it!** We know that the quality of care for PBC can differ hugely between countries and between centres within countries. This is not unique to PBC, but typical of the challenge faced by everyone with a rare disease. In the UK, most GPs will probably manage between 1 and 3 patients with the condition in their career and it is not reasonable for them to know current management approaches. They do, however, need to know where to find that information and to then adopt it. At the other end of the clinical spectrum, there are probably only 4 or 5 hospitals that have highly specialised clinics looking after only patients with PBC. Each of these centres will only have one or two consultants who are PBC experts. In practice, therefore, there are only 5-10 real expert PBC doctors in the UK. This limited number of expert centres, and their geographical spread, means that many, if not most, people with PBC are looked after by non-expert consultants (often general gastroenterologists) in general liver or gastroenterology clinics outside the expert centres. In our experience, the level of interest and knowledge of these consultants, and thus quality of care, can differ widely. How can you make sure that you get the best possible care? The answer is don't be shy! Another of my sayings is that in a consultation with a doctor about your PBC there are 2 people in the room, with one of them with much more invested in the conversation than the other! Make sure that you get what you want and need out of it. In simple and stark terms **don't die from not wanting to upset your doctor.** I always feel that this is one area where the UK can learn from America. American PBC patients are much more likely to push for what they want.

Our research has suggested that most PBC patients are happy to ask challenging questions about their care, but want guidance as to what they should be asking about. There are basic aspects of care for PBC that everyone must receive. **These are the things that you MUST discuss with your doctor**

1) Are you on UDCA therapy? UDCA is the bedrock of therapy for PBC. Partly because it is safe and effective (up to a point) and partly because it is the starting point for future therapy decisions (most second-line agents and trials need you to be on UDCA, or at least have attempted to take it, before you can move onto them). If you have not been offered UDCA ask your doctor why not and request it. If you have tried UDCA in the past, and struggled to take it, then ask to try it again and either split the doses during the day or try starting on a low dose and building it up over time. There is also the option of taking it as a suspension (a liquid medicine as opposed to tablet). One of these approaches usually works. It really is important to be taking UDCA if at all possible.

2) Are you on the right dose of UDCA? The optimal dose for UDCA is 13-15mg/Kg body (i.e. 780mg to 900 mg for a 60Kg person). This would need to be adjusted to fit with tablet size so 900mg would be the correct dose here. Going above 15mg/Kg isn't harmful (although we definitely would not go above 20mg/Kg) but it adds no additional benefit and can cause more in the way of stomach side-effects (as well, of course, as giving you more tablets to take). Under-dosing reduces effects and can get in the way of second-line therapy use. For people who really struggle to take the correct dose (i.e. it is the higher doses of UDCA that we now use that give side-effects) then it is better to take a lower dose than it is to take none at all.

3) Are you a UDCA-responder? This is where it gets a little more complex as there is no clear guidance as to which criteria should be used for assessing UDCA response (a failing in the field that we are working to rectify). A good starting point are the so-called POISE criteria (named after the POISE trial that demonstrated that OCA is effective and that led to its licensing for clinical use). Using these criteria you are a responder if your **Alkaline Phosphatase is below 1.67 times the upper limit of the normal range AND your bilirubin is below the upper limit of normal.** These criteria are evidence based and represent the absolute minimum of what we should be achieving with treatment. What they mean in practice for most UK patients is an **Alkaline Phosphatase below 217 AND a bilirubin below 20**. Note, however, that there are different measures for a small number of labs and different scales used in the USA for bilirubin so check with your local doctor or nurse. It is likely that, over time, we will move towards lower cut off values for acceptable response (rather as the target value for blood cholesterol has been reduced over time). If you are a responder using these values then that is good news. You need to continue to take the UDCA (it is best thought of as a life-long treatment in PBC) and to have your blood tests (and response status) checked every year. It matters less who does the checking (your GP or the hospital clinic) than that someone does and **looks and acts on the result**. The best person to know their numbers and their UDCA response status is, of course, you. If your doctor hasn't told you your alkaline phosphatase and bilirubin results numbers then ask for them. They are yours!

4) *Do you need second-line therapy?* This is a really important issue. If you are not a UDCA responder using the cut-offs above then you need to discuss with your doctor the options around second-line therapy. The use of second-line therapy is now standard practice and is proven to improve liver disease severity in UDCA non-responding PBC patients. Not everyone who is a UDCA non-responder will need to, or want to, go on to second-line therapy. The option always needs to be discussed, however. The currently available approaches for second-line therapy are OCA, Bezafibrate, trial therapy or watching and waiting. There are reasons to wait and see what happens (the tests are only slightly above the line and you have other ongoing health problems is a commonly encountered example) but the vast majority of people in this category should probably be treated. If you are not going to have second-line therapy this should be an active decision (it is considered, discussed between you and your doctor and an active decision made), not just because no one has thought about it! Our research suggests that most people, in the UK at least, who could benefit from second—line therapy but who are not receiving it have never had the option mentioned to them. This isn't good enough. If you have an alkaline phosphatase above 200 and/or a bilirubin above 20 ask your doctor what the options are. If they don't mention second-line therapy then ask them about it specifically. The question of which agent is, in a way, less important and the differences between individual agents are less than the difference between getting and not-getting at least one of them. That said, it should be normal practice to consider the licensed therapy (OCA) as the first option.

5) *Do you have symptoms?* Itch is a very treatable symptom in PBC with a number of effective drugs. Fatigue is not directly treatable with a specific drug but, there is an approach that can certainly improve quality of life in relation to it. The guidelines for PBC management clearly say that the doctor or nurse should be asking about your symptom level every year. If they don't, tell them anyway. With itch, having the symptom doesn't automatically mean that you should have treatment. That is for you to decide, however. In my clinic we ask people first if they have any itch. If they say yes we ask them how bad it is on a scale of 1 to 10 and whether they have problems with sleep from it. Finally, we ask them whether they feel that they need a change in treatment (either to begin treatment if they are not on any or to change or add treatment if they are being treated). For many people with milder itch simply knowing that there are treatment options if they want or need them in the future is sufficient.

SELF-MANAGEMENT FOR FATIGUE

In **Chapter 7** we discussed the approach to living with fatigue. A key component of this is the coping strategies to help minimise its impact. These are entirely in your hands and are really helpful. These are the key things to think about

1) Treat energy as a valuable commodity and use it wisely: Pacing of your activity is a critical element of managing fatigue. It is important not to "wrap yourself in cotton wool". By the same token, however, using energy wisely allows you to make sure you do the most important things. Think of energy as you would do money. Save it when you can and make sure you get the best value for money when you do spend it.

2) Understand and use the rhythm of the disease: Fatigue in PBC characteristically gets worse as the day goes on. This means that mornings are the best time to get things done. The corollary is that evening working, and, in particular, night shifts can be very challenging indeed. If you have important meetings or engagements try and organise them for mornings. If your work pattern involves evenings and nights then speak to your employer about changing your work pattern. The other aspect to disease rhythm is to accept that there will be good days and bad days. If you are having a bad day be philosophical, don't fight it and focus on the likelihood that tomorrow will be better.

3) Exercise is good: There is now trial evidence to suggest that exercise is associated with a significant reduction in fatigue severity. There are also good reasons to believe it should work based on our understanding of how the muscles are affected in PBC, and how exercise training might be expected to improve their function. The challenge for people is in getting started ("how can I exercise when I feel so tired"). There is also the perception that exercise is all about people with perfect bodies wearing lycra in gyms; an environment and an association that many people with PBC feel uncomfortable with. The good news is that there are lots of ways of increasing exercise as part of daily life. An activity increase of around 10-20% is thought to be enough to have a beneficial effect. Think how you could achieve this. If you can manage 30 minutes of exercise three times a week it will really make a difference. One area of real progress in this area has been the advent of digital technology that helps you keep a track of exercise. Tools such as "Fitbit" are very useful, and many smart phones have exercise trackers. This allows you to understand what you are doing and measure the changes you make. Simple steps to increase exercise are such things as walking rather than driving or taking the bus. If you do have to use transport, think about parking a bit further away or getting off a stop earlier. Sometimes people join walking groups (good for the social side as well), take up golf or get a dog! Gyms are, of course, a very good way of doing it and are not at all as most people imagine them to be. The vast majority of gym users, in this day and age, are ordinary people wanting to get fitter just like you. They are very welcoming and the instructors are really good at tailoring exercise regimes to what you are able to do and what you want to achieve. If you really get enthused then aim for 10,000 steps every day. This is the recommended healthy level of exercise. One piece of advice, particularly if walking is your chosen approach is to watch the speed. The benefit difference between slow walking and fast walking is huge. If you are too slow it is still a good thing to do but it may not be as beneficial as it could be.

One thing that people worry about is causing harm through exercise. This is absolutely not the case. You may feel more tired immediately afterwards (although the tiredness is a healthier feeling one) but as the days go by it will continually improve. Think of exercise as a long-term change. Make it part of your life and aim to be active most days. Always listen to your body, though, and if this is a bad day then don't force it. Tomorrow will be a better day and you can pick it up then.

4) Keep your social structures: One of the really striking findings from UK-PBC was that having fatigue wasn't automatically associated with poor quality of life. In fact, there is a group of people with significant fatigue who feel that their life quality is good despite their fatigue. What this group have in common is strong social networks. In contrast, people who have become isolated feel the symptom much more and their quality of life is worse. What does this mean in practice? What we often come across is people who try to save energy by changing their lifestyle; reducing or stopping their work, not going out and meeting friends etc. What our findings suggest is that this is almost always a false economy. This may save some energy but there is a price to pay in terms of overall life quality. The message we give to patients is to keep doing things! Adapt what you do to your capability but doing things remains really important. I know a patient who used to go rambling with friends. She found this increasingly difficult with her PBC and that she was being left behind. What she did, however, was not to give up going but to meet people at the end of the walk. Walk a short distance to meet them and then join them for coffee. A really sensible compromise.

Many patients also get benefit from digital media based social networking. This can be of great use to people with profound fatigue and, of course, became a lifeline during self-isolation during the COVID-19 outbreak.

PATIENT SUPPORT GROUPS

Around the world there are many patient support groups that do an excellent job in helping PBC patients with the practical and emotional problems that can arise with their diagnosis. They are also great champions for research aimed at improving understanding of PBC and its treatments and advocates for PBC patients and their rights. Real triumphs include the name change (a patient driven initiative) and the advocacy around getting new therapies such as OCA into normal clinical practice. Amongst the groups I have worked with are

- PBC Foundation (UK but with a global reach; www.pbcfoundation.org.uk)
- LIVErNORTH (UK; www.livernorth.org.uk)
- The PBCers (USA with a global reach; www.pbcers.org)
- Canadian PBC Society (Canada; www.pbc-society.ca)

This list is not meant to be exhaustive but is a good place to start if you want to get in touch with patient groups.

MEN WITH PBC

PBC is a condition where around 90% of patients are women. One effect of this is that much of the literature, and many of the patient groups, can feel female-focused. Our clinic waiting areas can also look like a very female environment. Ten percent of patients are, however, men and it is really important to be aware that the disease has its own specific impacts in men, to which is added the challenge that men with PBC can sometimes feel that they don't quite fit in. The biology of the disease in men and women appears to be the same, with the same autoantibody associations and biopsy findings. Our approach to medical therapy is, therefore, the same. There are, however, two important aspects to the disease which differ and should be borne in mind.

The first issue we encounter with male PBC patients is late or missed diagnosis. The disease is, typically, significantly more advanced in male patients at the point of clinical presentation and diagnosis. Men also tend to be diagnosed at a slightly older age. Both these observations point to the diagnosis being delayed. We suspect that this reflects the perception amongst many doctors that PBC is a disease of women, and the parallel assumption that liver disease in men is usually a result of alcohol. This will only be addressed by increased awareness and education amongst doctors. There may also be an issue around reduced accessing of medical screening opportunities by men in general.

The second aspect of men with PBC is that there are some subtle, but important, differences in the disease between men and women. Men appear to be slightly less likely to respond to UDCA therapy. This may be a consequence of the slightly later presentation, but a careful watch needs to be undertaken of response to treatment and timely progression to second-line therapy. A second difference is that the condition appears to be less symptomatic. Men with PBC appear to be, in particular, less likely to have fatigue. The lack of symptoms may also play a role in the later presentation (no symptoms means it is less likely that you will have investigations such as blood tests).

The differences between men and women with PBC are not profound. It is just useful for us to always remember that men with PBC can sometimes find it a little bit of a lonely struggle.

HEALTH, DIET AND LIFESTYLE

There are a number of other aspects of living with PBC which are not well covered in medical textbooks (and certainly not on the internet!) and where people can, as a result, end up getting the wrong information. I will cover a number of these in this section

1) What diet should I follow? The answer here is simple. A healthy well-balanced diet with very few changes specifically because of PBC. Sometimes people can be a little intolerant of fat (because of the changes in the flow of bile which is needed to help absorb fat) meaning that watching fat intake is helpful. Where people are intolerant they might get loose bowel motions and abdominal cramps after a fatty meal. Sometimes, PBC patients can have more profound problems with absorption of the food from their diet. This is less common than it used to be, in my experience, probably as a result of the widespread use of UDCA, but if you are struggling with too much weight loss this is definitely something to discuss with your doctor. Sometimes poor food absorption and weight loss can be a result of a linked bowel problem reducing food uptake (such as celiac disease). Sometimes this is the pancreas gland (which produces digestive enzymes) being reduced in its effectiveness as part of PBC. Sometimes it is just bile flow issues. Once anything worrisome is excluded the input of dieticians to explore supplements which may be easier for you to absorb than your normal diet is very helpful.

2) Are there any supplements I should be taking? Again the answer is if you get the diet right this shouldn't be needed. The natural anti-oxidants in the body, which reduce the impact of tissue injury, are reduced in PBC and many patients take an anti-oxidant vitamin preparation (easily available in pharmacies and supermarkets). The same effect can be achieved, however, by a healthy diet with, in particular, plenty of green vegetables. In terms of supplements that are best avoided our advice is to not take herbal medicines (in particular some of the unregulated traditional medicines). There have been cases of these being toxic to the liver.

3) Can I take my other tablets now I have liver disease? The issue of safety of medicines in people with liver disease is an area that causes real concern to both doctors and patients. There are, however, two potential sources of risk and not the single one that everyone worries about. The obvious risk comes from the possibility that, because of liver disease, the drug is handled differently (many drugs are cleared from the body by the liver) and this leads to either more toxicity from the drug or worsening of the liver disease. This leads to many doctors avoiding prescribing drugs to people with liver diseases such as PBC. There is, however, a counter-risk which is that people end up not getting the right treatment for important illnesses because of a mild additional risk due to their liver disease. The most extreme example I came across was someone who was told that they couldn't have chemotherapy for cancer because of mild PBC with normal liver blood tests on UDCA! We soon changed that decision as you might imagine. The other thing to be aware of is that the guides to prescribing, and patient information leaflets that come with drugs, very frequently talk about caution in liver disease. Sometimes this is based on examples of problems, but many times it is because we simply don't know whether there is a risk and, in the absence of being able to say there is no risk (and proving a negative is very difficult), drug companies are cautious. This can leave patients and doctors confused and worried.

So what are the implications for PBC? There are two important things to say. The first is that not all liver diseases are the same. PBC, as a disease where the bile ducts are the target for injury, with abnormality in the liver's ability to function coming much later, if at all, is a disease where we would not expect as many problems with drug handling as we might in diseases where the hepatocyte is the main injury target. The second thing follows on from this. In my experience, issues with drug toxicity in PBC are very rare indeed, and the risks of not getting the right treatment for another condition probably out-weigh significantly the risks of a drug reaction.

Sensible practical advice would be to avoid unnecessary drugs and always keep the tablets you are taking under review with your doctor (this is general good advice; doctors have a habit of starting drugs and not getting round to stopping them leading to over- and unnecessary treatment). Always remember, however, that not getting the right treatment can also be a risk. The other piece of sound general advice is that if you or your doctor suspect that a drug is causing significant side-effects the first step should always be to stop it until it is clear what is going on. If the drug is for a life-threatening condition then this decision clearly needs to be made quickly, but continuing with a drug causing significant side effects is a recipe for trouble. In my experience, where really bad issues have arisen with drug side-effects (in general, I have never actually seen one in PBC!) it is because this basic rule has been ignored.

4) Can I take HRT/Can I take the oral contraceptive: HRT and the pill both contain female sex hormones. These hormones, both naturally in the setting of pregnancy and in tablet or patch form in HRT (rarely) and the pill (more commonly), can cause cholestasis with elevation of liver blood tests and itch. This leads to a perennial concern that HRT or the pill might make PBC worse. They are, however, completely different processes that aren't additive. HRT and the pill both have their risks, as well as their obvious benefits, and that balance of risk and benefit isn't particularly altered by having PBC. My only observation is that if HRT is being considered for osteoporosis risk reduction there may be more effective treatments for you to consider (**Chapter 8**). If it is for more general menopause symptoms then it is something that I have seen be useful for improving overall life quality. As always, this is general advice and the pros and cons for you as an individual need to be discussed with your doctor.

5) Is pregnancy safe? **YES!** There is a pervasive myth (the internet plays its part here!) that pregnancy is dangerous in PBC. There is no evidence whatsoever for this other than in the very small group of people with very advanced liver disease (very uncommon in PBC). Even then it is a manageable risk. For the vast majority of patients with milder disease forms people don't seem to have an issue with getting pregnant, and don't have problems with the pregnancy or the birth (with no specific problems being seen in the baby). Our practice is to continue UDCA, although other units stop it because it hasn't been proven to be safe in pregnancy (there is no evidence that it is harmful, and in fact it is started in pregnancy in people getting obstetric cholestasis but it is that "can't prove a negative" issue again).

The only exception to the question of pregnancy risk in PBC is, as mentioned above, people with cirrhosis and portal hypertension. Later on in pregnancy the rise in pressure within the abdomen (a large baby in an abdomen with limited capacity to expand) can cause the pressure in the portal vein to rise. This can lead to a variceal bleed if varices are present. Standard practice is to do a routine endoscopy at around 6 months to check for varices.

6) Can I smoke and drink alcohol? NO and WITHIN REASON are the short answers here. Several studies have shown that smoking is, in fact, more common in PBC patients than in an equivalent age and sex group in the normal population. This often surprises people. Whether this suggests that smoking contributes to the risk of PBC, or whether people smoke as a result of their PBC (perhaps to calm anxiety or through boredom in people with fatigue) isn't clear. What is clear is that smoking is always bad for you in terms of heart disease and cancer risk and you should make every effort to stop. E-cigarettes haven't been evaluated in PBC and it is therefore difficult to give guidance. My only practical observation is whatever risk they may or may not have it is very likely to be lower than cigarette smoking.

The answer regarding alcohol is more nuanced. There is no association between alcohol consumption and PBC. The only liver disease associated with alcohol consumption is alcoholic liver disease! Telling people to stop drinking because they have liver disease is a knee-jerk reaction by doctors and serves to perpetuate the myth that there is some form of link between all liver disease and alcohol. Alcohol in small amounts is a normal part of life, and in a condition where disconnection from social structures can be an issue it can have tangible benefits for people. Our advice for people with early PBC (in essence people without cirrhosis) is that alcohol is fine but the liver probably can't handle it in the same way that it can in people without PBC. We therefore advise no more than half the normal safe drinking limits. This effect is exaggerated in people with cirrhosis and we would advise no more than 1 to 2 drinks per day. Many people with PBC choose not to drink alcohol. That is obviously fine but it should be their choice.

CHAPTER 10: WHAT HAS CHANGED SINCE 2020?

The 2-Minute Version

- The three years between the first and second editions of this book have been ones of rapid change in PBC. They are also ones in which the remaining challenges to delivering really effective treatment for PBC in practice have become ever clearer.

- The second-line therapy model (UDCA followed, where needed by a second drug such as OCA or bezafibrate) has become fully established in practice in most countries. Although we still lack formal trial outcome data to demonstrate an impact on survival to go along with the well-characterised improvement in liver blood tests, studies at a population level are now strongly suggesting that both OCA and bezafibrate improve survival.

- The real world use data have also highlighted some of the limitations of these drugs (and the way in which we currently use them). The degree to which they return liver blood tests to normal is, if anything, more disappointing than we had hoped. This has been observed at a time when the emerging evidence suggests that we really should be aiming for normal liver blood tests in PBC treatment. On the positive side, the issue of itch with OCA use has emerged as less as a problem than we had anticipated. Less positively, it is increasingly clear that bezafibrate use can be associated with kidney injury raising question marks about its long-term use. There is emerging clinical evidence to suggest that the combination of OCA and bezafibrate may be particularly useful for step-up therapy in PBC.

- Trials have suggested that a number of other drugs may be beneficial in PBC (all evaluated in the current treatment step-up model). Final trial evaluation is currently underway. I think it is likely that one or more will be licensed for clinical use. If so, the next challenge will be to work out where in the treatment pathway they fit in.

- There has been real progress in our understanding of the causes and treatments for itch and fatigue in PBC, both of which symptoms are the focus of clinical trials. It is likely that symptom-directed therapy will be the next major development in PBC.

- International groups have come together to look at the data on Fibroscan and this has really reinforced the value of it as a clinical test. It should now be thought of as the standard tool for assessing PBC severity.

- Large scale national audit has, unfortunately, pointed out the limitations of the reach of current treatments in PBC. Particular issues were identified with the use of second-line therapy and assessment of symptoms (both occurring in under 50% of patients) and in discussion of patients with the severest disease with liver transplant units (a third of patient are not being discussed). These findings emphasise the importance of getting what is now standard treatment out to everyone. New drugs are, and will continue to be, no use to people if those people don't get them! The best results were seen in the specialist centres with dedicated PBC clinics.

- COVID caused real issues with the delivery of care to PBC patients and may have contributed to some of the limitations seen in the audit. A simpler and thus potentially more robust model for treatment would be potentially very beneficial indeed. Paradoxically, COVID itself seems to have caused relatively few direct problems in PBC (although it may be that "long COVID" has been worsening PBC fatigue and cognitive symptoms.

Information about the advances in our understanding of the causes, management and treatment of PBC that have occurred since the publication of the first edition of this book has been incorporated throughout the preceding chapters. I thought, however, it might be helpful and interesting to include a new chapter that summarises these evolutions, as I see them, in one place. Think of it as a PBC "update" chapter. It is inevitable that, when looking at changes that have only occurred recently, some will end up being less important than they seen at this point, and other changes that look less significant take on a great importance. Please bear this in mind.

EVIDENCE TO SUPPORT SURVIVAL BENEFIT FOR SECOND-LINE THERAPY

As I outlined in **Chapter 5**, drugs need to be approved ("licensed") before they can be used in normal clinical practice. To get this approval, evidence needs to be presented to show that the drug is both safe (obviously) and effective. Evidence of effectiveness needs to be meaningful. Clearly, in PBC, a drug that reduced the risk of death would obviously be deemed effective. Given that many people at risk of dying from PBC will have a liver transplant before they get too unwell, reducing the need for transplant is, in essence, the equivalent of avoiding the risk of death. Reduction in need for transplant would therefore also be deemed to be evidence of effectiveness. The problem is, however, that even in the highest risk patients, PBC is a slowly progressive disease. Evidence of effectiveness in terms of reduction in risk of death or need for transplant would, therefore, take years, if not decades, to get. If the evidence of such long-term effect were being gathered in a placebo-controlled trial (one in which some people take a dummy tablet) it would mean that some people would end-up taking that dummy (from which they can get no benefit) for many years. This is not really acceptable or appropriate for most people. For this reason, we have used blood tests as what are called surrogate markers to support the approval of drugs such as OCA. In essence, higher levels of alkaline phosphatase and bilirubin are associated with worse outcomes (i.e. the higher they are the more likely someone is to develop severe PBC). A reduction in these values might reasonably, therefore, be expected to be associated with an improved prognosis. There is a need for caution, however. If transplant is used as an endpoint, and these blood test values (especially bilirubin) are used to time transplantation, then a treatment which artificially reduced the numbers through a mechanism unrelated to PBC would give rise to a totally false impression of benefit. This is why the licensing bodies are cautious about blood tests and other surrogate markers to approve drugs.

We are, therefore, left with a real problem in PBC. A trial to show meaningful benefit (death or transplant reduction) isn't possible as it will take too long, and a placebo trial wouldn't be appropriate or acceptable to patients. However, a shorter and more acceptable trial using blood test improvements as the target isn't enough to convince the licensing bodies. How can we square this circle?

In the last couple of years a really elegant solution has been pioneered in PBC which is a real breakthrough in the disease (and should lead to full approval of a number of drugs). The approach will also help therapy development in other chronic diseases. This is the use of "virtual" or "synthetic" controls. In a traditional trial the control group are the people not taking the drug (i.e. the ones taking placebo or dummy). The work of UK-PBC and the Global PBC study group over many years has given us unique insights into how PBC progresses and what happens to people over time. At the heart of this is lots and lots of case histories of people, with blood test information right throughout the disease course, treatment history and information on what happened to them (did they need transplant, are they alive and well etc). The thought experiment we did was to ask whether you could use the information from people who didn't go into a trial of a drug like OCA or bezafibrate (or take them in the normal clinic setting) as virtual controls. Identify the point at which they could have taken the treatment, but didn't, and track what happened over time exactly as would have happened had they been taking placebo in a trial. When this approach has been used to look at what happened to people in the Phase 3 OCA trial (POISE), compared to equivalent people in the population who didn't take OCA, the result is very striking indeed in two respects. The first is that when totally different populations are used to construct the control group (Global PBC and UK-PBC) exactly the same results are seen. This suggests that the approach is actually very reliable. The second, and key, result is that using both these populations, survival free of transplantation is found to be significantly better for people taking OCA. In essence, people taking OCA survive much longer than identical people who don't take it. This is the most convincing data to date to show that OCA really does improve survival and should be used in people who don't respond to UDCA. Let's hope the licensing bodies agree! A similar, if less elegant and robust approach has suggested that bezafibrate also reduces the risk.

It is very likely that this approach will be used in the evaluation of the newer drugs that are under trial at the moment, and that the approach will become standard. If so, it will play a major role in simplifying trials, making them much quicker and, given the reduced need for placebo groups, much more attractive to patients.

INCOMPLETE RESPONSE TO SECOND-LINE THERAPY AS CURRENTLY USED

Perhaps paradoxically, given the previous section showing how effective OCA and bezafibrate seem to be, there is also emerging evidence to suggest that there are limitations to these drugs. There are two aspects to this. The first is that both the trial and the real world data (the collected information from people taking the drugs in the normal clinic setting) suggest that a significant proportion of people don't "respond" using the same criteria we use for UDCA (although there is evidence to suggest that even people who don't technically respond get some benefit). In other words, they are UDCA and OCA/bezafibrate "double" non-responders. It has been suggested that UDCA non-responder who take bezafibrate are more likely to respond than people taking OCA. It is important to realise, however, that the drugs have not been directly compared in the same trial. Furthermore, when the trials in which they have been explored are compared (and the clinical use in practice) people taking OCA tend to have much higher levels of alkaline phosphatase to start with, and thus have much further to improve to reach the level needed for "response". The apparent increased in effectiveness of bezafibrate is just that, apparent not real.

The second aspect is the one that is going to become increasingly important in the future. We may have got the target for treatment wrong.......What do I mean by this? To date we have used a cut-off for blood tests values in response to UDCA based on a degree of ongoing liver function test. In simple terms, we have regarded some degree of abnormality as acceptable. Two strands of evidence have challenged this. The first is that the Global PBC study group have shown that any degree of elevation in alkaline phosphatase or bilirubin is associated with an increase in risk of death or need for transplant. People who are UDCA "responders" but who have ongoing slightly abnormal liver function tests have ongoing increased risk. It is not as significant as the people who are non-responder using these cut-offs, but it is still there all the same. More recent work from the UK has looked at the levels of inflammation in different patients, as assessed by the chemicals that the immune system releases into the blood and through which cells communicate. This has shown that, again, people with blood tests which make them "responders", but in whom the liver blood tests are not normal have ongoing evidence of PBC inflammation. The implication of these clinical and laboratory studies is that only people with normal blood tests have no active PBC and no increased risk. Our current approach of accepting some degree of abnormality is a compromise. A reasonable compromise in past years but a compromise none the less, and one that I suspect will not be regarded as acceptable for much longer. Our new mantra in the clinic is "only normal is normal". Does this matter and should we be chasing normal tests in everyone? The answer is, as always, nuanced. If the ongoing blood test elevation is marginal, and the patient is very elderly or has other health problems then it may not really represent a meaningful issue for them that warrants intervention. For a young patient who wants many decades of healthy life, and wants to avoid a transplant, it is potentially a significant issue and one that will increasingly be in our minds when we make treatment decisions.

POTENTIAL RISKS WITH SECOND-LINE THERAPY

All treatments in all diseases have risks associated with them (as well as benefits), and decisions about whether, and when, to use them involve a balancing of those risks and benefits. Perhaps inevitably, it takes use of these treatments in the "real world" (i.e. outside highly regulated trials involving selected patients) for the nature of the true balance to become clear. Second-line therapy in PBC is no different. When the first edition of this book was written, a reasonable consensus summary would have been that the main/only issue with OCA was itch, and bezafibrate was completely safe. For varying reasons, neither of these conclusions remains quite true.

In the case of OCA there are distinct positives and negatives. The positive is that the issue with itch appears to be much less significant than was originally feared. In our clinic, we have only had to stop OCA in a tiny number of patients because of itch. This is a real positive. There are several potential explanations for the seemingly lower impact of itch than was originally thought to be the case. The first is a simple dose issue. The original trials of OCA, in which itch really was an issue, used doses of up to 50mg a day. In practice now we start people on 5mg a day, 10% of the originally-trialled dose. If, as appears likely, the pro-itch effect is dose dependent this is likely to be a major factor. The second potential explanation may be patient selection. It may that clinicians are avoiding the use of OCA in people in whom they are worried about itch as an issue (i.e. people who already have itch). I think that itch is likely to be a factor in the use of bezafibrate rather than OCA as first choice second-line therapy in some patients. The third reason is patient preparation. In our clinic we assess itch in detail before using OCA, and where present, treat it before starting OCA (usually with rifampicin rather than cholestyramine because of the potential for the latter to bind OCA and neutralise it). Paradoxically, one of the agents we use to control itch in the context of actual or planned OCA use is.....bezafibrate making itch in a very high risk patient one of the settings in which the combination of OCA and bezafibrate is logical. A final reason why itch has less of an impact than might have been the case is the simple one of "fore-warned is fore-armed". In the original trials, when we didn't know itch might be an issue, we didn't warn patients. It therefore caught people by surprise. The simple act of making people aware that it is a potential issue makes it less of an issue if it does arrive.

The more negative aspect to OCA use is the emergence of possible risk in its use in patients with the most advanced disease. Ultimately, OCA (as with all the drugs we use) is best used as early as possible in the disease to prevent the development of cirrhosis. Inevitably, there are people in whom its use is considered who have already progressed to cirrhosis (either because they had already developed cirrhosis by the time they were diagnosed or because an earlier opportunity to treat effectively was missed (in many cases because OCA and other second-line therapies simply didn't exist at the point at which we would now consider second-line therapy use)). It appears that, in this setting, the damaged liver can't handle OCA and the drug can worsen rather than improve liver function. There have been a small number of deaths of patients in this setting, especially in the USA, and this has led the regulatory authorities to exclude patients with advanced cirrhosis from OCA use.

What on earth does this mean, and should you be worried if you are taking or are about to take OCA? The most important thing to say here is that for the vast majority of people taking, or likely to take, OCA this **does not have any impact at all**. I will try to explain and reassure. The first thing to say is that this isn't a new phenomenon. It has been known about for years in other liver diseases. Autoimmune hepatitis, viral hepatitis and Wilsons disease are all conditions that are fully treatable with drugs, and yet if those drugs are given in very advanced disease, they can make that disease worse rather than better. Hepatologists "know" this and factor it in to their treatment decisions. It appears, however, that they had "forgotten" it when it came to OCA in advanced PBC. The reality is that the patients who died with OCA were, almost without exception, far too advanced for this to have been a sensible treatment decision. A number should have been referred for liver transplantation not OCA use. It is interesting to observe that none of these issues were seen in the UK where there is formal treatment decision making process before OCA is prescribed. In essence, two clinicians need to rehearse the pros and cons and agree on a course of action. It's all about sensible decision making.

So who is safe to take OCA and who isn't? The only people in whom the drug needs to be absolutely avoided are people with cirrhosis complicated by what we call decompensation features (varices, jaundice, ascites, encephalopathy etc). These are actually really rare in PBC and, thus, the excluded group is very small. The vast majority of people taking OCA don't have cirrhosis (the whole point of the drug is to stop them developing cirrhosis) and are thus safe to take it. People with cirrhosis are also safe to take it provided they don't have complications. We have treated, and will continue to treat, people with early cirrhosis with OCA and in our experience it has been completely safe. We would evaluate people carefully, start on a very low dose and watch very carefully, however.

What about bezafibrate, the drug that we thought was completely safe? Here again there is reason to be cautious. It is very likely that the same issues of risk with very advanced disease use are seen with bezafibrate as with OCA. It is just as an off-label therapy the risks with bezafibrate have been subjected to much less in the way of scrutiny. This exemplifies the important of getting proper regulatory approval for drugs supported by proper, long-term evidence. In my practice, I would apply exactly the same cautions for the use in bezafibrate as I would for OCA. There is, however, a second and slightly more general issue (the advanced disease use issue only applies, at the end of the day, to a small group of patients). This is kidney injury. We are seeing growing numbers of patients treated with bezafibrate getting problems with their kidney function. For most people, this is a deterioration in blood tests that resolves once the drug is stopped. For a small number of people the problem has been more significant. The timing of the problem is also an issue. The problems, such as they are, with OCA (itch and deterioration of liver function in advanced disease patients, happen quickly after the drug is started, at the time when doctors are watching carefully. Kidney problems with bezafibrate can occur at any point after the drug has been started, including months or years down the line. This is often the sort of time period where attention has slipped and doctors aren't looking for issues. Certainly, in my experience, this has been a factor in more significant kidney problems. Kidney issues may be commoner in people given the slow release form of the drug (the 400mg once a day version). We would screen kidney function in all patients being considered for bezafibrate and would avoid the drug completely in anyone with significant issues. We would avoid the slow release version in anyone with any degree of impairment. We would then check kidney function regularly after the treatment has been started. The lingering question, however, is always why not just use OCA which has no kidney issues associated with it?

EMERGENCE OF ALTERNATIVE SECOND-LINE THERAPIES AND APPROACHES

We are in the midst of a treatment revolution in PBC and it is very likely that the range of treatments that we can use in the clinic in practice will expand significantly over the next few years. These treatments split into two groups. The combination of existing therapies and all new drugs.

When we think of combination therapy it is important to remember that we already use combination therapy in people needing second-line treatment as these drugs are almost always given in combination with UDCA. An emerging approach which shows real promise is, however, the **combination of bezafibrate and OCA** (along with UDCA). At the time of writing there is a clinical trial of the combination of these 3 drugs going on in UDCA non-responders. Triple therapy of this type is, however, being increasingly used in ordinary practice in specialist centres with good results (which have been published). My own experience has been really good. The main rationale for triple therapy is not, actually, better PBC control but to facilitate the use of OCA in people who are getting significant itch (and in whom there is a concern that OCA will worsen itch). In my experience, adding bezafibrate to control itch followed by OCA gives really good disease control with no ongoing itch issues. We certainly use triple therapy as the preferred approach in people who don't respond to a single second-line therapy rather than swapping to another single additional agent. There is also logic to the combination as OCA and bezafibrate have complementary modes of action on the liver.

The range of alternative second-line therapies under trial is growing. At present each is being evaluated as a single therapy in addition to UDCA, although in the future a number of these drugs may well have their greatest value as part of triple therapy regimes. The following is a summary of our understanding for each of the drugs in late 2022. Given that their development programmes are going at pace it is likely that this status will change so if you are reading this book in 2023 or beyond it might be worth checking on the internet as to the exact state of play.

The two most advanced alternative drugs are **seladelpar** and **elafibranor**. Both are what are called PPAR agonists and are thus in the same broad family as the fibrates. The PPARs (Peroxisome Proliferator Activated Receptors) are what are called nuclear receptors; proteins that regulate the production of other proteins specified by the DNA genetic code. There are a number of different types. In particular there is an alpha type (PPARα) and a delta (PPARδ). These work in slightly different ways and are found in different tissues. Different drugs activate the different PPAR types to differing degrees, and this may explain their varied degrees of effectiveness in PBC. In simple terms, fenofibrate is a pure PPARα agonist, bezafibrate is both α and δ (but more the former; interestingly they have in the past been used essentially inter-changeably when in fact they are quite different), elafibranor is also both α and δ (but more the latter) and seladelpar is pure δ. At this moment in time it isn't clear which specificity matters the most (and thus which drug is likely to be "best"), although there is a suggestion that significant δ activity is beneficial. On this basis it may be that elafibranor and seladelpar are better candidate drugs then bezafibrate which is, in turn, a better candidate than fenofibrate. What do the trials tell us? Is this theoretical difference born out in practice? As with all drug trials one key issue is that none of these drugs have been directly compared against each other in the same trial. We can compare different trials but, inevitably, there are differences in trial design and the types of people included meaning that we are often comparing apples and oranges. With that caveat in mind it is possible to draw two general conclusions. The first is that both seladelpar and elafibranor appear to be very effective at improving liver function tests in PBC. Certainly more so than bezafibrate, and potentially more so than OCA. There are no data yet on whether this translates into real benefit in terms of progression of the disease and avoiding death or need for transplant, however. The second conclusion is that, as is the case for bezafibrate, both appear to be really effective for reducing itch. In terms of the safety concerns with fibrates (decompensation with advanced disease and kidney problems) it is not, as yet, possible to say whether they also apply to the newer drugs. The trials done to date have excluded people with advanced disease so we have no data on the drugs in that setting. In terms of kidney injury, nothing worrying has been seen to date, however the trials have been small and the drugs not yet been given for long enough to know for sure.

One of the potential limitations of the current and emerging drug options described in the book so far is that they are all variations on the same theme. All are drugs that essentially work on the production of toxic bile acids and the constitution of bile. Are there options for other drugs that work in different ways? One such drug which has trial evidence to suggest benefit in PBC is **budesonide**. This is an interesting drug which probably has a number of different modes of action. The one that people tend to focus on is a steroid-like effect but without side-effects. Budesonide acts like prednisolone but, unlike prednisolone, is broken down in the liver and doesn't reach the general circulation. It thus has an effect on the liver but no side-effects beyond the liver (in theory at least). The whole issue of steroids and PBC is actually a complex one. We don't ever use them (other than in overlap), however there is trial evidence, from many years ago, to suggest that they are actually beneficial in PBC (albeit not sufficiently beneficial to out-weight the side effects). A drug which had the benefits of prednisolone without its downsides could thus be, in theory, useful. Budesonide may, however, have an additional action in the liver which is to increase the protective bicarbonate umbrella which reduces the injury to the bile duct cells caused by toxic bile. Given these 2 potentially attractive actions, does it work in PBC? The answer is yes and no. The primary endpoint of the recent trial of use in UDCA non-responders (the main question if you like) was around improvement in liver biopsy. This wasn't met, so technically budesonide was shown "not to work". However, and it is an important however, liver function tests (the primary end-point in all other recent PBC trials) did improve significantly. If biopsy hadn't been included (as it isn't in other trials) we would be saying that budesonide was an effective drug. A reasonable conclusion would be that budesonide has interesting potential applications in PBC and warrants further investigation.

A second alternative drug with a different mode of action is **setanaxib**. This represents a completely different approach to PBC treatment. It is an inhibitor of an enzyme called NADPH oxidase (and the only such drug in trial use at the moment). NADPH oxidase plays a major role in inflammation, contributing to free radical production and oxidative stress in diseases such as PBC. Given the importance of these mechanisms of tissue injury in the bile duct it is a logical therapy. The trials to date, again in UDCA non-responders, suggest that it has some LFT improving action but a more marked effect on Fibroscan. At face value this suggests that it may control or even reverse scarring or fibrosis in PBC. If so, it is the only drug yet shown to have this effect. This is currently being explored in further trials. Setanaxib also appears to have a significant impact on fatigue, something which I will expand on in the next section.

I strongly suspect that both budesonide and setanaxib will turn out to be beneficial in PBC. I also suspect that they may have their greatest use in combination with conventional anti-cholestatic therapy such as UDCA and OCA. How we will navigate the pathway to developing these combination therapies will be a key question in PBC.

ADVANCES IN SYMPTOM TREATMENT

An area where there has been real progress since the first edition of this book is, I think, the approach to symptoms in PBC. The first area of progress has been an increasing awareness and acceptance amongst clinicians and regulators about the importance of symptoms as an issue for patients (as I keep saying, patients have always known how important they are). Guidelines now clearly state the importance of asking about symptoms and managing them effectively (although there is far more we can do to make sure this actually happens in practice) and symptom assessment was included as an audit area in the recent UK national audit of PBC care. PBC symptoms should, therefore, be on the agenda for the management of all PBC patients.

A second area of progress has been an increase in data relating to the extent of the impact of symptoms on day to day functioning. If we "know" that symptoms have a big impact on patients why do data matter? It is all about context. If we talk about someone having mild, moderate or severe itch in PBC what does that mean? It tells us how that person might compare to other PBC patients, but it doesn't set the range of impacts in PBC in a broader context. How does the impact of PBC itch compare to, say, chronic pain from arthritis? This matters because, ultimately, decisions on funding for the development and then use in practice of treatments is based on degree of need, and the extent to which that need is met by existing therapies. High need (a big impact) not met by existing therapies (unmet need) gives rise to a high priority. The PBC symptom impact studies all indicate that, across the population of PBC patients as a whole, the impact on life from the symptoms of itch and fatigue is greater than from non-response to UDCA and the development of cirrhosis. Severe itch, in particular, is associated with a particularly marked impact on quality of life. What all this tells us is that symptoms really matter! Patients with PBC have known this for a long time. It is their doctors who have been slower to appreciate it. Hopefully this new knowledge will lead to a badly needed change in perception.

There are two aspects to the treatment of PBC symptoms. These are the specific treatments that we use, and the setting, and way, in which we use them. Both are really important. In terms of specific therapies the most progress has been made in relation to itch, with a number of potentially valuable therapies emerging. These split into two groups. The first is treatments for PBC itself which also have significant itch benefits. The second is specific itch-targeting therapies. In terms of disease controlling therapies, **bezafibrate**, **seladelpar** and **elafibranor** have all shown very promising itch reducing actions in addition to their effects on liver function. Of these, the only therapy currently licensed, and thus useable in practice, is bezafibrate. In terms of the specific itch treatment by far the most advanced is **linerixibat** which is now in phase 3 trial. It is taken orally but is not absorbed into the body (thereby reducing side-effects) and works by blocking the re-uptake of bile acids in the small bowel (it is an "iBAT inhibitor"). It has shown really promising effects in early trials and looks likely to make it through to approval.

Two other itch treatments are more experimental but look interesting. **Difelikefalin** is a highly specific opiate antagonists and promises to build on the already known about benefits of naltrexone (which is used in people who are not responding to other itch treatment but which is limited by side-effects). In essence, the drug targets the opiate receptors that are responsible for itch (outside the brain) but not those that are responsible for the side-effects. This greater targeting will, hopefully, enhance benefits and reduce side-effects. A very promising combination indeed. It is, however, yet to start clinical evaluation in PBC, and is therefore a number of years away from being used in the clinic. The final emerging drug is **EP547** (it is a drug that is very early in its development; so early that it doesn't even have a proper name yet!). This drug potentially works in a completely novel way. It is an MrgprX4 antagonist. MrgprX4 is thought to be a receptor on nerve fibres that is actually activated by bile acids. If this is the case, then it could potentially be the actual route by which bile acids cause itch. Blocking its response to bile acids could, therefore, be a uniquely attractive way to treat itch. It is, however, very early days indeed.

The final emerging treatment for PBC itch is not even a drug at all. It is **light therapy**. Light therapy (the approach of shining a very specific, high intensity, form of light on the skin) is a well-established approach to the treatment of skin diseases (in essence it builds on the observation that many skin diseases improve in the summer when the skin is exposed to sunlight). Light therapy has also been used to treat neonatal jaundice (jaundice developing in babies shortly after they have been born) for many years. It is thought to break down the jaundice pigment in the skin. What does this have to do with itch in PBC? It is not uncommon to come across PBC patients whose itch improves in the summer (just like in skin disease patients) and we have built on this by using formal light therapy in an increasing number of patients. We don't really know how it works, but presume that the light rays break down the molecules causing itch (possibly bile acids) in the skin. In my experience, when it works it works really well. It seems to work best in people with a low body weight (greater body surface area to absorb light per Kg of body weight). One of the main limitations in practice is the amount that it is safe to give in any year. There is a risk of skin cancer (small but there all the same) if people get too much light therapy. We have certainly seen people who "yo-yo" from no itch when they are getting the light treatment to high itch when they are having to have a break for a period of time to let the skin recover.

What about fatigue? Is the future as rosy as it seems to be for itch? Sadly not, although there are emerging treatment options. Again, existing second-line therapies show some promise. **Obeticholic Acid** reduces cognitive dysfunction and memory issues in mouse models of cholestasis and is undergoing clinical trial specifically for the treatment of central fatigue. Similarly, the PPAR agonists **elafibranor** and **seladelpar** show some signal in terms of reducing fatigue (although at present it isn't clear whether this is a potential direct anti-fatigue effect or an indirect one with reduced itch allowing better sleep and thus less fatigue). Interestingly, bezafibrate doesn't appear to have any anti-fatigue action, but does improve itch; observations that argue against a role for itch reduction in the anti-fatigue effects of the other PPAR agonists. Of the other disease-modifying drugs under trial, perhaps the most intriguing is **setanaxib** which, in addition to its effects on Fibroscan values (potentially through an anti-fibrotic effect) appears to significantly reduce fatigue. At present it isn't clear what the mechanism is but an obvious route to benefit would be through reduction in free radical production and inflammation impacting on the brain. In terms of specific therapy the drug **golexanolone** offers real potential. It blocks the action of neurosteroids (steroids that are produced in the brain in response to harmful or stressful situations, which cause sleepiness and fatigue, and which are known to be elevated in highly fatigued PBC patients. A trial of its use to reduce fatigue in PBC is to begin shortly. In terms of non-drug interventions there is further evidence now to suggest that exercise is very effective for reducing fatigue in PBC. This confirms earlier studies and is very much in keeping with our clinical experience. The challenge, as always, is getting started and maintaining the programme in the medium term.

Drugs and other interventions matter, but so does how we approach patients and support them to deal with their symptoms in practice. In Newcastle we had already taken this on board and developed our "TrACE" structured programme covered elsewhere in the book. We have now taken this a step further and have developed, and launched, a specialised symptom management clinic focusing entirely on itch and fatigue; how to treat them and how to live better with them. Feedback from patients is really good and lots of people are being referred. The next stage will be to put down on paper the structured care delivery model and its support tools so other interested clinicians can set up their own local versions.

NEW KNOWEDGE ABOUT THE VALUE OF FIBROSCAN

Transient elastography (most often referred to, as discussed earlier, by the trade name of the most widely used approach "Fibroscan") has been available for use in PBC for some time now and was introduced as a valuable test in the first edition of this book. It is a non-invasive method of assessing fibrosis severity in the liver. Why, then, does it now appear in this chapter focusing on new developments since the last edition. The answer is that there has been real progress in understanding its role and value in overall disease management, clarifying when and where it should be used. Fibroscan was originally shown to be highly predictive of the degree of fibrosis seen in the liver on a biopsy that was done at the same time as the Fibroscan and, on this basis, Fibroscan started to be used as an alternative to biopsy to get "stage" information. The data that have emerged since the first edition of the book, generated by a large international research consortium, show that Fibroscan is directly predictive of risk of death and complication development in PBC. This suggests it is perhaps an even more useful clinical tool than originally anticipated. This work identified three Fibroscan values as being important in understanding risk. The first is 7.8KPa. This value is a little higher than the one that would be seen in someone with a completely normal liver (where it would be 4-5), however a value below 7.8 is associated with a very low risk indeed of complication development. Between 7.8 and 15.1 the risk was elevated, but not dramatically so. However, values of above 15.1 were associated with significant risk of complication development. The third value is a slightly older one of 17.9 KPa. This was the value in the biopsy studies that was originally found to be suggestive of cirrhosis or stage 4 disease development. The reason why the 15.1 cut off for high risk is lower than the 17.9 cut-off for cirrhosis is probably that once the value has gone above 15.1, progression to 17.9 and cirrhosis is likely to be inevitable. What does all this mean for practice? In simple terms, we now know enough to suggest that Fibroscan should be included in the normal follow-up for all PBC patients, with frequency determined by the initial Fibroscan value (very low initial values indicate a low level or risk meaning that follow-up should be in 3-5 years, whilst higher values indicate higher risk and justify annual follow-up). In this setting, Fibroscan doesn't replace blood tests and UDCA response criteria. It instead adds an important additional dimension. For the largest group of patients (those with low Fibroscan scores and who are UDCA responders) the evidence we have now really does point to the fact that they have no risk form the disease at all (although symptoms may be a different matter).

LIMITATIONS IN THE DELIVERY OF TREATMENT FOR PBC IN PRACTICE

One of the less positive things that has emerged in the last few years is clear evidence to suggest that, unfortunately, PBC care in practice in the UK is patchy at best. Light has been shed on this by a national audit of practice in the UK which has included anonymous information on 9000 patients (probably about half of all UK PBC patients) being cared for in hospitals all across the country. Audit of this type tells us how we are doing in terms of care, and identifies areas where we need to improve. The audit only covers the UK but I am certain that the same issues would be seen wherever it were to be done. It is just that if you don't look you will never see problems.

One area that is positive is that it looks like PBC is being diagnosed efficiently these days (this wasn't always the case) and use of UDCA is seen in 92% of patients. Once care becomes more complex, however, it is delivered less comprehensively. Despite second-line therapy being the standard care approach, mandated in all guidelines, only 49% of UDCA non-responders were treated in this way. Also worrying was the fact that 36% of patients at high risk of deterioration, and for whom transplant would be a potentially really important option, had not been discussed with their local transplant centre. Very high risk PBC patients can deteriorate rapidly, and it is really important that anyone at risk in this way (usually because of a high and rising bilirubin level) is discussed with a transplant unit. Finally, for someone who puts so much thought and effort into symptom management in PBC, the fact that 40% of patients hadn't even be asked about symptoms is very disappointing indeed.

These figures are all national ones for the UK as a whole. When we look at different centres the picture becomes, if anything, more worrying. When we looked at second-line therapy use, this ranged from 65% down to 35%, despite there being no evidence to suggest that there is regional variation in the severity of PBC and the need for such therapy, and all centres being subject to the same use guidance. In terms of patients with very advanced liver disease, the variation in referral rates to transplant services was even more stark (100% to 20%; figures for under 70 year-olds). We can only speculate as to why there is such very stark variation in access to care and quality of care between centres that are sometimes only a few miles apart. What we can all agree on, however, is that there is no justification for such a post-code lottery. On the clinical side we will continue to do our very best to increase awareness and to push for uniform improvement in care quality. Patients and patient groups can also play a huge role in holding clinical care centres to account.

COVID AND PBC

It is a sign of the times that when I started writing the first edition of this book the world had never heard of COVID. Now it gets its own section in the second edition of the book! There are two broad aspects to COVID and PBC. The first is the risk that COVID presents to patients with PBC (in all its forms). The second is the impact that COVID has had on the care of PBC patients' liver disease. Although the former is the subject of most attention and concern, in reality the latter is likely to have the greatest long-term on the largest number of people.

In terms of the risk PBC patients face from COVID, it appears that this is low (albeit with 3 important caveats). There are only limited published data, however our own clinical experience suggests that there is little or no additional risk from COVID over and above that in the non-PBC population. Remarkably (and pleasingly) few of our patient population ended up in hospital or having real problems. Interestingly, shortly before this second edition was published, some data emerged to suggest that UDCA may in fact protect cells from being infected by the COVID virus. It could therefore be that our sense of low risk is accurate and is because of an un-heralded protective effect of a key PBC drug. There was concern about vaccination and its safety, although most people ended up being vaccinated. My advice throughout has been that the vaccine completely changed the nature of COVID and it is absolutely right to have it unless there are very specific reasons not to (and PBC is not one of them!). The vaccines do not appear to reduce transmission (plenty of people get COVID despite being vaccinated) but they do reduce the severity of the illness, especially in relation to the very problematic lung injury and clotting problems that were such a major issue in the first wave.

So what are the caveats? The first of these is that patients with advanced cirrhosis did and do appear to be more at risk, both of catching the virus and then getting real problems from it. Fortunately, this is only a small group in PBC. It is likely that this increased risk comes from the changes in the effectiveness of the immune response seen in cirrhosis (patients with cirrhosis are, basically, less able to mount an effective immune response than people who don't have cirrhosis) and this is manifest as an increase in the risk of a wide range of infection types. The second caveat relates to immuno-suppression therapy. The vast majority of PBC patients don't take immuno-suppression (correctly). Importantly, UDCA, bezafibrate and OCA (by far and away the most commonly used treatments in PBC) are not immuno-suppressants. This is probably the single reason why COVID has been less of an issue in PBC than in many of the other autoimmune conditions, treated with immuno-suppression, where infection and complication rates have been higher. Two groups of PBC patients do, however, take immuno-suppression and in these settings greater awareness and caution is needed. These are post-transplant patients and patients taking immuno-suppression for overlap syndrome. The increased COVID risk appears to differ according to the immuno-suppressive drugs used (with MMF perhaps having the greatest risk). Immuno-suppression also reduces the response to vaccines, including the COVID vaccine. Clearly, where people are taking immuno-suppression after a transplant this is an unavoidable situation. The advent of COVID reminds us, however, that new infections are always going to be there as a risk and immuno-suppression can only ever increase that risk, emphasising, yet again, the importance of developing better treatment regimens for PBC that mean we don't need to resort to transplant in the future... The other group of people taking immuno-suppression are patients with overlap syndrome. As we discussed in an earlier chapter, an overlap state can exist between PBC and AIH, with some patients having features of both conditions. If a PBC patient also has AIH then it is important that both aspects of the disease are treated. This includes appropriate use of immuno-suppression and with that comes, of course, the same COVID issues as in post-transplant patients. The really important point to re-iterate is that, whereas overlap clearly exists, it has been over-diagnosed in the past and isn't as common as has previously been thought. There are a number of people that come to our clinic who are on immuno-suppression for "overlap" when in reality they have bad PBC. This gives them the risks and side-effects associated with immuno-suppression without any benefits. This has always been an issue but COVID has dramatically increased the risk. It is really important that everyone with a past diagnosis of overlap has that diagnosis re-assessed in the light of current understanding of the disease, and appropriate adjustments to treatment made

The final aspect of PBC and COVID is one that I don't really have an answer to. That is the question as to whether PBC patients are more susceptible to, or experience worse symptoms from "Long COVID". The issue is that many of the clinical features described for Long Covid are very similar indeed to PBC symptoms (brain fog being the most obvious, but not the only one). I have certainly seen PBC patients whose symptoms have been worse after COVID.......in many ways the issue is one of semantics, however, as structured support to reduce the impact of long COVID symptoms is, in essence, the same TrACE approach as we use in the management of fatigue in PBC.

CHAPTER 11: **THE FUTURE**

I have now worked in the field of PBC, and with PBC patients, for over 30 years. It is striking how much progress has been made, in particular over the last 10 or so years. This has accelerated over the last 3 years as outlined in the previous chapter. My early years in the field were marked by the advent of a single therapy, UDCA, and the failure of all other attempts to treat the disease with drugs. In retrospect, there was a message in all those failed trials, which used immuno-suppressive drugs. The message was that PBC is, fundamentally, a disease of the bile ducts and of bile flow, and that the target of treatment should, as a result, be the bile ducts. Sometimes the answer hides in plain sight! The early success of UDCA was followed by a slower realisation that it was actually relatively limited in its effectiveness, and that we need new and better treatments. This was the realisation that led to the current revolution in PBC therapy. This revolution is still ongoing. But where do we go from here? What are the remaining challenges? Even more so than the rest of this book, this chapter is a very personal view of what we need to do and what we might reasonably hope will come to pass. Let's see what the future holds! As the last chapter shows, the future is coming towards us very fast. Let's hope that when I write the 3rd edition of this book some or all of these "wishes for the future" will have been delivered.

A TREATMENT FOR FATIGUE

I don't think it particularly contentious to say that the biggest need we still have is for an effective treatment for fatigue. This symptom blights peoples' lives and, at present, all we can do is support them to live their lives as best they can. This can be a real help for people, but it would be fantastic to make the approach entirely redundant by having a treatment that reverses fatigue in the first place. I think a critical first step is to know what we are treating. This is partly to guide treatment development, and partly to make sure that in trials of new therapy (and new therapy won't get into clinical practice without trials) we are treating the right people. Almost certainly, fatigue comes in different forms in PBC (central and peripheral being the obvious first split). It is likely that a treatment for one will not be a treatment for others. If we are developing and testing a treatment for central fatigue then the trials need to be done in people with central fatigue. Central fatigue is certainly the area where we have made the most progress in terms of understanding the problem and, crucially, finding ways to measure the brain processes underpinning it in ways that can be incorporated into clinical trials. This is an area where I think there will be real progress in the near future. Peripheral fatigue is likely to be more difficult, and it may be that there is no specific treatment as such if it is all part of de-conditioning. Exercise as part of a rehabilitation programme is likely to be key, and the recent clinical trials show real promise. The next stage is to really understand what types of exercise people should be looking to do (as well as how frequently and for how long) and to find ways of making exercise programmes fit in with peoples' lifestyles. Less about the concept (which is well supported) and more about the detail as to what it looks like in practice.

There is another major challenge with regard to fatigue, however. We need to address the real issue of clinicians not recognising it for the problem that it is. We were aware of this issue before, but the UK national audit has made the scale of the problem all too clear. It will be no good having an effective treatment if patients then do not receive it because their doctors think the problem is not real. I have spent over 15 years trying to understand and treat fatigue in PBC, and yet every time I talk about it I have to respond to "experts" saying it does not exist (or even worse, that people only feel that they are fatigued because I tell them that they are; a truly bizarre thought). I thought that when the first brain imaging results emerged, demonstrating that fatigue in PBC is associated with clear-cut brain changes, this would solve this problem but seemingly not. Do these doctors not listen to their patients? The strong voice of patients and patient groups will be key here.

"TREAT AND FORGET" OPTIONS FOR ITCH

This may seem like a slightly strange ambition, given that we already have treatments for itch, but it would actually make a huge difference to people in practice. Although we have effective treatments, data from UK-PBC suggest that the extent to which they actually get to patients in practice is limited (a significant proportion of people with severe itch, for example, are not on any treatment at all). I do not think there is a single reason for this. It is lots of issues with lots of treatments that make the whole area complex (cholestyramine is difficult to tolerate, rifampicin can cause liver toxicity (an obvious worry in patients who already have liver disease) and needs lots of monitoring, naltrexone can worsen pain etc). What we need, more than anything in the area of itch, is a simple treatment that can be given to everyone with itch and which can, in essence, be forgotten about because it carries on working and is perfectly safe and easy to take. Is this something that could happen? Rather like fatigue (especially central fatigue) itch is an area where there are a number of emerging new treatment options. Will any of them be my "treat and forget" agent? I am not sure. That will take use in practice, but I suspect one or more will certainly make it through into clinical practice. The other reason why the itch studies are important is that they make trials of treatment aimed at improving symptoms normal for doctors, patients and, of course, the regulatory bodies who approve treatments for use. This will clearly be important in itch as an end in its own right but will also really help with the fight against fatigue.

BETTER CARE FOR EVERYONE

This may sound like an unambitious goal but it is really important. As mentioned above, UK-PBC has shown that the treatments we have for itch are not reaching all the patients who need them in practice. This is not, however, restricted to itch. UK-PBC data (up to and including the recent audit) suggest that even something as simple to use and universally recognised as UDCA is not being used in all patients. When UK-PBC started, only around 80% of PBC patients were being prescribed UDCA. Now the figure is over 90% (92% in the audit). Interestingly, guidance for doctors has not changed over that time, suggesting the power of a simple and consistent educational message to doctors, delivered by PBC experts, patient groups and patients themselves. The experts do have an important role to play in "getting their house in order" however. We have been guilty of taking a simple message (use UDCA followed by checking to see if it is working after a year) and over-complicating it. This was firstly by endless rather arcane arguments about whether it "works" or "doesn't work". This always was a flawed argument; one that sought a global answer to a question that does not have one. The reality was, and is, that UDCA works a lot in many people, a little in quite a lot, and not at all in a very small number; the critical issue as we now perceive it is that it works most in the lowest risk people, and least in the highest risk. We could have avoided losing many years of progress by accepting that UDCA has an important role to play, but that there always was a need to look for additional or alternative approaches to treatment.

The other area where we the experts have sought to take something simple and make it complex is in relation to the criteria we use in practice to decide if someone has responded or not to UDCA. These all relate to liver function tests, and all are variations on different cut-offs and combinations of bilirubin, ALT and, universally, alkaline phosphatase. The basic concept behind each on its own is fine (the lower the biochemical values the better response), although the introduction of a cut-off to define response creates an instant problem. If the cut-off for response is an alkaline phosphatase of below twice the upper limit of normal (say 250 for a local laboratory where the upper limit of normal is 125) does this mean that someone with a value of 249 is fine but someone at 251 is not? If someone's value falls from 251 to 249 then technically they have responded to UDCA even though their value has barely changed. In contrast, if their value has fallen from 1000 to 251 they are deemed to have not responded, even though the fall has been dramatic and must have some clinical relevance. The reality is that measures like these have value across large populations where these anomalies tend to even themselves out, but are less and less valuable as you get down to the individual patient. They are tools which should be used to contribute to understanding disease and its progress, but should not be thought of as absolute standards.

There is a second challenge around UDCA response criteria, and that is the large number of different versions used by different clinicians. These criteria have been developed by clinicians around the world and are frequently named after their own centre (which instantly introduces an element of parochialism into them). They usually work best in the populations in which they are derived (which shows that the statisticians have done a good job!) and are still valid in other populations (although usually working a little less well). Across a large group of patients they will give the same basic picture (all "work" but some are more stringent than others). The challenge is, again, at the level of the individual patient. It is perfectly possible for a patient to be a responder by 4 criteria and a non-responder by 3. What on earth does that mean to the doctor and the patient? To me that would mean that someone has had a marginal response and we should be looking to improve on it. To someone who is not an expert, and is not really interested in PBC, this would suggest that we the experts "do not know what they are talking about" and that this is "all nonsense" (these are direct quotes!). The field should have agreed on a single cut-off years ago, and then audited to see whether we had chosen the right one once it became clear how well patients had actually done.

There is, of course, another way of approaching response to UDCA (and indeed all the other drugs we use to treat PBC) and that is why not aim for normal? This is a question that I am asked by patients who think and read about PBC a lot. Why do we use strange multiples of the upper limit of the normal when we know exactly what normal is? Are we not, in fact, "normalising" ongoing abnormality in the liver by accepting long-term test abnormality (and ongoing elevation of alkaline phosphatase undoubtedly means ongoing cholestasis)? There is also a lesson to be learned from autoimmune hepatitis where there was a similar argument for many years. An ALT elevation of twice the upper limit of normal (ALT is the most sensitive blood test in AIH) was, for decades, regarded as an acceptable response to treatment). It is now universally accepted that such "responders" had progressive disease and ended up being transplanted (or worse). Now, nothing less than normal will do. We should be doing the same in PBC. So why haven't we? The cynic in me might suggest it is because if we did that our treatments would all of a sudden look much less effective. UDCA only returns LFTs to normal in around 25% of patients. There is little doubt in my mind that a move to normalisation of LFTs as the goal of therapy would make everything much clearer in the minds of both patients and doctors and would sharpen our focus on the need for better treatment approaches.

The first step towards better treatment for everyone is, therefore, a simpler and more consistent message regarding treatment. "UDCA for everyone, for ever" is a phrase I use all the time and is one that is simple and unambiguous. It makes the point that everyone should get UDCA (it either will work for them or it will need to have been tried if they are to get second-line therapy). I think it is also essential that all patients are given the opportunity to talk about any symptoms that they have, and be offered treatment, especially for itch where there are easily useable and effective therapies available. This should be simple. All patient also have a right (and I mean a right) to second-line therapy if they are likely to benefit from it. There may be reasons why someone with ongoing abnormalities in their LFTs at the level of "UDCA non-response" might not go on to take second-line therapy. In all cases, however, this should be active decision. By this I mean that the potential value of second-line therapy should have been considered, and discussed with you, and a joint decision made to monitor the disease and review the need for therapy in the future rather than moving to second-line therapy now. The alternative, where the decision is arrived at by default (no one has thought about second-line therapy or the decision not to use it has been made by a doctor on behalf of a patient without discussing it with them…..) happens all too often at present. How do we get to a position where all these things happen? I think there are three ways.

1) *Conventional clinician education:* We continue to chip away at the lack of awareness of optimal PBC treatment amongst clinicians, using clinical guidelines and educational opportunities. The challenge, however, is the "don't know that they don't know" group who tend not to access education because they do not know there is an issue.

2) *Care pathways:* If we are driving somewhere and we don't know the route we use satellite navigation. We used to use maps, but they were not as useful as we thought they were. Looking at a map before a journey explains the overall route, which then makes sense; the problem is when you reach the end of the road and the options are left or right, with neither way being sign-posted for your destination. At that point the map isn't really very useful. The beauty of satellite navigation is that it tells you which way to turn when you reach that end of the road with the option of a left and a right turn (and at the turning after that and so on). We have the equivalent of maps for clinical care (guidelines which, like maps, aren't as useful in practice as you think they should be). What we actually need are care pathways that actively guide clinicians and patient through the whole disease journey from first diagnosis onwards. At each stage there would be simple options to guide you. Like turning left or right. There is much discussion of "apps" and other digital technologies and their potential value in patient care. Much of this is, to me, exaggerated. Where I think the technology may be hugely useful would be in just such a patient "sat nav".

3) *"Reverse education":* Many patients I know describe consultations with doctors where they feel that they know more about the disease than the doctors do. Why do we not use this to help get information across to doctors? At the end of the day, the patient has more vested in the consultation than

the doctor does. Maybe the way to get all patients on to the patient pathway in the future (the "sat nav" outlined above) is through empowering patients through the patient groups to ask for the approach to be used. In the UK at least we can sometimes be too polite for our own good.......

PREVENTING OR CURING PBC

May there ever come a time when everything I have written in this book about treatment is redundant because we can cure the disease, or, even better, prevent it in the first place? In terms of cure, for many years I would have said no. The reason being that we thought that by the time PBC is diagnosed the cells lining the bile duct, the biliary epithelial cells, had already apoptosed or died with no way of them being replaced. We now know that this is not actually the case. It is now clear that the cells go through a phase of senescence (my "zombie state" described in **Chapter 3**) before they die. We also think that if you catch it early it may be possible for us to reverse the state of senescence. So might we be able to cure PBC? The answer for me is a resounding......possibly! To achieve this we will, however, have to approach the treatment of PBC in a completely different way. The current model of waiting to fail treatment is probably the completely wrong one if we are looking to cure. To cure we will need to be aggressive with treatment from the very beginning, completely controlling cholestasis and senescence as soon as possible after diagnosis. This is possible, but will need a completely different mind-set amongst patients. I think this is an achievable goal. We should "reach for the stars". The "OPERA" trial to address just this question will open across the UK in early 2023.

What about prevention? In general terms, across the whole population, I think this will be very difficult indeed. It is just too hard to spot who is likely to get PBC before it develops. The genetics of PBC do not help. Most people who have the gene types that predispose to PBC do not get PBC and most people getting PBC do not have those gene types. They are only associated at the level of the whole population. The one group where it may be possible is the relatives of people who get PBC. The daughters of mothers with the disease. In this setting avoiding some of the environmental triggers that we are recognising maybe, just maybe, could help us to prevent PBC. A longer shot than cure to my mind, but definitely worth exploring in a group for whom the concern of PBC can be a significant problem.

APPENDIX 1: **FREQUENTLY ASKED QUESTIONS**

In this appendix I have collected a set of the questions that I am asked most frequently in clinic and attempted to answer them.

How come I got liver disease when I don't drink? There is a very unfortunate, and completely incorrect, view in society that all liver disease is caused by excess consumption of alcohol. In the UK these days alcohol isn't even the commonest cause of liver disease (that is fatty liver disease related to obesity and type 2 diabetes). Despite this, all too often both members of the public (and, sadly, doctors and their receptionists) can assume that someone with liver disease must have been an excess drinker and therefore brought their disease upon themselves. Let us be absolutely clear. **Alcohol has got absolutely nothing to do with PBC**. Alcohol consumption is typically much lower in PBC patients than in the non-PBC population. Furthermore, the patterns of blood liver function test abnormality (and liver biopsy appearance if a biopsy has been done) are completely different in alcohol-related liver disease and PBC. In the former the injury is mainly to the liver cells themselves (the hepatocytes), and the characteristic elevation is in alanine transaminase (if there is any blood test abnormality at all). In the latter the injury is to the bile duct cells and the characteristic elevation is in alkaline phosphatase. There is really, therefore, no reason whatsoever why PBC and alcohol-related liver disease should be confused. The answer to this is for all of us (patients, patient groups and doctors) to explain and educate.

I have read about primary biliary cirrhosis and primary biliary cholangitis. Which do I have and do I have cirrhosis? I am confused. This, in a nutshell, is why the name of PBC was changed a few years ago from primary biliary cirrhosis to primary biliary cholangitis. There are several important points to make here. The first is that the two terms actually refer to the same condition. Older books written before the name change will talk about primary biliary cirrhosis. More recent ones primary biliary cholangitis. There are also doctors and others whose awareness is perhaps not as up to date as it could be who still talk about primary biliary cirrhosis. So why was the name changed? There are two main reasons. The first is that the term cirrhosis was, for the vast majority of PBC patients, inaccurate. They didn't actually have cirrhosis at all! The term cirrhosis refers to the combination of liver injury and scar formation. It develops when liver injury (of any type) occurs for a long period of time with the effect that the body tries to recover, by forming scar tissue, whilst the process of liver injury is still going on. The term primary biliary cirrhosis was first coined in the 1940s when PBC only tended to be diagnosed very rarely, and once advanced liver disease had developed. The reason for this was that in those days we didn't have access to the antibody tests such as anti-mitochondrial antibody (AMA) which are now freely available, and which allow us to diagnose the vast majority of PBC patients long before cirrhosis develops. The advent of effective treatments such as UDCA and Ocaliva also means that early diagnosis can allow early treatment, further reducing the likelihood of cirrhosis ever developing. At any one time, in the UK at least, probably fewer than 1 in 10 PBC patients actually has cirrhosis. Hence the term primary biliary cirrhosis really isn't appropriate in this day and age.

The other reason for the name change was to avoid the word "cirrhosis" which causes its own specific problems. As outlined earlier in this answer, it is purely a technical, pathological term referring to the combination of injury and liver scarring. There are over 100 different liver diseases that can result in cirrhosis and the term itself holds no implication for the aetiology of the underlying liver disease. However, although ill-informed, there is a lay population association between the word "cirrhosis" and alcohol-related liver disease. Many many PBC patients have had the experience of being asked, repeatedly, about how much alcohol they drink (even though most PBC patients don't drink any alcohol at all). This was, and can still be, a very negative experience for people. Avoiding the word cirrhosis has helped to reduce this point of tension.

The term "primary biliary cholangitis" was chosen so that the abbreviation PBC could still be used. The abbreviation is a useful one, and all patients, and most doctors, are familiar with it. To have gone to a completely different term, would have meant that people would have had to explain that it was the "new term for primary biliary cirrhosis" thereby going back to discussing the word cirrhosis. Completely counter-productive if you think about it. The name change for PBC has been really successful and the old term is rapidly disappearing. The change was driven by the patient community, with the support of the doctors and it is a really positive example of patient practical action.

Why did I get PBC? Did I cause it myself and is there anything I could have done to prevent myself getting it? I will answer the second question first. No! There was nothing you could have done to prevent yourself from getting PBC. Think of it as "one of those things" that happens in life that is unavoidable. One of the sayings that people in my clinic are familiar with is "in life we have to play the hand we are dealt". What I mean by this is that there is nothing to be gained by looking back over events in your life and thinking about how you could have done them differently and not got PBC. There is nothing you could have done. There is no point in being fed up about the diagnosis. There is so much that we can now do to deal with PBC and its symptoms. It is far better, therefore, to get on with making sure that the future is addressed rather than looking to the past. Another saying, which will recur throughout both this book and its companion volumes, is "own the problem, own the solution". Owning the problem as a concept relates to accepting the situation and, rather than looking backwards accept that you need to look forwards.

Accepting that there is nothing that you could have done to prevent yourself from developing PBC, why did you get it? Current thinking is that there are two broad factors that combine to give rise to disease risk. These are a genetic susceptibility and an environmental (in the broadest sense of the word) trigger. This combination is absolutely not unique to PBC and is thought to underpin pretty much all chronic diseases. The genetic contribution to PBC risk is actually rather small, and there most definitely isn't a "PBC gene". Rather, genetic risk appears to be through the combination of a large number of individually small genetic variations, all of which are perfectly normal, and each of which contributes to a very small degree to a particular type of immune response. In essence, PBC patients appear to have an immune system that is a little too easy to turn on and a little too reluctant to turn off. This contributes to a tendency to over-react to any particular immune target. Clearly, if this is a harmful virus this high degree of response is actually an advantage as it helps you to clear the virus effectively. In the context of an autoimmune response such as that seen in PBC, where the body is incorrectly recognising one of the body's own proteins as being harmful, this tendency to over-respond (and in particular to not turn off the response) can be a real disadvantage. The fact that the genetic "mix" that is associated with PBC relates to the regulation of the immune response in general rather than anything PBC-specific (and it is interesting that the gene variations associated with PBC appear to be exclusively related to the immune system and not anything that is related to, for example, the liver) explains why PBC patients have an increased risk of developing other autoimmune diseases.

The genetic variants that seem to contribute to PBC are all, in reality, common and yet the disease is rare (only about 350 people per million in the population have it at any one time). Why is this? I think there are two reasons. The first is that although each of the genetic variations is common, the combination of multiple ones will get rapidly less common. Imagine, hypothetically, there is a gene variant that you "need to have" to develop PBC that is present in 50% of the population. As we have discussed above, however, the key thing for disease development appears to be a combination of gene variants. Assume the next gene variant you also "need to have" is also present in 50% of the population. Assuming it isn't linked to the first, only 50% of 50% of the population (i.e. 25%) will have it. If there were a further 7 also at 50% only 0.098% of the population will have all these "necessary" variants. About 1 in a 1000 people. This is despite each gene variant being seen in half the whole population. Given that we think that upwards of 30 different gene variations contribute to PBC in one way or another we can begin to see how common gene variants can contribute to rare diseases without there being an inherent contradiction. It is all about the combinations.

The second reason why seemingly common gene variants contribute to a disease that is rare is that the main factor in the development of the disease is probably not genetic at all. It is something in the environment that is needed to trigger the disease in a person who is at risk through their genetic make-up. We always talk in the clinic about "the ploughed field and the seed" and the analogy is, I think, a useful one. The ploughed field is the genetic make-up that makes disease development a possibility. Without a ploughed field the crop won't grow and without the "wrong" combination of genetic variants PBC won't develop. It is the seed or the environmental trigger that directly leads to the crop growing and the disease developing. The main evidence for the existence of an environmental trigger comes from the science of epidemiology; the study of populations. Research from the UK and USA have shown that there are "clusters" of PBC. These are areas where the rate of PBC is higher than it should be based on the normal population rate (up to 3 or 4 fold increase in some places). This suggests, although doesn't prove, that there might be something present at elevated levels in the environment in those cluster areas that is able to trigger the disease (with higher levels leading to greater triggering). If there is an environmental trigger of this type then the genetic background might explain why you developed PBC rather than the person who lived next door (same exposure in both of you but only you have the risk genetic background). Likewise, the absence of the environmental trigger at elevated levels elsewhere in the country would explain why you developed PBC but someone living in another part of the country, but with the same set of disease risk gene variants, didn't.

The "64 million dollar question", of course, is what that environmental trigger might be. Is it an infectious agent such as a bacteria or virus (at the end of the day the immune system in programmed to respond to infections) or a chemical that, perhaps, gets concentrated in the bile explaining why the injury in PBC is to the bile ducts. At the moment we don't know. Eric Gershwin in the USA has identified a specific bacteria that might be a trigger. Other work from the USA and the UK has pointed to a chemical trigger of some sort. The most intriguing data come from Jess Dyson in the UK who has looked at how disease clusters in the North-East of England are linked to other geographical variations. She found that there was a strong association between PBC rate and a past history of local coal mining activity. There was also an association between the disease and levels of the metal cadmium in the environment (with the effects of mining and cadmium being additive (i.e. cadmium levels were extra-high in areas where mining previously took place)). Interestingly, heavy metals such as cadmium are concentrated in the bile and are known to alter the immune response......

The reality is that these hypotheses are intriguing, but remain just that; intriguing hypotheses. We truthfully don't know what the PBC trigger is, and, indeed, whether it is one trigger or a number of factors able to have the same effect (although we are very confident that there is a trigger of some sort). What I strongly suspect, however, is that whatever the trigger is it is likely to be something that we can't eliminate exposure to (ultimately we can't significantly change our environment). Therefore, given that we can't change our genes (our parents are our parents), and it is unlikely we could stop environmental exposure, there is almost certainly nothing we can do to prevent PBC.

Is PBC getting commoner and if so why? This is a really interesting and topical question. There is a widely held view that PBC is, indeed, getting commoner, with published research seemingly confirming this. Is this true or is it an illusion? At one level this is simple. There are certainly more and more people being diagnosed with PBC and, given the effectiveness of current treatments and their capacity to lengthen life, more and more people in the population living with the disease. The key question is whether the increase in the diagnosis rate reflects more people developing PBC or the fact that clinicians are more aware of it, and better at diagnosing it. There is certainly an element of the latter. The PBC community (clinicians and patient groups have been very active indeed at increasing awareness of the disease and how easy it is to look for it with simple blood tests. Increasing awareness of PBC symptoms has also driven diagnostic activity (the classic example being chronic fatigue; once you are aware that PBC can cause fatigue as a doctor you start doing the AMA test in all your patients with fatigue and, lo and behold, you find people with PBC.......). We are confident that at least part of the increase in the PBC rate is down to diagnosis for the simple reason that the spectrum of disease severity at diagnosis has been evolving over time as well, with more and more people being diagnosed with early disease. The implication is that in the past these people wouldn't have been diagnosed until later in the disease course, meaning that the number of the people recognised as having the disease at any one time would be lower (but that important opportunities to treat it better would have been lost).

Is better diagnosis the whole explanation for the increase in apparent PBC rates? Probably not. If you look at areas that have been studied in detail in relation to PBC for many years (such as the North East of England), and where clinician awareness hasn't really risen because it was always high, there has also been a rise in patient numbers.

The conclusion is, therefore, that PBC is definitely being diagnosed more frequently (and earlier with real benefits for treatment). This reflects a combination of a true increase in disease numbers and better diagnosis.

My doctors use the term liver function tests all the time. What does this term mean? The short answer is the blood tests that are easily available, and which are very useful (but not infallible) in understanding the progression and severity of your liver disease. There are a number of ways that doctors can monitor your liver disease. Each adds its own form of information, none is perfect and each has its own strengths and weaknesses. Other answers in this section will look at two of the main ways of assessing liver disease, namely liver biopsy and Fibroscan. Here we are going to talk about blood tests. Blood tests have the obvious advantages that they are universally available, easy to do, non-invasive for patients and cheap. The disadvantage is that the information that they give is somewhat indirect, and thus always needs to be interpreted in the context of potential limitations. The term "liver function tests", often abbreviated to "LFT" is widely used in the UK. In North America alternative terms such as "liver labs" or "liver biochemistry" are often used. Each refers to a group of blood tests that are done at the same time to look at different aspects of how the liver works. Paradoxically, the archetypal tests in this set (alkaline phosphatase (ALP) and alanine transaminase (ALT)) don't even measure liver function. They are, in fact, markers of liver damage. They are enzymes (a type of protein) that are released into the blood by cells when they are damaged. ALT is present at the highest levels in hepatocytes or liver cells, and is thus a reasonable marker of damage to these cells (higher levels suggest more cells being injured) whilst ALP is present at the highest levels in bile duct cells. As these are the target cells for injury in PBC this makes ALP a reasonable marker of cholestasis or bile duct damage. Hence, this is the most useful test for monitoring PBC severity and is the basis of assessing the need for and response to treatment with, again, higher levels suggesting more injury. The panel of liver function tests includes two other markers which actually do (to a reasonable approximation) measure liver function. These are bilirubin (the pigment produced from the breakdown of haemoglobin from red cells that are "past their sell by date" in the spleen) and albumin, an important blood protein. As bilirubin is cleared from the body by the liver, whilst albumin is made by the liver, reduced liver function is associated with a rise in bilirubin and a fall in albumin. If the levels of bilirubin are high enough then the pigment becomes visible in the eyes and skin (jaundice). Low albumin can lead to the leak of fluid into tissues (including the abdomen (ascites) and the ankles (ankle swelling)). When doctors look at the liver function test panel they are, in fact, thinking about two aspects of the disease. The levels of ALP and ALT relate to how much ongoing liver and bile duct cell injury there is, and how the liver might work in the future. The bilirubin and albumin relate more to how much damage to the liver there already is (i.e. how much injury there has been in the past). When I see a person in the clinic for the first time the really key question is what the alkaline phosphatase level is. This is because this tells me what is going on in the liver in terms of injury right now. This is the thing I am able to address and therefore do something about.

I have a daughter. I am worried that I will pass PBC on to her. Will I?
This is one of the most frequently asked questions in the clinic. The answer
is no (but with a caveat). PBC is not an inherited condition (there is no "gene"
that causes PBC that can be passed on to your children; similarly, there is
almost certainly no infectious or other trigger that could be passed on). PBC
is, however, related to the way that your immune system is constructed;
something that does have a genetic component to it. In simple terms some
people have an immune system that is more vigorous than other peoples.
Like height, these basic characteristics are passed form parents to children
(tall parents tend to have tall children). What this means is that the type of
vigorous immune system that predisposes to PBC is more likely to be seen
in the offspring of PBC patients than in people with no PBC in the family.
The overall risk of getting PBC is, however, still very low (the daughter of a
mother with PBC probably has a lower than 1 in a 100 risk of developing the
condition). Because PBC is uncommon in men (around 90% of patients with
PBC are women) the risk in sons is that much lower (less than 1 in a
thousand). What does this mean in practice? It means that the risk is very low
and as a result we don't recommend screening of relatives for the condition
(you have to declare it on insurance forms). If, however, a son or daughter
has abnormal liver blood tests, or develops the symptoms we all associate
with PBC such as itch or fatigue, then it is the right thing to do to perform
an AMA test and consider UDCA therapy.

*I hear people talking about PBC itch, but I have never had it! Does this
mean I don't have PBC?* The short answer is no, not having itch absolutely
doesn't mean that you can't have PBC. It just means that you have non-
itching PBC! The UK-PBC study has looked at patterns of itch over the years
in PBC patients. It showed that people fall into one of three equally sized
groups. A third of people literally never experience itch. A third have itch
"now you come to mention it" and a third have significant itch that needs
treatment. What is very interesting is that, with the exception of people with
significant itch who respond well to treatment, people rarely move from one
group to another. What this means in practice is that if you are in the group
of people who have never had itch it is probably unlikely that you will go on
to develop itch in the future. Good news! We don't, at the moment, really
understand why people get itch in PBC. We therefore also don't really know
why some people get itch and some people don't. We suspect that, rather like
PBC itself, itch in PBC is a result of the combined effects of genes (probably
controlling the transporter molecules that control the passage of bile acid and
other bile components of bile out into the bile duct) and environment
(something present in the body at elevated levels that might contribute to
itch). If people don't have the "wrong" gene or environmental exposure they

don't get itch. Given the black and white nature of PBC itch it is probably more likely to be genes than environment, but this is conjecture.

My doctor has said I need a liver biopsy. Do I really need it? The question of liver biopsy is one of the most contentious ones in the whole of PBC management. No one wants an invasive investigation such as a biopsy unless it is really necessary. The questions, therefore, are is it necessary and does any risk outweigh the benefits from having it. Biopsy is, if done carefully, perfectly safe. Is it necessary, however? As with many of the questions I have attempted to address in this section, the answer is complex and depends, to a significant degree, on the context. At the simplest level, for the vast majority of people with PBC, biopsy is not needed to make the diagnosis. We diagnose PBC based on the presence of three key findings, with 2 out of the three conventionally being regarded as sufficient to make the diagnosis. The first of these key diagnostic findings is elevation in the liver blood biochemistry tests (usually known as liver function tests (LFT)) most directly related to PBC (in particular alkaline phosphatase but also gamma glutamyl- transferase (usually known as "gamma-gt")). The second is the presence of anti-mitochondrial antibody (AMA) or one of the anti-nuclear antibodies (ANA) that are characteristic of PBC (watch out for a trap here, however, as the ANA that suggest PBC are very different to the ANA type classically seen in autoimmune hepatitis; one of the other autoimmune liver diseases and a condition that always needs to be through about in people who may have PBC). The third finding is a liver biopsy that is "suggestive or diagnostic of PBC". In practice, most people reach the required 2 findings through their LFTs and the presence of AMA, meaning that biopsy is not needed to make the diagnosis. In fact, although biopsy is sometimes thought of as being the definitive test for PBC it can also mislead. The really diagnostic, "classic" biopsy appearances are frequently not seen. Furthermore, it is possible to have areas of normal liver tissue on a biopsy from a PBC patients as the disease is patchy. Given that if someone had elevation of alkaline phosphatase and AMA, but the biopsy was reported as normal, we would always treat with UDCA you can see that the biopsy is adding nothing.

A second area where biopsy is no longer appropriate is to look for the presence of cirrhosis (or "stage IV disease"). The advent of non-invasive tests such as Fibroscan (a form of ultrasound), and an increased understanding of the value of blood tests such as the platelet count, mean that there are much safer and more patient friendly ways to check whether cirrhosis has developed.

There are, however, four settings where liver biopsy remains an important diagnostic tool. The first is for the diagnosis of AMA negative PBC. Whereas 95% of PBC patients have AMA (or an equivalent ANA) in their blood 5% do not. Their disease appears to act in the same way, and responds to the same treatments. Clearly, however, it is not possible to reach the two positive diagnostic tests needed to make the diagnosis without a biopsy in someone who is antibody negative. The second setting where biopsy remains important is in people with more than one liver disease. The commonest combination we see is of PBC accompanied by fatty liver disease (non-alcoholic fatty liver disease or NAFLD). The possibility usually comes to light through the presence, in the same person, at the same time, of AMA and fat deposition in the liver on ultrasound. Without a biopsy it is not possible to determine which the dominant disease process is, and thus what treatment approach to take. The third setting is a variant of the second. This is overlap syndrome where both PBC and autoimmune hepatitis are present. Both are autoimmune forms of liver disease, and thus co-exist in some patients. Understanding whether autoimmune hepatitis is present alongside PBC makes a really big difference to management, as the standard treatment for autoimmune hepatitis is with steroids; drugs that I would never want to start (because of their side-effects) without being certain that autoimmune hepatitis was really present. In the past, overlap has probably been over-diagnosed (although it does undoubtedly exist in some patients). Many of the features of the more aggressive form of PBC, which is treated with drugs such as OCA, mirror those of overlap and, in the days before awareness of the existence of these more aggressive forms of PBC, these features tended to always be interpreted as autoimmune hepatitis. Anyone with a long-standing diagnosis of overlap should probably have their case looked at again in light of this evolution of our understanding of PBC; all the more so if they have ended up being treated with long-terms steroids or other immuno-suppressants. The final setting is treatment resistant disease where, increasingly, we will be looking to use bespoke treatment regimes. The treatment options for PBC are expanding rapidly and with this our ability to treat the disease effectively has increased dramatically. We are now starting to understand why some people don't respond to certain treatments (especially UDCA), and, thus, the nature of high risk disease. The direction of travel in the treatment of PBC is towards "earlier and better" therapy to stop the disease in its tracks before it becomes established. To do this we will increasingly need to know the precise nature of the problem in individual patients. To try and treat without this information is to attempt to "fly blind". In the future, therefore, biopsy will continue to be a really important test in PBC. Its use will, however, evolve away from diagnosis and towards treatment planning

My advice, if your doctor is suggesting a biopsy, is that you ask them why they are suggesting it. They should be able to clearly explain which of the four settings apply to you. If none do then ask why the biopsy is being suggested.

Is liver biopsy safe? Yes, liver biopsy, if done properly, is very safe (although, self-evidently, there must be more risk attached than if it wasn't done at all. Thus, in deciding to do a liver biopsy the risk must be weighed against the improvement in care that might arise from the extra information the biopsy has given. The word biopsy refers to the taking of a very small piece of liver tissue using a hollow needle that is then examined under the microscope. There are three main routes by which the biopsy can be taken. These are directly through the skin, via the blood vessels that act as a route into the liver, and in the context of an operation on the abdominal cavity allowing a biopsy to be taken directly. The first two are by far and away the most commonly used in practice. The original way developed to take biopsies was through the skin. This is still, in most centres, the most frequently used approach. Nowadays it is always done with ultrasound guidance and with a biopsy "gun" (a device that allows the actual biopsy to be taken very safely and accurately). The liver itself has no nerves, meaning that once the needle reaches the liver it doesn't cause pain. The skin and muscle that the needle needs to go through to reach the liver, as well as the lining around the liver (the capsule), do have nerve fibres meaning that they need to be frozen using local anaesthetic to make the procedure as comfortable as possible. Whilst the biopsy is taken you will be asked to breathe in, then breathe out and then hold your breath whilst the biopsy is taken. This is to make sure the liver (which moves up and down with the diaphragm as you breathe) is stationary when the biopsy is taken. After the biopsy you will be asked to lie flat for a few hours whilst clot forms in the part of the liver the biopsy was taken from. The main risk of doing a biopsy in this way is bleeding. The liver has a large number of blood vessels in it and if one of those is caught by the needle a small bleed can result. This can cause some pain, going through to the right shoulder tip. To minimise the risk of bleeding your clotting will always be checked before the biopsy, and if it is abnormal then this approach won't be used. You can't have a liver biopsy done this way if you are taking either aspirin or warfarin (or other blood thinning drug). If you do get abdominal or shoulder pain after a biopsy, or your blood pressure drops, the doctors will organise an ultrasound scan to check there isn't significant bleeding. Very occasionally, other organs, such as the bowel, can be caught by the biopsy needle. This was an issue in the past when biopsies were done blind and is much less common now that ultrasound guidance is used.

If the risk of bleeding is high because your clotting isn't normal, or there is concern about difficulty reaching the liver through the skin (because of the presence of a bowel loop next to the liver, or ascites) the biopsy can be done via the jugular vein ("a trans-jugular biopsy"). In this approach the blood vessels are used to provide a "route" by which a biopsy needle on the end of the wire is manoeuvred into the liver, and a biopsy is taken through the wall of the vein into the liver tissue. Because the approach is made from a blood vessel into the liver, any bleeding from the liver tissue is also into the blood vessel, meaning that it is perfectly safe. The approach is also usually pain free as the skin is frozen before the wire is inserted into the neck and there is no passage of a needle through the liver capsule (the origin of most pain in a conventional liver biopsy). There can, however, be a little bit of "pulling and pushing" as the wire with the biopsy needle on it is positioned in the liver. This can sometimes feel a little bit disconcerting. The downside of a trans-jugular biopsy is that it takes longer to do and the size of the biopsy is often smaller. It is also possible for the vein that the wire and needle is passing down to be punctured itself giving rise to risk.

The exception to biopsy only being occasionally needed in PBC is in the post-transplant setting. Here it is likely to be needed in most people on one or more occasions. This is normally to look for evidence of rejection (which needs its own form of treatment), although it is increasingly used to look for evidence of recurrent PBC.

The conclusion with liver biopsy is that it can be a really important part of understanding your PBC, helping to guide therapy. For most people it isn't needed but if it is, it is very safe.

I have fatigue with my PBC and have been advised to exercise. Is this safe? Yes. Not only is this safe but it is an important part of managing fatigue in PBC. There seem to be two different forms of fatigue in PBC. One is very much a brain type fatigue, with people often talking about experiencing "brain fog" and describing real problems with concentration and short-term memory. The other type is a much more physical or muscular type of fatigue, with patients often talking about how they feel as if their "batteries have run down". This form of fatigue appears to be very much linked to a loss of power in the muscles, and thus an ability to sustain activity. A few years ago, fascinated by the ways in which people talked about this form of fatigue, we did a number of studies. The first one was a really simple one. We asked people to use a grip strength meter to measure how strong their hand grip was. We asked them to do that every 5 seconds until their strength had halved through repeat use (or 5 minutes, whichever was shorter). We studied a group of PBC patients with fatigue, a group of PBC patients without fatigue and a group of healthy non-PBC people. Interestingly, all had the same base-line grip strength suggesting that it isn't the case that PBC patients in general aren't as strong as non-PBC people. What we found, when we asked people to grip repeatedly, was that the healthy people rapidly lost about a third of their strength on repeat exercise, but after that could pretty much keep going without any further problems. The fatigued PBC patients, in contrast, ground to a halt very rapidly indeed, with most of them unable to even use the meter after about a minute. Interestingly, the non-fatigued PBC patients behaved exactly like the healthy controls, with no abnormality in their muscle function. If people rested they all recovered to the same strength as they had originally. If they repeated the whole exercise pattern, then the same phenomena emerged with the fatigued PBC patients showing a rapid decrease in their muscle strength.

It took us a few years to follow this up because of the lack of the technology to do so. This was changed by the advent of magnetic resonance scanning technologies which allowed us to "look inside" muscle whilst it is exercising, measuring energy levels and the consequences of exercise. What we found was very striking, and really surprised us. When we asked healthy individuals to exercise to 35% of their maximum capacity (actually a relatively low level of exercise that wouldn't normally cause people any problems) their muscle pH (the measure of how much lactic acid builds up in their muscle) hardly changed at all. PBC patients, in contrast, showed a highly significant level of lactic acid build up, reaching levels that people would normally only see after a bout of really significant exercise (one of the patient experiences that led us to do the study was the lady who said that she "felt like she had just finished a half-marathon" after minor exercise; it turns out that she was right……..that was exactly what was happening in her muscle). Interestingly there was no difference between fatigued patients and non-fatigued PBC patients. Pretty much everyone was abnormal. Where the fatigued and the non-fatigued patients differed was in the speed of recovery. Non-fatigued PBC patients showed a recovery in their pH back to baseline that was very rapid indeed (exactly as was the case with the healthy controls). The fatigued PBC patients showed only very slow recovery with a long and lingering presence of lactic acid in their muscle.

What does all this mean for our understanding of fatigue in PBC and the value of exercise? The first thing to say is that it suggests that there is a very real energy-based reason for muscle fatigue in PBC. For whatever reason, PBC patients over-use anaerobic metabolism, building up lactic acid in their muscle. This allows them to exercise (as I always say to people in the clinic, their muscles work; if there was a fire in the clinic they could run out as fast as anyone else). They just do so at the price of a metabolic "debt" that needs to be paid back. The degree of lactic acid production in muscle is very likely to result in stress signals being sent to the brain to tell people not to do any more exercise (as it would cause further acid build up and muscle damage); hence, a muscle issue can result in the brain perception of fatigue. The really interesting group is the PBC patients without fatigue who appeared to have found a way to compensate for the excess lactic acid production (they still produce it but it clears really quickly). This suggests that the body has the potential for "work-arounds" that can compensate for lactic acid build up. If we could find a way to trigger that compensating work-around it would be a potential treatment for fatigue.

This, of course, is where exercise comes in. Athletes have known for years that training (i.e. exercise) increases the capacity of muscle to lower production of lactic acid and to clear it where it does form. Exercise training does exactly the same thing in PBC, helping the body to learn to cope with lactic acid build up and preventing the fatigue stress signal being sent to the brain. There are now two different studies of exercise therapy in PBC, both of which clearly show a reduction in fatigue (and no down-sides). Hence the answer to the question is not only that exercise is safe, but that it actually, over time, protects the muscles and will reduce fatigue. Our research also shows, however, that people with PBC can really struggle to get going with exercise and to work out what form of exercise is best. This will be covered in the next question and answer.

I want to take up exercise to help with my fatigue. What should I be doing? There is a whole science about different types of exercise and things can very rapidly get more complicated than they need to. Paradoxically, not feeling confident about knowing what they should be doing can sometimes lead to people not taking up exercise at all. My feeling is that it is very easy to over-complicate this whole area, and it is really helpful to simplify it whenever possible. There are three basic rules to exercise in PBC. The first is that exercise really helps (and is proven to help) with fatigue, as well as improving general health (diabetes risk, heart disease risk etc). In essence, exercising is a really good thing for PBC patients. The second is that it probably doesn't matter greatly what you do as long as you do something and do it at a sufficient level to have a biological effect. The problem with exercise programmes is that they tend to take time and that is what people often don't have. It is easy to design a "perfect" programme, but a less perfect programme that people end up following is, at the end of the day much more valuable than a perfect one that you don't do. One of my colleagues coined the term "movement as medicine" in relation to exercise in health and I think it is a great term. Make every bit of activity you do part of a daily programme. Park a bit further away from work and walk the final bit, get off the bus a couple of stops earlier and walk the rest of the way, walk to the shops rather than driving. These sorts of changes add relatively little time to your day but can, cumulatively have a big effect. If you want to get serious about exercise then a programme that combines cardiovascular exercise (walking, swimming, cycling, running etc) with resistance training (weights, leg bands, sit up etc) is ideal. Three sessions of 30 minutes a week at a reasonable intensity (enough to make you slightly out of breath) is perfect. Don't, however, let worry about going down the resistance line get in the way of doing cardiovascular exercise. The final rule is, whatever you are doing at the moment, do more. I once asked my colleague who talked about movement as medicine what "increasing exercise" meant in practice. His answer was doing 10% more than you are doing now. If you have a standard walk that you do, look to gradually extend it whilst taking the same time (thus having the double benefit of more exercise and greater speed) and then keep gradually increasing it. The best advice I can give is to try and make exercise a part of your life. That way, when time pressures occur, and the onset of winter means a walk is suddenly less attractive, you continue because it is in-built. Do it! It really makes a difference.

Can I take HRT? This is a really important question given the age and sex of the typical PBC patient (a woman in her 50s). There are two broad reasons why HRT is considered in PBC patients. The first has been, historically, as a way of preventing osteoporosis. The second has been for the treatment of post-menopausal symptoms which can add significantly to the impairment of quality of life seen in PBC. The answer to the question is that I wouldn't use it for osteoporosis prevention in this day and age as there are much more specific and effective interventions now available. I would, however, actively consider it as part of a package of interventions to address as many of the factors that go into quality of life impairment as possible. Post-menopausal symptoms aren't a specific issue in PBC or even linked to the disease. They are, however, much easier to treat than many PBC-specific symptoms and are, therefore, a "quick win" around quality of life.

A different way to look at the question is, in fact, to ask "why not use HRT in PBC"? Again, this is a really good question and it relates to a bit of confusion and even folklore. We know that, very rarely, women taking the pill or HRT can get liver function test abnormality. This is to do with a chemical effect of the synthetic hormones in the tablets interacting with transporters in the bile duct. This has no connection at all to PBC and doesn't occur more frequently in people with PBC than in anyone else. The blood test change is, however, similar to that seen in PBC and can be associated with itch. This has led to the erroneous view that this is linked to PBC. Over the years I have seen many PBC patients treated very safely and effectively with HRT.......and have never seen liver blood test worsening!.

There are, of course, concerns about the use of HRT in anyone in relation to blood clot formation and the risk of some hormone responsive cancers. In truth these are a little over-blown and, in reality, the risk is low. As with any treatment, however, you need to be absolutely clear what the likely benefits are to weigh up against any risk. This should happen both before starting the treatment and, importantly, after it has been in use in a person for a while. How much better do they really feel and have they had any problems? Any decision to continue should be based on this evaluation. If HRT has really benefitted your symptoms, and you have no personal or family history of clotting or relevant cancers, then the decision is usually easy. The only thing we tend to do is to recommend that patches are used rather than tablets because that reduces the drug level that the liver is exposed to. If there is any enhanced risk to the liver that we don't as yet know about this will minimise it.

What is UDCA and why do people with PBC take it? Ursodeoxycholic Acid (UDCA or "urso" as most people call it) was the first treatment shown to improve the outcome in PBC patients and, as such, it was, and is, universally used. Unless there is a very good reason not to, all patients with PBC should take UDCA. It is a non-toxic form ("hydrophilic") of bile acid which probably has its main effect by displacing the more toxic ("hydrophobic") types of bile acid from PBC patients' bile acid pool. It is these toxic bile acids which probably cause bile duct injury in PBC and displacing them reduces the toxic effect. UDCA is also an anti-oxidant, meaning that it reduces the impact of free-radicals; a further factor in bile-acid induced injury to the bile ducts and another mechanism for UDCA to reduce tissue damage in PBC. UDCA reduces the levels of liver function tests in PBC in essentially everyone who takes it. In around a third of people (in my experience) it returns them to normal. Long-term follow-up studies now show, quite clearly, that UDCA reduces the rate of progression of PBC to cirrhosis, complication development, need for liver transplant and even risk of death. There are, however, limitations to its effectiveness that always need to be borne in mind. It has minimal, if any, beneficial effect on itch (and in a small number of people it can make itch worse). It almost certainly has no beneficial effect on fatigue. It is, also, effective in different people to different degrees. In simple terms, although across the whole patient population it is effective, at an individual level there are winners and losers; those who respond fully and those who have an insufficient response. The lack of effect on symptoms, and the existence of people with an inadequate response to UDCA, mean that there is an ongoing need for additional treatments in PBC.

What is a Fibroscan? Do I need one and does it hurt? Fibroscan is a relatively new technology and one that is very useful (but not infallible) in PBC management. It is based on ultrasound technology and when you have the scan it looks and feels very much like have a normal ultrasound scan. It involves some jelly on the skin, and some pressure as the probe is pressed over the liver. It doesn't hurt, and there are no risks associated with it. What it does is, rather than build a picture of the liver as would be the case with a normal ultrasound, measure how much of a signal that is sent out by the probe bounces back and can be measured by the probe. It therefore works very much like active sonar used by warships to detect submarines. In sonar a "ping" is sent out. If there is nothing hard for the ping to bounce back off (water doesn't cause this bounce back as it is not solid) then there is no return signal. If there is a submarine there the ping bounces back off the metal and is picked up. Returned signal=submarine there, no returned signal=no submarine. In the case of Fibroscan and the liver, the more solid the liver is the more signal is returned. Normal liver has a very soft consistency (almost fluid-like within the liver capsule). The more scar tissue there is the harder it becomes and the greater the signal reflection. It is therefore, in practice, a way of estimating how much fibrosis is in the liver without the need for a liver biopsy. It is therefore a very good, non-invasive way of screening for cirrhosis.

One of the advantages of Fibroscan as a screening approach is that it is quick and easy to so. If you have the machine in your clinic then you can do the test "there and then" (it takes about 10 minutes). We tend to Fibroscan everyone the first time we see them (if they haven't had it done already) and then repeat it every 1-5 years depending on how active or aggressive the disease is.

There are some limitations to Fibroscan, however, and it is really important to keep them in mind. The first is that it is operator dependent and is a "real time test". What I mean by this is that there is no physical record of the findings that can then be checked (it doesn't produce a picture in the way a scan would). If the person doing the scan isn't experienced (and there is a learning curve), and a rogue value is recorded, there is no way of going back after the test and checking it (other than by repeating the Fibroscan). A second is that, of course, it doesn't actually measure fibrosis. It measures liver density, an important cause of which is fibrosis. A subtle distinction but an important one. There seems to be a degree of natural variation in liver density (the way you are built). There are also other reasons why liver density might go up, including, I suspect, active liver inflammation of cholestasis. What this means is that although a low value is pretty good evidence that there isn't fibrosis or cirrhosis (scar tissue always pushes up the density) the converse, that a high value means fibrosis is there, isn't as clear cut.

What this means in our practice is that Fibroscan is a really useful part of our assessment of disease state but it isn't the "be all and end all". We always interpret the findings in the context of the full clinical picture. If the value doesn't quite make sense in terms of the overall picture we look to repeat the study and to cross-check its findings against other parts of the clinical picture. If the Fibroscan suggests cirrhosis then we would expect to see other, subtle, signs that support that finding. With this caveat it really is a very useful test and should, and will, become a completely standard part of how we watch PBC patients in the future.

Urso makes me feel sickly. Any suggestions? It is not uncommon for people to feel a little sickly when they first start UDCA. I suspect that this is simply the result of its chemical make-up. It is a bile acid itself and, although one of the least irritant or toxic ones, all bile acids can irritate the stomach (think of the horrible feeling you get if you ever vomit bile). In my experience it usually passes in a relatively short period of time as the body starts to adapt to it. There are, however, some tricks that can help. The first is to start on a much lower dose and "wean it in". UDCA has its beneficial effects through long-term use. You don't need to be on the full dose right now. Better to take time and manage a full dose than to go too quickly and fail. On occasions I have gone back to a single tablet on alternate days (or even every three days) with a plan to increase the dose as we can. This usually works (although isn't necessary for most people). The other trick is to try out different ways of taking it. We tend to suggest to patients that they take it in a single dose in the evening, as that seems to be the way it is tolerated best. Some people, however, find it better to take it during the day along with food. Again, the key thing is getting to the point of being able to take the right dose rather than the speed of the journey to get there.

There are a small number of people who really can't take UDCA because of these types of issue. I have probably, however, only come across a handful over the years. What are the options then? The first question I would ask is do you really need treatment. If you have normal liver blood tests, or the tests are only mildly abnormal off UDCA, then the sensible thing is to wait and see. If the risk is higher, and the blood tests are more abnormal, then the licensed treatment option is Obeticholic Acid (OCA). This is mainly used in addition to UDCA in people showing an inadequate response to UDCA, however its other use is in people who can't tolerate UDCA (there is no evidence to support bezafibrate as an alternative to UDCA). In my experience the tolerance issues such as nausea that stop people taking UDCA rarely recur with OCA. It does, however, have its own side effects such as itch which really need to be weighed up and balanced in any treatment setting.

Does urso cause you to gain weight? The short answer here is yes, but only a little. Clinical studies of UDCA use have suggested that, on average, PBC patients put on 1-2Kg when starting UDCA. It is useful to be aware of this, to watch out for weight gain, and to be ready to watch your diet. This gives rise to the obvious question which is why would PBC patients gain weight with UDCA? The important thing to say is that this isn't a direct metabolic effect as would be the case if you were taking steroids. Instead, my feeling is that it is more of a return to normal. What do I mean? We know from past years, before we could treat PBC, that people can tend to lose weight with the condition because of the changes in bile production. Bile is essential for absorbing food from the diet (especially fat because of the role of bile acids in making fat soluble and thus absorbable by the bowel). The net effect is that the body becomes used to a lowered level of nutrition and adapts by adopting a "starvation mode" approach. When UDCA is started it has a number of effects, reducing any toxic actions on the liver. It also, however, replaces the bile acid in the bowel that is missing because of poor bile flow in PBC. It therefore has the effect of returning food absorption capacity to normal. The problem is that the body is still in "starvation mode", meaning that suddenly there is too much, rather than too little, nutrition uptake. Hence an element of weight gain. UDCA, however, is at the heart of effective treatment for PBC and worries about weight gain absolutely shouldn't get in the way of taking it.

My doctor has said that I am an "urso non-responder". What does this mean and should I be worried? & I am an urso non-responder. What are my options for treatment now? I will take these questions together because they make a natural pair. They also lie at the very heart of the current approach to the treatment of PBC: the escalation of treatment to meet the needs of the individual patient. Until recently, PBC had a single therapy in the form of UDCA. We prescribed it to most patients and then watched them. In essence, however, all we could do was to keep our fingers crossed as, if it didn't give people the effect we wanted to see, we had no other treatment options. The revolution in PBC treatment (and it is, I think, not an exaggeration to call it a revolution) over the last 10 years has two critically important, and inter-linked, elements to it. The first is the recognition that the response to UDCA varies from person to person and in some people the response is not sufficient to significantly reduce the risk of PBC progressing. The people showing this insufficient response are conventionally called "UDCA non-responders" although, in reality, the vast majority of patients show some response to UDCA and the "non-responders" would therefore be more accurately described as "under-responders". The term non-responder is the one that has entered into widespread use, however, and we will stick with the term in this book. UDCA non-response is defined in terms of the liver function test ("liver blood test") values after UDCA has been used at the correct dose for a sufficient period of time to have had its effect. Conventionally, the correct dose is regarded as 13-15mg/Kg body weight and a sufficient period of time is a year. I don't think the dose will change in the future, however I think we may move to a shorter period of use (say 6 months) before we make a judgement as to whether someone is a responder or not. This move towards a shortening in the UDCA treatment period before response is assessed is for two reasons. The first is that, in practice, all the response that is going to be seen to UDCA is seen by 6 months. In other words, there is no need to wait another 6 months as you will already have the answer by 6 months in the vast majority of people. The second is that, of course, if you are a UDCA non-responder it implies that there is ongoing liver injury and you would rather not wait another six months on failing treatment when there are new treatments that can be added. This introduces the second element to the PBC therapy revolution, that of second-line therapy.

UDCA is first-line therapy in the sense that it is the treatment that is given first to all patients. We are now, however, in a world where there are additional therapies that we can use. It is the current convention (although I suspect this may change over time) to use them only after people have been shown to have an inadequate response to UDCA (i.e. in "UDCA non-responders"). In this sense, these treatments are currently used as second-line. It is conventional to add them to UDCA rather than use them to replace UDCA although this is, if you think about it, a little illogical. It is standard practice however. The second-line therapy options in PBC can be split into two. Licensed therapies that can be used now in normal practice, and new therapies that are currently under clinical trial and which can't be used outside those trials. Over time, of course, therapies being explored in trial will, hopefully, be proven to be safe and effective and become available as normal treatments in practice. The split into approved treatments and those under evaluation outlined here is correct for 2023, however if you are reading this book in later years this may have changed.

The best evaluated second-line therapy (and the only such treatment specifically licensed for use in PBC is obeticholic acid ("Ocaliva" or OCA). This is now in widespread use in patients who are UDCA non-responders (it is also licensed for use in PBC for people who are intolerant of UDCA as first line therapy). Experience suggests that it is a very safe and well-tolerated therapy. The only issues with it are to do with some worsening of PBC itch in some patients early after the treatment is started, and some worsening of liver function in patients with very advanced disease, especially if they are treated with too high a dose. In my experience, however, these issues impact only a small minority of patients and are largely avoidable by thoughtful drug use. Itch is minimised by being aware of the potential impact, and optimising itch therapy before OCA is started. The worsening of liver function in advanced liver disease has been fully addressed by dose adjustment in all cirrhotic patients, and avoiding the drug altogether in patients with liver disease of a certain severity. The reality is that patients with severe liver disease (cirrhosis with complications) are the ones who should be being considered for liver transplantation not drug therapy. The other widely used treatment is a drug called bezafibrate (its close cousin fenofibrate is the version used in some countries). It is used in a similar fashion to OCA. It doesn't worsen itch (in fact it reduces it), however it can worsen liver function more frequently than OCA does and, importantly, it can cause kidney damage. The kidney aspect is a real issue, and the drug shouldn't be used in people with impaired kidney function to begin with (something that is far from uncommon in people with the age profile of PBC patients) and kidney function needs to be carefully watched with blood tests. The issues with kidney function do slightly highlight the pitfalls of using a drug designed for one purpose (in this case reducing cholesterol) for another condition, without evaluating it properly in that new condition. People think of drug trials as being about whether a drug works or not. This is part of the process, but in many ways the key part of a drug trial is assessing safety. The reality is that much more is known about the long-term safety of OCA (essential when the drug is going to be used long-term) than bezafibrate.

Of the drugs under trial as second-line therapies in PBC (other drugs are under trial for symptomatic management) the furthest advanced are seladelpar and gemfibrozil (elafibranor). They are related to bezafibrate in terms of their mode of action, but more targeted to the mechanisms of liver injury important in PBC. Both have shown clear evidence of benefit and both reduce itch. It is a little too soon to know their long term safety profiles (do they also cause kidney problems for example?) and to understand where they will ultimately fit in to the list of second-line treatment options.

I have been prescribed obeticholic acid ("Ocaliva"). Do I still need to take urso alongside it? This is a really good question. It is conventional practice to continue UDCA if you are started on OCA. This is, in a way, paradoxical because the rationale for starting OCA is usually that UDCA hasn't worked (then why continue it!). We do know that OCA therapy on its own is highly effective (this question has been looked at in specific clinical trials). One reason why still taking UDCA might be logical is that OCA works by significantly reducing the amount of bile acid that your body makes (the logic being that those bile acids build up in the liver in PBC because they can't get out of the liver and cause further injury to the bile duct). One potential issue is, of course, that bile acids are there for a reason (to help absorb fat from the diet). If someone has no bile acids, therefore (because production has been stopped by OCA), they could struggle to absorb fat and have nutrition issues. Taking UDCA in tablet form provides bile acid into the gut (UDCA is a bile acid, just a non-toxic one) which could in theory normalise fat absorption.

So what do I do in practice? I continue UDCA in most OCA patients as it seems to work in practice. If, however, people are getting UDCA side-effects that are worsened by taking OCA I have a very low threshold for stopping the UDCA and just continuing with the OCA. A very pragmatic solution.

How long do I need to take UDCA for? This is a really simple question to answer. In essence, you will need to take it life-long. Urso doesn't change the underlying disease process in PBC, it just reduces the degree of damage to the liver occurring at any time-point when the drug is being taken. As soon as you stop taking it the damage will return and your liver function tests will most likely return to the level they were at before you started the urso. The analogy I always use is with blood pressure tablets or cholesterol lowering treatments such as statins. They are really effective at reducing blood pressure and blood cholesterol levels respectively; 2 effects that really reduce the risk of heart disease. The moment you stop taking the tablets the blood pressure or cholesterol will go back up. These drugs control but don't cure and UDCA in PBC is exactly the same.

My doctor has said that I need to increase my dose of UDCA. Why is that? UDCA was originally introduced as a treatment to dissolve gallstones (and thus avoid the need for surgery). It isn't terribly effective in this role (although its long-term use in PBC has probably contributed to a reduction in the frequency with which PBC patients get problems with gallstones). The initial observation that it helped in PBC was actually a chance one that followed this gallstone dissolving use. The dose that is recommended in the UDCA guidance still relates to the optimal use for dissolving gallstones. Over time, it has become clear from research and from observing what happens to people given UDCA in the clinic, that we need to use slightly higher doses than were typically used for dissolving gallstones (and thus originally used for PBC treatment). All the evidence points to a dose of 13-15mg/Kg body weight as the correct dose for PBC and if you are starting UDCA in this day and age there is no reason not to start on this dose. There are, however, a number of people in the population who were started on UDCA a number of years ago at lower dose levels. The question now is whether the dose should be increased. I take a very pragmatic view of this. If your liver blood tests have returned to normal on a lower dose of UDCA then that is clearly all you need and I wouldn't arbitrarily increase the dose (full response is full response). However, if you haven't responded fully to a lower dose of UDCA, then before any consideration of second-line therapy, you should increase your dose to within the 13-15mg/Kg range. In many cases this is all that we need to do to get better control.

There is one other trap with the dose of UDCA. That is to remember that if your weight changes then the dose needs to follow it. As time goes by we all run the risk of putting weight on. If this happens to you remember that, if you keep the actual tablet dose of UDCA the same, you may fall to below 13mg/Kg and will need to increase the dose a little (after, of course, discussing it with your doctor).

The pharmacy says I should take my UDCA three times a day but my PBC specialist says to take it all at night. Which of these should I do? This is one of the things that causes more confusion than anything else…..and it needn't. The dosing advice for UDCA in the packet relates back to the older use of UDCA as a treatment for gallstones. In this setting spacing during the day works well. For PBC, single dosing at night actually works better and that is why we advise doing that. There are 2 further points. The first is that once a day dosing is, obviously, a lot easier for people and, given that you will be taking UDCA life-long, ease of use and the accuracy of taking the drug that can follow from that are really key. The other is that a number of PBC patients also take cholestyramine (Questran) and UDCA and cholestyramine bind to each other. If you take UDCA and cholestyramine at the same time this will happen in your gut. This isn't harmful, but it does mean that you lose the benefit of both. Given that people often take cholestyramine spaced out 3 times a day, and you need to leave 4 hours between UDCA and cholestyramine to stop the interaction, there just aren't enough hours in the day to take both three times a day. Cholestyramine three times a day, with the last dose at tea time, and UDCA in the evening works very well as a practical regime.

I have just been diagnosed with PBC. Will I need a liver transplant? It is really important to say that for the vast majority of patients with PBC, a transplant will never be needed. Think of it as a safety-net and nothing more. A good thing to have if it is needed, but even better is to never require it. This observation, of course, applies to people who developed PBC and were treated for it in the past, in the days before the increasingly effective therapies that we now have became available. If we are correct in our understanding of these treatments and their effectiveness it should be the case that transplant becomes ever less necessary.

It is really key, however, to not be complacent and to make sure that everything that possibly can be done is done to avoid the need for transplant in the future. The first crucial thing is to make sure the disease is diagnosed early. In our clinic the majority of people going on to transplant have been diagnosed with PBC at an already advanced stage. In this setting, of course, there is much less capacity to treat it, as our treatments work better the earlier in the disease process it is started. By definition, if you are reading this book you have already got your diagnosis, so that is a good start. The second crucial step is to avoid delay in starting UDCA and then avoid interruptions in its use. All too often we come across people who have been diagnosed with PBC, but who don't start UDCA for a year or two. Why not? We know from research that delay in starting UDCA is associated with a reduced chance of responding to it. There is, therefore, absolutely nothing to be gained from delaying starting it. I start UDCA at the first clinic after the diagnosis of PBC has been made......The need to start UDCA in a timely fashion is accompanied by the need to get the dose right (13-15mg/Kg of body weight) and then to continue it life-long. Short interruptions are OK (if a prescription runs out for example) but the way UDCA works means that you have to continue it. It controls the disease rather than curing it.

The next key part in good management (and the one that is improving most rapidly) is the use of second-line treatment if your response to UDCA is inadequate. Everyone who is a UDCA "non-responder" (an issue covered in another question) should be actively considered for second-line therapy, and the presumption, from my perspective, is that it should always be used. These are safe and effective drugs. Why not use them if they would help improve your chances?

There will always be people for whom all this good news doesn't work out the way they would want it to. We can minimise the risks that treatment doesn't work, and that transplant ends up being needed, but we can't eliminate them completely. The question relates to a new diagnosis. What are the "danger signs" at the beginning of PBC that increase the likelihood of transplant eventually being needed? There are, in essence, two. The first is a presentation with a very high alkaline phosphatase level. This is the most accurate marker of PBC activity and tells us "how far we need to go" with treatment. Our upper limit of normal is 130. Most people with PBC present with levels of 150-250. We see people with levels of 750-1000 occasionally, however. We Know that it can be much more difficult to bring these under control (and will essentially always need second-line therapy in my experience). The second red flag at presentation is if fibrosis or cirrhosis is already present (nowadays usually detected using Fibroscan). This suggests that the disease has already been present for a while, and that it is aggressive. We also know that the treatments we have are much better at stopping fibrosis developing than they are at reversing it so getting treatment on board before fibrosis has developed is key.

The key fact is that the vast majority of PBC patients have only slightly elevated alkaline phosphatase at presentation and no fibrosis. If this is the case, then the likely need for transplant in the future is vanishingly low.

Are vaccinations safe in PBC? YES! This was probably the question I was asked most during COVID and I will give the answer that I gave each time then. Vaccination is, along with access to clean water, one of the most important health intervention development of the last 300 years (more so than antibiotic development). What changed the trajectory of COVID was the development of safe and effective vaccines which, although they didn't seem to reduce the risk of catching COVID, significantly reduced the risk of becoming unwell with it. Long before COVID we had the many many vaccines that have eliminated diseases that were, only 50 or 60 years ago major killers. When I started as a doctor we still had the "iron lung" ventilators that were used lifelong for people who had been paralysed by polio and would never be able to breathe on their own again.......something we literally never see any more after the advent of the polio vaccine.

There is no evidence at all that PBC patients respond any differently than other people in the population to vaccines, or that vaccination has any impact on PBC. The only (tiny) caveat is in relation to post-transplant patients on high levels of immuno-suppression. Vaccines split into two broad types, live attenuated organisms and killed or synthetic vaccines. The original vaccines were the former (think of Edward Jenner and the cowpox). They rely on giving people a mild version of the infection in order to mount an immune response and prevent a more serious form. In people with very high levels of immuno-suppression the mild infection could theoretically become a more aggressive infection, as the immune system can't control it as effectively. For this reason, it is better to avoid live vaccines after transplant. The vast majority of modern vaccines (up to and including COVID) are either killed organisms or fully synthetic. Because there isn't a live organism, and thus no infection, they can't get out of control and are therefore perfectly safe. The types of vaccines used in different settings slightly differ from country to country so local policy is something to discuss with your doctor or nurse.

What is alkaline phosphatase and why does the level in my blood matter? Is it harmful? Alkaline phosphatase measurement is a really important test in PBC, and is the standard way in which we monitor how well treatment is working. Alkaline phosphatase is an enzyme (a type of protein) that is released by the cells of the bile duct when they are injured (as is the case in PBC). The more cells are injured, the more alkaline phosphatase is released. The more the disease is controlled, the less injury there is and the lower the level. It is really important to say, however, that alkaline phosphatase is **not in itself harmful**. Higher levels in the blood do not lead directly to higher levels of tissue damage and, therefore, reducing the levels of alkaline phosphatase (as would be possible through dialysis) does not, in and of itself, reduce risk. It is a marker rather than a mediator of injury. An analogy might be with a raised temperature in the context of an infection and a raised potassium level in the blood in renal failure. We all know that temperatures go up infection. It is not, normally, however, a key part of any injury that might happen with infection. It is just a suggestion as to what may be going on. Therefore, and here the analogy is highly relevant, artificially lowering the temperature through using cold towels or taking paracetamol won't reduce the risk of the infection (although it will make people feel better). Alkaline phosphatase in PBC is like a temperature in infection. It is a marker of what is going on and nothing more. A raised potassium in renal failure is the complete opposite. It is both a marker of what is going on and an integral part of the disease process. A higher potassium both provides a marker of renal failure, and is an important aspect of risk in the disease, warranting reduction as an important part of treatment.

It is also important to realise that although a lot of store is placed by alkaline phosphatase levels in PBC it is actually not that great marker of disease severity (and we badly need better ones). This is for three reasons. The first is that the actual concept of higher levels of release being related to more injury is, itself, a bit of an over-simplification as levels of production by the bile duct cells can also increase. The second is that all elevation is relative as alkaline phosphatase is always being released as a result of the natural life cycle of bile duct cells (they divide, grow old and die (releasing alkaline phosphatase) throughout life). No-one ever, therefore, has no alkaline phosphatase in their blood. The final one is that it isn't just the bile duct cells that produce alkaline phosphatase. The other main tissue is bone with high levels being released from bone during bone growth in childhood and puberty and in some bone diseases. As with so many other tests in PBC, the context of the test is really critical. No test is absolute enough to dictate the management plan in isolation. Everything needs interpretation and judgement.

What can I do to help myself fight PBC? This question is probably better re-phrased as "what can I do to live the best possible life with PBC". For the majority of patients PBC is actually a mild condition and, as such, doesn't really need to be "fought". It needs to be respected and taken account of but not "fought". There are three really important elements to living the best life you can with PBC (and always remember the mantra repeated throughout this book which is "own the problem/own the solution"; it's your life, take control of it)

1) **Live your life**: Don't spend you live regretting that you have PBC, or wishing that you didn't have it. You are where you are and you need to look forward. Accentuate the positives looking forward and don't dwell on what happened in the past. There is nothing that you can do about the past.

2) **Get the best possible treatment you can:** We are in the great position that treatment options for PBC are increasing, and getting better, all the time. However, and it is an important however, a treatment that you aren't getting cannot possibly be effective. The UK national PBC audit shows, very clearly, that half of all patients who might benefit from additional therapy beyond UDCA aren't getting it. This just isn't good enough. We are working nationally on increasing doctor education, but ultimately you need to take control of the clinic discussion. What is your Fibroscan score and what are your blood test values? Based on your specific values, would you benefit from additional therapy? The more specific the questions you ask the more specific the answers you will get. If your specialist doesn't know about second-line therapy, or says you don't need it without reference to your own test values, get another specialist.......

3) **Find a way to co-exist with fatigue:** Clearly, this aspect only applies to people who get fatigue! We currently don't have a specific treatment for fatigue, meaning that adapting to it and minimising its impact is absolutely critical. We talk about "coping strategies" (which are covered in detail earlier

in the book) but in reality it goes far beyond this. Understand your body and the levels of energy that you have and use them wisely.

I am a man who has just been told they have PBC. Everything I read about PBC talks about it being a disease of women. I am very confused (and a little embarrassed). Can you help? PBC is a condition that is commoner in women than men (around 90% of patients are women). This can lead to a perception that it is a female disease. It very definitely, however, occurs in men. There are, however, some subtle differences between PBC in men and women. The first difference is that UDCA response appears to be a little lower in men than women (i.e. men are a little more likely to be UDCA non-responders than women, and to therefore potentially need second-line therapy). Conversely, men are less likely to experience symptoms with their PBC, and where symptoms are present they are typically less severe. Men tend to have more advanced disease at diagnosis (and this may contribute to the lower UDCA response rate). In my experience, this tends to be because of an assumption amongst doctors that PBC doesn't occur in men, meaning that the potential diagnosis isn't thought about.

Although it is obvious it is worth pointing out that the fact that PBC most definitely occurs in men implies that the apparent female skewing can't be a result of something that only happens in women (a triggering event related to pregnancy, for example). My own view is that the gender difference is likely to result from differences in the function of the immune system in men and women relating to the actions of sex hormones.

I certainly recognise the sentiments in the question. In PBC clinics most patients seem to be women. Patient support groups have a majority female membership. Patient literature often focuses on issues like pregnancy. All this can, and does, sometimes make men feel that none of this seems to be "about them". It is beholden on all doctors and patient support groups to recognise this issues and make sure we remember it when we talk about PBC. The PBC family needs to include everyone.

Can I go on holiday with PBC? One of the bits of advice I always give to people with PBC is to go and live their lives (we only get one chance at it at the end of the day). Be aware of any risks, mitigate them but don't over-limit what you do for no good reason. I will split the answer to this question into a number of sections. The first is, what are the additional risks of my PBC being made worse by the act of travelling? The second is, what are the issues that could co-incidentally arise to complicate my PBC whilst I am on holiday (but which could lead me to need to seek medical care whilst abroad) and the third is what steps can I take to reduce any risk?

The first is really easy to address. There is almost no way in which travelling could worsen your PBC. Where complications arise they typically do so because of progression of the disease rather than any extrinsic factor that might be encountered when travelling. I often hear concerns from patients about pressure changes when flying increasing the risk of variceal bleeding. I think this is, to be honest, an urban myth (a bit like mobile phones interfering with electronic equipment in hospitals) and I have not seen any evidence of it happening (or experienced it with any of my patients). Also, of course, remember that the vast majority of PBC patients don't have varices and therefore obviously can't bleed from them!

The second aspect is a little more complicated. What is the risk that you might get unwell with PBC whilst you are away on holiday and need to seek medical attention? The issue of needing that attention obviously relates to whether it is going to be available, and how much it potentially might cost. Both of these aspects are massively impacted upon by the question of where you are travelling to. Overall, this risk is actually very low. I don't think I have ever looked after a PBC patient who has needed to seek medical care for their liver disease whilst on holiday. What risk there is really relates to how complicated your disease is. If you have non-cirrhotic or early stage PBC, and are managed with UDCA with or without one of the other available drugs, the chances of any sudden change in the disease or complication is essentially zero. If you have cirrhosis or have been transplanted, or have overlap syndrome and take immuno-suppression the risk is higher (although still not high). In these settings it is sensible to discuss with your own doctor about your own individual risks.

So what can you do to reduce any risk (and therefore also help your holiday by stopping you from worrying)? There are some simple but important things that you can do. The first is to make sure your disease is well controlled. This applies to everyone with PBC, at all times, but it is particularly important with travel. If you have just been diagnosed, and are starting on treatment, then save it for next year by which time you will be on therapy and everything will be stable. The second thing is to use some common sense about where you travel to, based around healthcare availability. If you have varices and have bled in the past then do you really want to go trekking in the Himalayas, a week's trek from a hospital? I wouldn't. I know a lot of PBC patients who go on cruises simply because high quality medical care is always available immediately on the ship. They find this hugely reassuring. Remember, also, your own country will have great holiday destinations that you haven't explored. You don't have to travel the world to have a good holiday. The final tip is, obviously, to make sure you have insurance. This is really important. If you are ill on holiday it is unlikely, as we have discussed, that it is a PBC problem. Having PBC, however, might easily worry a doctor in your holiday country who isn't familiar with it, and lead to you being sent to a hospital, or even, admitted to one, when anyone else would not be managed in this way. If you don't have the right insurance this could cost you a lot of money. The absolutely key thing is to be completely transparent with your insurance company about your PBC. They should be asking questions about issues like cirrhosis and varices risk so have that information at hand before you talk to them about cover. If you feel that they aren't hearing anything after you mention liver, or appear to have never heard of PBC, then think about going to one of the more specialised insurance companies who specialise in patients with medical conditions. Patient group such as the PBC Foundation are a really good source of advice about things like insurance companies. Remember, if you don't tell them about your PBC and you then make a claim it won't be valid **even if the claim is nothing to do with PBC**. One way around this is to take cover that excludes claims related to PBC (i.e. if you have a car crash it is still covered). Given the actual risk of a PBC-related emergency is very low this is often a very practical (and cost-effective) approach.

I want to start a family but have read some really worrying things on the internet about pregnancy and PBC. Is it safe to have children? The internet has been a real source of good, taking information out to people who would previously have struggled to access it. It can, however, be a double-edged sword, providing disinformation as well as information. A particular area that causes problems is in extrapolating from an individual's personal experience to other people in the population. If one person experiences a problem or complication in a disease setting, then that experience is, of course, important to them. What that individual experience means, however, to other people with the condition is, of course, the critical question. If they had that experience, will you? Are they the only person to have that experience (in which case the relevance to you is limited)? On the other hand, does everyone get it, but they are the only person to write about it? Remember, also, that media such as the internet tend to exaggerate issues, as people who don't have problems tend not to write about their experience of having no problems! The key point is that, in getting your information about PBC, be really cautious about your sources. Go to places you trust like the PBC Foundation website (as well, of course, as this book)!

Pregnancy is one of the areas where the actual information we have is very limited, and this vacuum in knowledge has been rather filled by the internet. The following is my experience of managing PBC for 30+ years, together with what is "known" from the literature. The number of pregnancies in PBC patients is relatively limited. This is, however, more a reflection of the age distribution of PBC patients than anything else. Most women only develop PBC in the years after they have finished having their families. Where women with PBC do want to get pregnant there do not appear to be any in the way of significant issues (with one exception, that of premature ovarian failure which is a rare form of autoimmune disease and is, thus, seen slightly more frequently in PBC patients). As a rule of thumb, as for all chronic conditions, the mantra of "healthy mum=healthy baby" comes into play. The better controlled the disease the more straightforward getting pregnant is likely to be and the easier the pregnancy. In my experience, pregnancy has no significant impact on the disease itself (if anything, liver function tests will slightly improve, although they can be difficult to interpret as the alkaline phosphatase level will naturally go up during pregnancy for reasons unrelated to PBC). If the disease does improve during pregnancy then it may worsen again once the baby is born so it is worth watching carefully.

One area where people are always concerned in pregnancy is in relation to drug use. UDCA is, we think, perfectly safe in pregnancy (indeed it is routinely used in cholestasis of pregnancy as a therapy), and it is our practice to continue it. Much less is known about bezafibrate and obeticholic acid, with the numbers of pregnancies reported amongst people taking them being very limited indeed (I think this is a reflection of the relatively recent introduction of the drugs, and the infrequency of their use, rather than any issue with getting pregnant). What experience we do have suggests that they are safe, however. The one drug relevant to PBC that absolutely must not be used in pregnancy in any circumstances is MMF (mycophenolate mofetil) which is an immuno-suppressant that is sometimes used in people with PBC/AIH overlap (and after liver transplantation for PBC and other conditions). It can directly damage the development of the baby and must never be used in people seeking to get pregnant.

The one form of PBC where pregnancy can have a real impact is where cirrhotic disease is present and is complicated by portal hypertension. The pressure in the abdomen goes up during pregnancy, especially towards the end (it's very simple, a large baby inside a relatively small abdomen is going to squeeze anything else in there). If portal hypertension has caused varices to be present then this pressure rise can increase the risk that they may bleed. This is very easy to manage, but we do need to know if the risk is there. For this reason, any woman with cirrhosis who is pregnant should have an endoscopy at about 6 months of pregnancy to assess the risk and plan management. Cirrhosis absolutely should not stop people from having a family. It just needs to be thought about and managed a little more.

For fairly obvious reasons this answer has focused on women with PBC. What about men? Is there any evidence that fertility drops with PBC increasing the risk of male factor infertility. The short answer is no!

The value for my AMA test has gone up. Should I be worried? The short answer is no! Anti-mitochondrial antibody (usually know by the abbreviation AMA) is present in the blood in almost everyone with PBC. However, and it is an important however, it doesn't actually play any part, as far as we are aware, in actually causing the disease. A small number of people (around 5%

of the whole population) get PBC but don't seem to have AMA. Furthermore, a number of people seem to develop AMA (usually in the setting of an infection) but don't go on to get PBC. Taken together, this all suggests that there is no direct link between AMA and PBC. Why is it there then? We don't really know. What it shows is that the immune system has "seen" and recognised a protein that is present in mitochondria (the battery packs of the cell providing it with the energy it needs to power itself). The resulting immune response has several different forms to it. These include antibodies (proteins produced by lymphocytes (the cells of the immune response) that bind to target proteins in the blood) and T-cells (the true "immune cells"). It is likely that the key immune response in PBC is the T-cell response which is the one that can actually damage the cells of the bile duct. The antibody response is probably just "noise in the background", which suggests that an immune response is happening, but doesn't actually cause any harm. The levels of all antibodies in the blood will go up and down depending on how activated the immune response is (a bit like the thermostat for your central heating). AMA is no different. Thus, if the level goes up it doesn't mean that the immune injury is getting worse. Likewise, if the levels go down it doesn't mean that the immune response is any less. In fact, for this reason, we tend not to re-measure the AMA level once PBC has been diagnosed.

There is one exception to this "AMA levels don't matter" rule. This is the rare occasions when AMA disappears and stays absent. This doesn't happen often in my experience in PBC (even after liver transplant when AMA seems to remain present, again not causing any problems to people). There are rare occasions, however, when it does happen. The immune system does have the capacity to lose its memory. This is why we need to have boosters after vaccination. Just occasionally, PBC will burn itself out. Any damage which has already happened (fibrosis development or cirrhosis) will typically stay but there won't be any progression of the disease. Liver function tests normalising with UDCA **does not** mean that that the disease has burned out; it just means that the UDCA has controlled the disease well. The bottom line is that you should continue taking the UDCA (think of the analogy of your blood pressure being normal on anti-hypertensive drugs.....not a reason to stop the treatment!). If the liver blood tests are normal and AMA has disappeared it may just mean that burn-out has occurred. What does all this mean in practice? The short answer is not much. I never really talk about this as a potential *denouement* of PBC because it is so rare (I don't want people to have unrealistic visions of what might happen to them in the future). What it does tell us is that it is perfectly possible for the immune response in PBC to be "turned-off". If we could find a way to trigger the off-switch using drugs it could, one day in the future, herald a whole new approach to treating the disease. One day!

APPENDIX 2: A DICTIONARY OF PBC

Albumin: A protein made by the liver and released into the blood. It is the protein with the highest level of liver manufacture, meaning that the level (which is easily measureable in the blood) is a useful test of liver function (and as such forms part of the panel of **_liver function tests_**). The albumin in the circulation plays two important roles (neither of which is, paradoxically, the one everyone thinks of which is as a source of nutrition). The first role is as a transporter for other molecules in the blood that are not soluble in water. One example, of many, is **_bilirubin_** which is transported to the liver in its insoluble form (prior to conjugation or "tagging" which renders it soluble) bound to albumin. The other important role is to help keep fluid in the correct place in the body. Although we think of the blood as the major fluid compartment in the body the tissues themselves have fluid within them to help "perfuse" the cells (carry nutrients to them). Where too much fluid gets out of the circulation and into the tissues oedema or swelling can result (the classic example is swelling of the lower leg ("swollen ankles")). This can reduce the blood volume, causing blood pressure falls, and can cause damage to the swollen tissues (skin stretching and ulcer formation as well as "heavy legs" that can reduce mobility). The balance between fluid in the blood and in the tissues arises because of the net result of a number of processes. A key one is the pressure within the blood vessel (in the swollen ankles analogy the fluid is pushed out from the veins by the high pressure in the lower leg that occurs when people stand up). Although there is some degree of reverse effect by the pressure within the tissue, the main factor keeping fluid within the circulation is osmotic pressure; the tendency for fluids containing a large number of molecules to attract water and dilute themselves. As albumin stays in the circulation because of its size (unlike ions such as sodium and chloride it cannot easily get across the blood vessel wall and out into the tissue) it is the key factor in exerting osmotic pressure to keep fluid in the circulation. This is why a low albumin (typically from liver disease but it can also occur with a very poor diet and through certain diseases of the bowel and kidney) is almost always associated with oedema or tissue swelling.

Alanine Transaminase (ALT): A blood test that forms part of the normal **_liver function test_** panel. It is released predominantly by injured **_hepatocytes_** and is therefore more associated with hepatitis in its various forms than with PBC (PBC is a disease primarily of the cells lining the **_bile duct_**, the **_biliary epithelial cells_**, rather than the hepatocytes). ALT can, however, be elevated in both **_overlap_** and **_UDCA non-responders_**. Where ALT is significantly elevated in PBC it always warrants investigation to determine whether additional treatment is needed. ALT elevation can also occur with toxicity of drugs such as *rifampicin*. ALT is, therefore, used as a safety test when monitoring drugs such as rifampicin.

Alkaline Phosphatase (ALP): An enzyme released by the *biliary epithelial cells* (the cells lining the *bile duct* amongst other organs)). Release of ALP by bile duct cells is a marker of stress or injury and an indicator of *cholestasis*. It can be released (in slightly different forms) by other tissues, in particular the bone, so caution must always be taken in automatically ascribing its elevation to liver disease. If in doubt the level of the specific liver form can be measured or, alternatively, the presence of cholestasis can be cross-checked by also measuring *gamma-glutamyl transferase (GGT)*, another enzyme released by stressed/injured bile duct cells. ALP forms part of the standard *liver function test* panel. The combination of elevation of biliary ALP and *anti-mitochondrial antibodies* is normally sufficient to make the diagnosis of PBC. The level of alkaline phosphatase is an important marker for disease severity, and guides therapy use in practice. This makes it a key marker in the disease. It is important to say that elevation in the levels of alkaline phosphatase is not harmful per se; it just indicates what is happening more generally in the disease. The question of what constitutes the ideal alkaline phosphatase level is a complex one. In practice, the lower the better is the mantra. Currently, targets are for a value between 1.5 times and 3 times the *upper limit of normal* depending on national practice. I suspect that over time the target value will fall (rather as has been the case for cholesterol values) until the point at which the target is normal tests, achieved as quickly as is possible.

Anti-mitochondrial Antibody (AMA): The classic *autoantibody* type seen in PBC. These antibodies are reactive with the body's own *pyruvate dehydrogenase complex*, an energy-generating enzyme complex which is located on the inner membrane of mitochondria (the batteries of the cell). As is the case with many autoantibodies, there is no clear evidence to suggest that they are themselves harmful to the body. They are, however, a very important marker for the disease and form the bed-rock of diagnosis. The combination of AMA with raised *alkaline phosphatase* (a component of the *liver function test* blood test panel) is over 95% accurate for the diagnosis of PBC.

Apoptosis: A process of programmed cell death, and one of the three key mechanisms by which the body loses functioning cells in disease (the others are necrosis and *senescence*). Necrosis is where a cell literally falls apart. This happens in situations such as ischaemia (where the blood cell is cut off to a tissue) and burns. As well as the loss of the cell itself, necrosis is a harmful process because cell contents are leaked which can themselves stimulate more inflammation and tissue damage. Apoptosis is a "cleaner" way for a cell to die. In essence, it turns in on itself, neatly packaging itself up for disposal. This avoids the harmful consequences of necrosis. The cell is, typically, signalled to undergo apoptosis by an external signal, usually sensed through a receptor on the surface. The stimulus can come from a *T-cell* or other form of killer cell. In PBC apoptosis can arise through the actions of T-cells as part of the autoimmune response or through the actions of toxic *bile acids* which can be harmful to the cell, especially when they build up in the disease setting.

Ascites: Collection of fluid in the abdominal cavity leading to swelling of the abdomen. It can be caused by a number of processes, including heart failure and the presence of tumour cells in the abdominal cavity in the setting of cancer. The commonest cause by a long way is, however, *cirrhosis*. The mechanisms by which fluid accumulate are complex and include *portal hypertension*, low *albumin* levels in the circulation and retention of the steroid hormone aldosterone. Ascites is relatively uncommon in PBC, and is only a feature of advanced disease. If the fluid volume is very high it can restrict movement and compromise breathing through pressure on the diaphragm. Ascites can occasionally become infected by bacteria from the gut to cause spontaneous bacterial peritonitis. This is a potential cause of further deterioration in liver function in people with cirrhosis. As with ascites in general, however, it is rare in PBC. When ascites is a problem it is usually controlled with diuretics ("water tablets" such as frusemide and spironolactone). Occasionally it needs to be drained through the abdominal wall using a needle and plastic drain; a relatively harmless procedure.

Autoantibody: Antibodies that react with the body's own proteins. Antibodies are a key part of the normal immune response to foreign proteins. They are themselves proteins that are both present on the surface of immune cells (the *B-Cells*) and free in the circulation. They bind to specific proteins (the protein that they match up to which triggered their production in the first place) blocking their function and helping the immune system to clear them. Normally, antibodies are specific for proteins that are foreign to the body. As part of the miss-targeting seen in autoimmune disease, however, they can end up reacting with the body's own proteins. Antibodies of this type are known as autoantibodies (from "auto", the Greek for self). PBC, as is the case with other autoimmune diseases, is characterised by the presence of autoantibodies in the serum. The commonest PBC autoantibodies are the ***anti-mitochondrial antibodies*** which are seen in over 95% of PBC patients. As is often the case with autoantibodies they are probably not directly responsible for tissue damage in PBC. The most obvious exception to this lack of direct effect is the thyroid stimulating autoantibodies seen in thyrotoxicosis which actually drive thyroxine release.

Autoimmune Hepatitis: An autoimmune liver disease in which the target for immune injury is the ***hepatocytes*** rather than the ***biliary epithelial cells*** which are the target in PBC. Autoimmune hepatitis presents very differently to PBC (more often an acute illness with jaundice) and responds to different treatments (steroids are still the mainstay). There is, therefore, usually no difficulty in distinguishing PBC and AIH. There is, however, a relationship between AIH and PBC. PBC associates with a number of other autoimmune conditions and AIH is one of them. There are therefore, undoubtedly, a group of people (albeit a small one) who have both conditions. This state is called PBC/AIH ***overlap***. In overlap the activity of the two disease components can fluctuate independently (I have seen people move from 100% PBC to 100% AIH and back again), and each component disease needs to be treated on its own merits. The challenge is that most people labelled in the past as having overlap do not, in fact, have it! Instead, they have the more recently recognised aggressive form of PBC, which is often characterised by some AIH-like features.

"Batteries Running Down": The term patients frequently use to describe the peripheral type of ***fatigue*** that is probably the commonest symptom in PBC. In this type of fatigue people know what they want to do, and can clearly plan it, but the power in their arms and legs lets them down. The imagery is very powerful. Recent research has shown that there are changes in the way that muscles work in PBC, with a build-up of lactic acid after even relatively low levels of exercise. This may explain the mechanism for peripheral fatigue.

B-Cell: A key part of the immune system responsible for antibody production. B-cells are lymphocytes (the cells that generate specific immune responses (i.e. those targeted at specific molecules/cells rather than acting more generally)). The role of B-cells is to produce antibodies; proteins that are released into the circulation where they can bind to and help eliminate bacteria and viruses in a targeted fashion. Each B-cell produces a single antibody of a unique specificity. Although antibodies are typically directed against proteins foreign to the body (viruses, bacteria, fungi, vaccines etc) miss-targeting can occur, giving rise to antibodies specific for one of the body's own proteins. These are known as ***autoantibodies.*** The autoantibodies most commonly seen in PBC are the ***anti-mitochondrial antibodies***. Once B-cells arise they can be very long lived, reverting to a dormant or memory phenotype. If the body is re-exposed to the same target then they can be rapidly activated to produce antibody. This is the mechanism that underpins immunological memory, the process by which we can avoid being infected twice by an identical virus, and which is, of course, critical for how vaccination works. Immunological memory also explains why autoimmune diseases are typically long-lived. If the organ that the immune system started to recognise is still there then the immune system will never be able to "forget" it has seen it.

Bezafibrate: One of the agents that has entered clinical use as **second-line therapy** for PBC patients who are **UDCA non-responders**, typically given in addition to UDCA. It is an anti-cholestatic agent that appears to modify the production of the **bile acids** that are responsible in part for cholestatic injury to the **biliary epithelial cells.** It is one of a class of drugs called the **PPAR agonists.** Unlike **obeticholic acid,** the licensed second-line therapy, it is not itself a bile acid. There have been a number of small reports of its benefits in PBC and a single clinical trial (the BezUrso trial). This showed that around 30% of PBC patients who were UDCA non-responders normalised their **liver function tests** with bezafibrate. The definition for UDCA non-response was very broad, however, and included a number of people with really quite mild (and thus easier to treat) disease, raising questions as to how generally applicable the finding is. Issues with liver and kidney toxicity were also seen. Bezafibrate, however, improved rather than worsened itch which is in contrast to obeticholic acid which can cause worsening of itch in a small number of people. A trial specifically looking at its actions on cholestatic itch showed benefit and the drug is increasingly being used for this indication in PBC. Bezafibrate is licensed for use in the treating of hyperlipidaemia (it is an old lipid lowering drug which has been largely superseded by statins in this role). It is not, however, licensed for use in PBC. When used in PBC instead of the licensed drug, obeticholic acid, it should be for a specific clinical reason such as potential itch improvement. At present, it isn't clear whether bezafibrate is useful as monotherapy in PBC (i.e. in people unable to take UDCA as well). In countries, such as the USA, where bezafibrate is not licensed for any indication **fenofibrate** is often used in its place. Emerging data suggest that bezafibrate can cause issues with kidney damage in some people. It should be used in caution in people with kidney dysfunction (and the slow-release form avoided completely). Kidney function should be checked in all PBC patients after they have been started on bezafibrate.

Biliary Epithelial Cells (BEC): The cells that form the lining for the **bile ducts.** These cells are integral to PBC as they are the target for damage in the disease. There appears to be a combined action of the immune system and the toxic effects of **bile acids** which accumulate in the disease. This gives rise to a progressive cycle of bile duct damage, and eventual loss of the bile ducts (**ductopenia**). Two processes appear to be key in BEC injury and loss. The first is **apoptosis,** a form of programmed cell death that occurs in response to an external "death signal". This mode of BEC injury in PBC is induced by both autoreactive **T-cells** and by the toxic actions of bile acids. More recently, it has been recognised that a second mode of cell loss is also important. This is cellular *senescence*. This mode of cell loss appears to be the key one in high risk PBC (BEC senescence is strongly associated with *UDCA non-response*). It probably arises, in part, as a consequence of the BEC losing the capacity to cope with injury in PBC. Preventing BEC senescence is likely to be seen as an increasingly important goal of treatment in PBC in the future.

Bile: The drainage fluid of the liver. It is actively produced by the *hepatocytes*, and then modified by the cells of the *bile duct*. It performs two key functions. The first is to facilitate outflow of the by-products of metabolism by the liver. The second is to transport *bile acids* into the bowel where they perform their critical normal function of helping the uptake of fat from the diet into the body by making it soluble.

Bile Acids: Cholesterol-based molecules synthesised by the *hepatocytes* and actively transported across into the *bile canaliculi* where they form an important component of *bile*. The physiological role of bile acids is to act as a detergent, emulsifying lipids or fats in the bowel to make them water soluble. This allows them to be taken up across the bowel wall. Bile acids are, therefore, key for normal nutrition. There is emerging evidence to suggest that bile acids have, however, a broader role in regulating metabolism in the body, as well as aiding absorption of fat from the diet. Bile acids, although natural to the body, have the potential to be irritant to cells. They do, however, vary in the degree to which they can have this effect. In PBC there is a shift towards hydrophobic or fat soluble bile acids which are more irritant, and away from hydrophilic, or water soluble forms, that are less irritant. There are normally protective processes to mitigate against bile acid irritation, including production of a "bicarbonate umbrella" that shields the surface of the bile duct. These appear, however, to be dysfunctional in PBC patients. Whether this is a cause or a consequence of the diseases is not, at present, clear. Once bile acids are in the bowel, having reached it via the bile duct, they do not go on to pass out of the body in the stool. They are re-absorbed in the end section of the small bowel and return to the liver to be re-used (the "entero-hepatic circulation"). This re-cycling has probably evolved to avoid the significant energy/nutrition loss that would result if bile acids had to be continually synthesised. One area of bile acid biology that is controversial is the role played by them in the genesis of itch. One of the effective treatments, *cholestyramine*, works by binding bile acids in the bowel and preventing their re-uptake in the small bowel. This implies a role for bile acids in itch. Newer drugs in trial (the IBAT inhibitors) directly block bile acid re-uptake and show real promise for the treatment of itch. Bile acids, therefore, must play some role in itch in PBC. It may be that this is as itch triggers rather than the actual direct skin irritants. Both *ursodeoxycholic acid* and *obeticholic acid* are themselves bile acids.

Bile Canaliculi: The space between the sheets of **hepatocytes** where the constituents of bile form together. The bile canaliculi, which represent the upper-most part of the biliary tree, drain into the small **bile ducts.**

Bile Duct: The tubular system that drains bile from the liver into the bowel. Bile constituents are actively transported into the **bile canaliculi** where flow towards the gut begins. "Downstream" of the canaliculi, the bile enters a structure of increasing size tubes, all lined by **biliary epithelial cells.** The bile duct drains into the **duodenum** (the part of the small bowel immediately after the stomach). The traditional way of describing the bile duct network is as the biliary "tree". This is actually a good description. The bile ducts start as very small structures, equivalent to the twigs to which the leaves are attached. Follow the twigs down and you get to branches that eventually join together to form two or three main branches which join the tree trunk. PBC is a disease of the small twigs. The larger bile ducts (the branches if you like) are never affected in PBC.

Bilirubin: The pigment chemical that gives rise to **jaundice** (the yellowing of the skin seen in advanced liver disease). Bilirubin is produced naturally as part of the recycling process for red blood cells that have reached the end of their useful life (around 150 days). Ageing red cells lose their shape and function and are taken up and broken down by the **macrophages** in the spleen. Haemoglobin, the complex structure that actually carries oxygen within the red blood cell, is partly recycled and partly disposed of. The actual oxygen carrying part of haemoglobin is called haem and contains the iron essential for oxygen transport. The iron is stripped out to be recycled, but the rest of the haem group cannot be used and must be disposed of. It is this that goes on to form bilirubin. At this initial stage it is not water soluble and needs to be carried to the liver for disposal by **albumin.** In the liver, the insoluble bilirubin is taken up by the **hepatocytes** and is "tagged for disposal" by a process called conjugation, in which another chemical group is attached to it by conjugating enzymes. It is then actively transported out into the **bile canaliculi** and carried out in the **bile.**

"Brain Fog": A term frequently used by patients to describe **cognitive symptoms** and central **fatigue**; two of the key symptom types in PBC. The imagery is very powerful and describes the sense that people have to actively think their way through problems.

Budesonide: A form of tablet steroid that has some of the beneficial actions of prednisolone in the liver but is then broken down by the liver reducing the risk of systemic side-effects (such as weight gain and skin thinning). It is used in **autoimmune hepatitis** as a replacement for prednisolone, and therefore is a logical agent to use in **overlap** to reduce the need for prednisolone. More recently it has been trialled as a *second-line therapy* for PBC in patients without overlap. The trial showed no significant improvement in *liver biopsy* abnormalities, but did show significant improvement in *liver function test* values. It therefore has potential value in PBC and warrants further evaluation. One area of interest is whether it has an additional beneficial effect outside its prednisolone-like effect. There is some evidence that it can help restore the bicarbonate umbrella that helps protect the *biliary epithelial cells* from damage by toxic *bile acids*. Budesonide should not be used in people with *portal hypertension* (usually, but not always in the setting of PBC, people with *cirrhosis*). In this setting the protective capacity of the liver to break it down is lost, meaning that it can get into the general circulation causing the steroid side-effects its use is designed to avoid.

Cholangiocytes: The alternative (and technical) name for the *biliary epithelial cells*. They line the *bile duct* from the small intra-hepatic bile ducts (the ones affected in PBC) all the way to the bile duct outflow into the *duodenum*.

Cholestasis: A state of impaired *bile* production and/or bile flow and its consequences. The term does not imply the mechanism responsible, which can range from blockage of the bile duct through a *gallstone* or pancreatic tumour, all the way to a failure of the transporter molecules in the liver which produce bile in the first place. Cholestasis has characteristic clinical features including itch (very prominent in PBC and some of the genetic transporter conditions) and jaundice. In terms of investigations, *liver function tests* tend to show elevation of *alkaline phosphatase* and *gamma-glutamyl transferase* (GGT) out of proportion to any elevation in *alanine transaminase*. *Bilirubin* will only be elevated in more severe forms of the condition. Imaging is crucial to determine whether there is a physical blockage to bile flow and, if so, what the cause might be. Initial imaging is always done using *ultrasound* which allows the structure of the liver to be examined. The sign of a blockage to the bile duct on ultrasound is often not the blockage itself but a widening of the bile ducts above the blockage because of the obstruction to bile flow.

Cholesterol: A form of lipid or fat present in the body. It is used as a fuel source and as the precursor for *bile acids* and steroid hormones such as cortisol, oestrogen and progesterone. The association between elevation of cholesterol and risk of atherosclerosis and heart disease has led to a widespread perception that cholesterol is a "bad thing". It is, however, essential for life and is only an issue if it is at the wrong level, in the wrong form or is in the wrong place. Cholesterol forms a key part of lipid transport complexes called lipoproteins. These shuttle lipids between the gut (where they are absorbed from the diet aided by the dissolving actions of *bile acids*), the liver where they are modified and synthesised (the focus on diet control for high cholesterol rather misses the point that most of the cholesterol present in the body is in fact created in the body) and the cells of the body where the lipids are taken up and used. It is the nature of the lipoproteins that determines the risk they pose to the blood vessels. Very low density lipoprotein (VLDL) and low density lipoprotein (LDL) at elevated levels do result in blood vessel damage and atherosclerosis and are termed "bad cholesterol" in the lay press. High density lipoprotein (HDL), in contrast, is protective for the blood vessels ("good cholesterol" which actually removes cholesterol from the cells of the vessel wall). An absolute cholesterol number is therefore difficult to interpret. This is a particular challenge in PBC where total cholesterol values are frequently elevated; something that causes concern to both doctors and patients. Typically, however, this is elevation of HDL cholesterol and PBC patients in fact have a lowered or normal LDL and VLDL cholesterol level. If the elevation is in HDL only then patients absolutely do not need cholesterol lowering treatment. Understanding cholesterol in PBC really needs what is called a differential cholesterol measurement (i.e. individual lipoprotein levels) with treatment only used if VLDL and or LDL are elevated.

Cholestyramine: The first line treatment for itch in PBC. In use since the 1960s, it is thought to bind bile acids in the gut and remove them from the body (they pass through and out of the bowel bound to cholestyramine). Some patients respond well to it, but it is very much towards the milder end of the spectrum of treatments for itch in PBC. One issue with it is tolerability. It has an unusual texture that many patients struggle to tolerate. Adding fruit juice, or chilling it in the fridge overnight before taking it, can help. Care needs to be taken taking it along with either ***ursodeoxycholic acid*** or ***obeticholic acid.*** These are both bile acids and so will bind to cholestyramine if taken at the same time (leading to reduced effectiveness). A minimum of 4 hours should be left between taking either of these drugs and cholestyramine

Cirrhosis: This is the single word that causes more problems for PBC patents than any other. Amongst the public it is synonymous with alcohol-related liver disease. This is incorrect, however, as it is a pathological description describing the end-state of chronic liver injury of all causes. The erroneous association is a highly unfortunate one, however, as PBC has nothing to do with alcohol. Indeed, PBC patients typically drink little or no alcohol. A tendency for ill-informed members of the public and, regrettably, health care workers to make a false connection between PBC and alcohol can be a very negative factor for PBC patients. This was a major driver behind the world-wide initiative to change the name to primary biliary cholangitis, a name that more accurately describes the actual disease process in the average patient and avoids the term cirrhosis whilst retaining the familiar, and useful abbreviation PBC.

Clinical Trials: The bedrock of the testing of new drugs and approaches to treating any disease. Clinical trials allow us to understand the extent to which a drug is helpful, and also the potential side effects that it may cause. From this, the risk and benefit can be determined. Regulatory bodies such as the Food and Drug Administration (FDA) in the USA and the European Medicines Agency (EMA) in Europe use this information to decide whether a drug is safe and effective enough to be granted a licence (i.e. be approved to be prescribed by doctors). In diseases, or versions of diseases, with no current treatment, the drug under investigation will normally be compared with a dummy treatment or ***placebo***. If the question is whether a drug improves on the current best treatment (or "standard of care" as it is termed) then it is this that the new drug is compared with.

Cognitive Symptoms: Symptoms of reduced short-term memory and/or concentration. People often struggle to follow plots in books or films or to do puzzles. This symptom set is seen in around 30% of PBC patients and can, if severe, cause real problems for people at work (especially if information processing is a key part of their job). As is the case with ***fatigue*** and ***itch***, the other cardinal symptoms of PBC, the cognitive symptoms can be seen at any stage in the disease process and are NOT a feature specifically of advanced disease. There is often confusion between these symptoms and those of ***encephalopathy*** which also exhibits memory and concentration problems. Encephalopathy is a feature of advanced cirrhotic disease and is very uncommon in PBC. The cognitive symptoms of PBC, which overlap with fatigue, do not improve with current disease management approaches (***UDCA*** as first line therapy and ***obeticholic acid*** or ***bezafibrate*** used as second-line therapies, in combination with UDCA, if first-line therapy has been insufficiently effective). PBC patients with cognitive symptoms often worry that they are developing dementia. I suspect this is one of the reasons why people do not discuss their memory problems in clinic. It is important to know that there is no evidence at all to link dementia and PBC.

Cytokine: The chemical mediators of the immune and inflammatory response. They are produced by activated ***T-cells, macrophages*** and other inflammatory cells. They can activate immune cells to function, or even cause ***apoptosis*** directly. Targeting cytokines such as TNF-alpha has been an effective approach for the treatment of a number of inflammatory and immune diseases. This approach has not, as yet, been tried in PBC in ***clinical trials***.

Ductopenia: Loss of the bile ducts within the liver. This is seen in a number of conditions, including severe PBC, and it represents an adverse state. Typically accompanied by worsening itch and jaundice, the severe impact on bile flow makes treatment very difficult and patients with extensive ductopenia frequently need transplantation. One of the major goals of treatment in PBC is to prevent ductopenia from arising in the first place.

Duodenum: The first part of the small bowel, immediately down from the stomach. The **_bile duct_** drains into the duodenum.

Elafibranor: An experimental **_second-line therapy_** in PBC which is currently undergoing **_clinical trial_** evaluation in patients who are **_UDCA non-responders_**. It is one of the family of **_PPAR agonist_** drugs. It has a slightly different profile of activity to **_bezafibrate_**, the first PPAR agonist used in PBC. In early phase clinical trials it has been shown to significantly improve both **_liver function tests_** and **_itch_**.

Encephalopathy: A blanket term for a state of toxic brain dysfunction. In the context of PBC, this is an abbreviation for hepatic encephalopathy. This state occurs in advanced cirrhosis when the liver fails to clear the toxic by-products of metabolism. These can then build up and cause a reversible toxic state affecting brain function. This can range from minor changes in memory, concentration, personality and sleep pattern, through to coma. This can be a very disabling (and distressing) complication of cirrhosis. Fortunately, it is very rare indeed in PBC. If it does occur then it is an absolute indication to consider liver transplantation as a potential treatment. It is also important to distinguish hepatic encephalopathy in PBC (very rare) from the much commoner mild **_cognitive symptoms_** seen in many PBC patients as part of the fatigue problem set, and which can be present at any stage of the disease.

Endoscopy: Known colloquially as a "telescope test". Flexible endoscopes are one of the key medical technology inventions of the last 50 years, transforming the management of bowel and bladder disease. Upper endoscopy is the examination of the oesophagus (gullet), stomach and duodenum under direct vision. The endoscope is a flexible tube with a fibre optic light source that allows the doctor or nurse to directly examine the inside of the bowel. An instrument port allows biopsies to be taken (important for the diagnosis of celiac disease in PBC) and to pass instruments down. These allow, for example, the direct treatment of **_varices_**. Guidelines recommend that PBC patients with **_cirrhosis_** have regular endoscopies to check for the presence of varices. This is a minor procedure normally done with just an anaesthetic throat spray. It takes a few minutes at most.

Fatigue: The commonest symptom described by PBC patients, and one that is often neglected by doctors. Approximately 50% of PBC patients will experience noticeable fatigue at some point in their disease, and half of these will have significant fatigue (fatigue that is bad enough to have an impact on day to day living and quality of life). There appear to be two "types" of fatigue in PBC, although it is important to understand that we do not, as yet, fully understand the causes of fatigue, meaning that the relationship between these two "types" may be a lot more complex than we currently appreciate. Peripheral fatigue is a sensation of weakness in the muscles which affects a person's ability to carry tasks out (the motivation to do something is there but the arms and legs let people down; people often describe the sensation as being like their *"batteries running down"*. Central fatigue is a sensation of difficulty in initiating activities. People just cannot get going. They also feel like their thought processes are slowed down, and often use the term *"brain fog"*. This type of fatigue overlaps with the *cognitive symptoms* which are increasingly being recognised in PBC. Fatigue can cause significant reduction in the quality of life of PBC patients and does not seem to improve with any of the current treatments (either UDCA or second-line). A systematic approach to reducing its impact can have real benefits. It is really important for patients to "own the problem" and find ways to adapt and minimise the impact of fatigue. One really important thing is to avoid social isolation which can be one consequence of energy-saving lifestyle modifications. These can improve fatigue, but often do so at the cost of worsening of overall life quality.

Fenofibrate: An alternative to *bezafibrate* as a *PPAR agonist second-line therapy* in PBC. It is mostly used in countries where bezafibrate is not licensed. The evidence supporting its use is less than for bezafibrate and it may be less effective.

Fibroscan: An important, and now established, technology in liver disease that allows us to examine for the presence of liver *fibrosis* or *cirrhosis* without needing to do a *liver biopsy*. The technique is a variant of *ultrasound*. The principle is very much like sonar on a submarine. A "ping" is sent out and the machine measures how much is returned. The more of the ping that returns the more solid (i.e. fibrotic) the liver is. The test can be done in real time as part of a clinic review and is painless. It has almost completely replaced biopsy in the monitoring of PBC patients for cirrhosis. Originally, Fibroscan was used to predict the presence and degree of fibrosis in the liver. More recently it has become clear that Fibroscan can directly predict the risk of complication development in the future (varices, need for liver transplant and death from liver disease). A value of less than 7.8 KPa suggests a very low risk, a value between 7.8 and 15.1 suggests a moderate risk, and above 15.1 a higher risk. The combination of Fibroscan with *liver function assessment* of *UDCA response* is likely to be the most accurate way of monitoring PBC risk progression and response to treatment.

Fibrosis: The development of scar tissue. The natural response of the body to injury is to attempt to repair and return the tissue to a normal structure and function. Where this is not possible, scar tissue forms to at least retain the physical integrity of the tissue. An example is the skin where a burn, if shallow, will normally heal, returning the skin to normal appearance and function. If the burn is very deep then it cannot heal and, instead, a scar forms. This is not as effective as normal skin, but at least keeps the integrity of the body surface intact. Similarly, following most forms of acute liver injury the liver will recover to normal size and structure. If the injury is chronic, however, the rate of injury can exceed the capacity to repair meaning that chronic injury builds up. The response of the body to this is to form scar tissue. Once scarring becomes extensive the state of **_cirrhosis_** develops.

Gallstone: Accretions that form in the bile duct and/or gallbladder from the crystallisation of bile contents. These soft "stones" are typically formed from either cholesterol or bilirubin ("pigment stones"). Gallbladder gallstones are the commonest type and usually cause no problems (the days of automatically having your gallbladder removed because stones had been found have, thankfully, long gone). They can cause intermittent pain ("biliary colic") which, if severe and frequent, is in indication for gallbladder surgery. Occasionally, gallstones form in, or move from the gallbladder into, the **_bile duct_**. These are much more problematic, potentially causing obstruction of the bile duct (characterised by pain and **_jaundice_**). Infection can develop in the obstructed bile duct because the bile can no longer drain. This is a real medical emergency. In this situation, the first step is to treat the infection with antibiotics, drain the bile duct (either through an **_endoscopy_** approach called ERCP or through a drain inserted into the liver and through into the bile duct). Then the bile duct stone is removed at ERCP. It is almost always appropriate to later remove the gallbladder to prevent recurrence. A gallstone blocking the very bottom of the bile duct, just as it joins the **_duodenum_**, can also block the duct draining the **_pancreas_** (which usually joins the bile duct very low down). This can cause an acute inflammation of the pancreas called pancreatitis which is, again, an acute medical emergency.

Gamma-Glutamyl Transferase (GGT): An enzyme that is released by **_biliary epithelial cells (BEC)_** when they are injured. It is very similar in this regard to **_alkaline phosphatase_**. It is not, however, part of the **_liver function test_** panel in most hospitals. It can be a little more erratic in its pattern than alkaline phosphatase (it can go up and down on a day by day basis; something that alkaline phosphatase tends not to do in PBC) which is one of the reasons it tends not to be measured. It can also be problematic in PBC patients as its elevation is (erroneously) thought by many doctors to suggest the presence of alcohol-related liver disease. Its main use in my practice is in confirming that elevation of alkaline phosphatase is from the liver rather than the bones or gut. If the origin is the liver GGT will be elevated as well. If it isn't liver it won't be.

Global PBC: An international consortium of researchers who have used data from many centres to build up a research picture of PBC. Along with *UK-PBC* the Global PBC Study Group have been responsible for major advances in our understanding of PBC which have transformed clinical practice.

Golexanolone: A novel drug which is entering clinical trial for the treatment of *cognitive symptoms* (*brain fog*) in PBC. It blocks the actions of a steroid produced in the brain (allopregnanolone) which we know is elevated in PBC patients with brain fog. Elevation of allopregnanolone is associated with an increase in daytime sleepiness (a hallmark of PBC). Golexanolone appears to reverse this effect.

Hepatic Artery: One of the two sources of blood flowing into the liver (the other is the *portal vein*). This dual perfusion type is unique to the liver. In fact, the majority of the blood flow into the liver actually comes from the portal vein, although all the blood supply to the *bile duct* comes from the hepatic artery. Hepatic artery problems only arise in PBC after *liver transplant*, when thrombosis of the artery can be an early complication.

Hepatic Vein: The vein (actually usually several veins) that drain blood from the liver out into the *inferior vena cava* for return to the heart. It is not to be confused with the *portal vein* which is one of the sources of blood flowing into the liver (the liver has two sources of blood flowing in, the portal vein and the *hepatic artery* but only a single outflow, the hepatic vein).

Hepatocellular Carcinoma (HCC): A cancer of the *hepatocyte*. Most cancers in the liver are metastases (secondary cancers) arising from primary cancers elsewhere in the body (commonly the colon or large bowel). Primary cancer of the liver can, however, arise and it is growing in frequency. It typically arises in an already injured liver. This is usually *cirrhosis*, but in the case, in particular, of viral hepatitis in can be in pre-cirrhotic liver. HCC is therefore, correctly, viewed as one of the complications of cirrhosis. It is unusual in PBC (although the risk is slightly higher in men as testosterone appears to favour its growth). We screen everyone with cirrhosis, or probable cirrhosis, with a specific blood test called an alpha-fetoprotein and an ultrasound scan on a 6-monthly basis. If HCC is suspected, a second type of imaging, usually a CT or an MRI scan will be used to confirm it. HCC management is a complex area and beyond the scope of this book (not least because of the rarity of HCC in PBC). As is the case with all complications of cirrhosis in PBC, HCC is something that is far better managed by the prevention of the development of cirrhosis by effective disease treatment, than it is treated once it develops.

Hepatocytes: The cells of the liver. A normal adult male will have up to 1.5Kg of liver cells. Each hepatocyte performs all the functions of the liver (i.e. there is no sub-specialisation of the cells). Each hepatocyte performs multiple functions. Liver failure arises when there is an insufficient mass of functioning hepatocytes to undertake all key functions.

iBAT Inhibitor: A novel class of anti-*itch* drugs in PBC. They block the re-uptake of **bile acids** from the bowel at the end of the small intestine (the terminal ileum). In essence the mode of action is a more efficient version to that of **cholestyramine** which binds bile acids within the gut to prevent them being taken back up into the portal vein. The most advanced drug in the family is **linerixibat** which has been very effective in early phase clinical trial and is now entering phase 3 evaluation.

Immunoglobulin G (IgG) & Immunoglobulin M (IgM): The immunoglobulin fraction in the blood is a technical term for all the antibodies of all types measured as a protein level (i.e. including both ordinary antibody and **autoantibody**, and includes antibody of all specificities). The IgG fraction represents the mature, finely-tuned, antibodies that are produced long-term after an immune stimulus. In contrast, the IgM fraction is the early, immature and less specific "first" response produced to a stimulus. The Igs can be measured in the laboratory and are useful additional tests to **liver function tests**. In PBC, the IgM measure is almost always raised (for reasons that no-one has yet explained). The presence of an elevated IgM (which has almost no other causes) can be a useful additional factor in making the diagnosis of PBC if other tests are equivocal (although it does not form part of the standard diagnostic panel). The level of IgM does reduce with treatment in PBC, but it does not really have value as a prognostic marker. IgG is typically not elevated in PBC other than in **overlap** where elevation is normal (IgG is classically elevated in **autoimmune hepatitis** (AIH)). A normal IgG level makes a diagnosis of overlap very unlikely. Unlike IgM in PBC the level of IgG is quite a sensitive marker of disease activity in overlap (and indeed AIH).

Inferior Vena Cava: The large vein that takes blood from the lower half of the body back to the heart to be re-oxygenated in the lungs. The **hepatic vein** drains into it. The inferior vena cava actually passes through the liver, meaning that in liver transplant surgery a section of it has to be removed. Current practice is to use bypass to connect the portal vein and the inferior vena cava below the liver with the venous circulation above the liver to allow normal venous drainage during surgery.

Interface Hepatitis: An inflammatory reaction reaching into the plates of *hepatocytes* adjacent to the *portal tract.* It is not seen in mild or uncomplicated forms of PBC. Where present, it suggests a more aggressive disease and it is typically seen in *UDCA non-responders.* It may arise in aggressive PBC as a consequence of *senescence* of the *biliary epithelial cells*, with the cells sending out a "distress signal" of chemokines and *cytokines* as a result of chronic injury in *cholestasis.* Interface hepatitis can also occur in *autoimmune hepatitis* and, until recently, when it was appreciated that it can also occur in aggressive PBC, its presence was thought to indicate PBC/autoimmune hepatitis *overlap.* We now think that overlap is actually quite uncommon and that most PBC patients with interface hepatitis have more aggressive PBC. This is not as arcane a point as it sounds, as it makes a key difference to the approach to treatment that should be used.

Itch: An important symptom in PBC which can have a significant impact on life quality. The characteristics of itch in PBC are different to those of allergic skin reactions. In PBC, the sensation is very much one of irritation deep under the skin (a sensation of "creepy crawlies" under the skin is commonly described) whereas allergic itch is more superficial in nature. The distribution of PBC itch is characteristic, often affecting the palms of the hand and the soles of the feet, the scalp and the back. It is not associated with the presence of rash (other than as a result of scratching). It is often worse at night and can disturb sleep, thereby contributing to fatigue. Unlike the other symptoms of PBC it is relatively easy to treat, with *cholestyramine* used as first-line treatment and, in most centres, *rifampicin* as second-line. *UDCA* typically does not worsen or improve itch. *Obeticholic acid* can worsen itch. When this does happen rifampicin is usually the agent of choice. *Bezafibrate* does not worsen itch and seems to actually improve it. It is increasingly being used as an anti-itch therapy. Effective treatment of itch is the major contribution clinicians can make to quality of life in PBC. It is worth noting that the itch seen in PBC patients is not strictly a PBC feature. It can be seen in any *cholestasis*-causing disease process.

Jaundice: The clinical consequence of elevated *bilirubin* levels. Clinically, it is a yellowing of the skin. Initially this is very subtle and usually only visible in the whites of the eyes (for obvious reasons it is easier to see in the only truly white tissue in the body). Bilirubin levels can rise because of liver disease itself (a failure to conjugate and transfer bilirubin into the *bile duct.* It can obviously also occur if the flow of bile itself is impaired (it backs up into the *hepatocytes* and leaks back into the blood). Jaundice can also occur if the breakdown of red blood cells is greater than normal in a haemolytic anaemia. Thus, although jaundice is usually a feature of liver disease it does not have to be. In PBC, jaundice is only seen in the very end-stages of disease and most patients will never be jaundiced. As with hepatic *encephalopathy* the advent of jaundice is a significant event in PBC and should always lead to consideration as to whether transplant might be appropriate. There is one significant trap with jaundice in a PBC patient, as in anyone else. This is a phenomenon called Gilbert's syndrome. This is a genetic variation in one of the transporter molecules that carries bilirubin out into the bile duct. It leads to a less effective transporter, which leads to a higher background bilirubin level. It is not an illness (it is best thought of as a variant of normal) and does not cause problems, but it does mean that the bilirubin level is elevated and jaundice can be seen. To make it even more complicated, the bilirubin level can go up even further if people are stressed or ill. The important point is that if we use bilirubin and jaundice level as a risk marker in PBC, then the presence of Gilbert's can make people look like they have more severe disease than they actually do. This is why we do not only look at bilirubin and jaundice as severity markers, but look at the whole picture.

Kupffer Cells: The population of ***macrophages*** found in the liver. The scavengers of the immune system, the Kupffer cells play a key role in eliminating bacteria that get across the bowel wall and into the ***portal vein***.

Light Therapy: An emerging potential treatment for difficult to control ***itch*** in PBC. It is likely that the light energy breaks down the irritant (possibly ***bile acid***) in the skin that causes the itch sensation. It works best in people with a low body weight (as they have a greater body surface area in relation to their body weight). There is a limitation as to how much light therapy can be given in any one course because of the risk of skin cancer.

Linerixibat: One of the ***iBAT inhibitor*** family of anti-***itch*** drugs in PBC. It has now entered phase 3 evaluation having shown significant effects in early phase trials.

Liver Biopsy: One of the more controversial issues in PBC. Liver biopsy is the technique by which a very small sample of liver is taken to examine under the microscope. These days, it is done either under ultrasound control through the skin, or via the hepatic vein through a line inserted in a peripheral vein (usually in the neck). There is often great concern about biopsy amongst patients, however some of these concerns are perhaps a little over-stated. In reality, it is a simple process. There can be a little bit of discomfort, and there is a small risk of bleeding, but it is actually very safe and well-tolerated. It was undoubtedly over-used as a test in the past, both for the diagnosis of PBC and to stage it (to work out how bad the disease is). Although it is useful, the combination of ***anti-mitochondrial antibody*** and ***liver function tests*** is just as accurate, meaning that biopsy is not really needed to prove a diagnosis of PBC. In terms of disease stage, ***Fibroscan*** is, again, just as effective and is obviously non-invasive. One of the issues with biopsy, as opposed to, say,

Fibroscan, is that it takes a single tiny sample from what is a large organ. PBC can be a patchy disease meaning that different areas are affected to different extents. A single biopsy from one site may, therefore, not be representative of the whole liver. Fibroscan assesses a larger volume of the liver, making its findings more representative. There are two situations where biopsy is essential, and two where it is very useful. The two essential situations are in people who are *autoantibody* negative and in potential *overlap* cases. In the absence of autoantibody, PBC can't be distinguished from other causes of elevated liver function tests without a biopsy. In overlap, it is critical to distinguish this from more severe PBC (both overlap and more severe PBC can be characterised by greater than usual elevation of *alanine transaminase* (one of the liver function test panel)). The reason for the need to distinguish them is that it makes a real difference to treatment. Overlap is typically treated with steroids, and I do not think it is appropriate to give anyone with PBC steroids without being absolutely certain of the diagnosis of overlap. This needs biopsy. The two areas where biopsy is useful are *UDCA non-responders* and in people with more than one liver disease. Although UDCA non-response is usually diagnosed on blood tests, the number of treatment options is growing rapidly. Increasingly, the choice of the right one will make a big difference to patients. Biopsy will help us with this. As we move towards curing PBC (a realistic long-term aspiration in my view), so this individual targeting will become key. In terms of other diseases, we are seeing increasing numbers of patients with features of both PBC and another liver disease. This is most typically NAFLD. Working out which disease predominates, and which should be the main treatment target is key and often requires biopsy.

Liver Function Tests (LFTs): This is the colloquial terms for a number of blood tests relating to the biochemical function of the liver which are normally performed as a panel (i.e. if you order one you get them all). The term is actually a misnomer as they largely measure liver damage rather than liver function! This is the key test set that will be carried out when you go for liver check-ups in the clinic. The panel normally consists of *alkaline phosphatase* (ALP), *Alanine Transaminase* (ALT), *Bilirubin* and *Albumin*. Some centres also measure *gamma-glutamyl transferase* (GGT) and *aspartate transaminase* (AST). ALP, ALT, AST and GGT are largely markers of injury rather than liver function as they are all enzymes released by injured cells. The higher the blood level the more cells are being injured. Alkaline phosphatase is predominantly produced, in the liver, by the cells of the *bile duct*, and elevation is therefore used as a marker for bile duct injury or *cholestasis*. Elevation of ALP is the classical biochemical abnormality in PBC and the combination of ALP elevation and *anti-mitochondrial antibody* presence is sufficient for the diagnosis of the disease. Across the whole population, the higher the ALP the more aggressive the disease but, as with many of these tests, extrapolating that to the individual can be much less accurate. We do, however, use improvement of ALP as a key marker of response to therapy. ALP is not, however, only produced by the bile ducts and elevated levels can also be seen in both bone and bowel disease. It is possible to measure the specifically liver form to confirm liver origin if in doubt. An alternative (and more easily available) option is to also measure GGT. If that is elevated as well as ALP it strongly suggests a bile duct origin. ALT and AST are present in high levels in *hepatocytes* so elevation of these is suggestive of hepatocyte injury in the first instance (although AST in particular can also be released by injured muscle). In PBC, the ALT is typically ether normal or only minimally elevated. It can be more significantly elevated in two situations. These are *overlap* and aggressive PBC. Very elevated ALT (over 5 times the *upper limit of normal*) is suggestive of overlap. Lesser elevations are more typical of aggressive PBC. In the past, before the nature of high risk or aggressive PBC was fully understood, overlap tended to be over-diagnosed, and steroid therapy over-used. It is good practice to revisit the diagnosis in everyone labelled with overlap in the past to make sure that the correct treatment is now being used. Many of the patients treated with steroids in the past, often with little or no response, have done very well when treated with *obeticholic acid* or *bezafibrate.* GGT is an enzyme produced by both damaged and proliferating bile duct cells. It can be susceptible to more in the way of short-term fluctuation than alkaline phosphatase making it slightly less useful as a marker of cholestasis. Its main use is in confirming that ALP elevation is of biliary origin. In contrast to ALP and ALT, albumin and bilirubin are true markers of liver function. Albumin is a protein made by the hepatocytes and released into the blood, meaning that a normal level in the blood suggests normal protein synthesis. A low level could suggest poor liver function, but care needs to be taken because it could be low as a result of dietary short-fall or increased loss from the circulation (seen in renal disease, burns and some forms of bowel disease). Bilirubin is cleared by the liver in an active process of conjugation and transport, so elevation can be a feature of reduction in that functional capacity. Remember, however, that elevated bilirubin can also arise as a result of increased production in the first place (an increased rate of red blood cell breakdown by the spleen) and obstruction to bile flow down-stream of the liver. Ironically, perhaps the most useful blood test of liver function is one that is not even included in the liver function test panel. This is the prothrombin time, often converted into a measure called the INR or International Normalised Ratio (a test familiar to anyone who has taken warfarin to thin their blood as it is the standard monitoring test for getting the dose of the drug right). A number of blood clotting factors are produced by the liver, and their levels can fall very quickly if the liver starts to malfunction. A number of these contribute to a measure called the prothrombin time. The longer this time (beyond a normal of around 12 seconds (which varies from lab to lab)) the more the liver is malfunctioning. The INR is the same value but expressed as a ratio to a reference normal sample (i.e. an INR would be 1 for a PT of 12 with a reference of 12, 2 for a PT of 24 seconds with the same reference). Because PT (and INR) can change very rapidly they are sensitive monitors of actual liver function. In PBC, prolongation of both the PT and INR are very unusual indeed, demonstrating, again, how well hepatocyte function is maintained in this condition.

Macrophage: The scavenger cells of the immune system that are critical for mopping up bacteria and cellular debris in the context of infection or tissue injury. Macrophages in the spleen are responsible for the breakdown of red blood cells which have reached the end of their useful life, generating *bilirubin*. Macrophages in the liver are called *Kupffer cells* and play a key role in protecting the body from bacteria that have leaked out from the bowel and entered the portal vein.

Mitochondria: Structures present within the cytoplasm of human cells (organelles) that are essential for the generation of energy by the cell. They are often talked about as the "batteries" of the cell, although "generators" might be more appropriate as a description. They contain a number of different enzyme types including *pyruvate dehydrogenase complex* and related enzymes. The classical *autoantibodies* of PBC are directed against mitochondria, and are most commonly specific for pyruvate dehydrogenase complex. These are the *anti-mitochondrial antibodies*. As far as we can determine these antibodies have no direct effect on the capacity of the mitochondria to function in the body.

MRCP: A type of body scan which can examine the *bile ducts* in great detail. The approach uses magnetic resonance imaging (MRI). Prior to the advent of MRCP, investigating the bile duct for the presence of gallstones or other blockages needed a telescope based test called an ERCP. This required the injection of dye into the bile duct and brought with it the risk of damage to the *pancreas* in the form of pancreatitis, or the introduction of bacteria causing sepsis. MRCP represents a major step forward as it uses a computer reconstruction approach to image the bile duct, removing the need for dye to be physically injected into the bile duct. If MRCP suggests a gallstone or blockage in the bile duct then ERCP is still the next step. MRCP pre-assessment means, however, that this only ends up being done in patients who really need it.

Naltrexone: A tablet used for the treatment of itch in PBC. It blocks the actions of natural opiates. These are the body's own pain killing molecules that are also thought to play a role in giving itch signals to the brain. It is effective in many people and for some of them it has been life changing. It can, however, have two different side effects that can limit its use in practice. The first is that, perhaps predictably, it can worsen any pain which people may coincidentally have. Examples include, in my experience, shingles pain and toothache. The other issue is a form of withdrawal reaction to the, now blocked, natural opiates. This can include nausea, vomiting, shivers and nightmares. This usually settles after a few doses, but in some patients it can be ongoing. The issues with naltrexone in practice mean that we tend to use it only after **_cholestyramine_** and **_rifampicin_** have been tried. Alternative opiate antagonist drugs which don't have the side effects of naltrexone are about to enter into clinical trial in PBC.

Non-Alcoholic Fatty Liver Disease (NAFLD): A common form of chronic liver disease characterised by the deposition of fat in the liver cells. When accompanied by inflammation it is known as non-alcoholic steatohepatitis (NASH). It is an increasingly common complication of obesity and type 2 diabetes (both of which are increasing rapidly in their population frequency). It is not associated specifically with PBC but, given its frequency in the population, it is increasingly being seen in PBC patients as an additional disease process. The presence of NAFLD in a PBC patient can complicate assessment of blood tests and limit the effectiveness of PBC therapy.

Obeticholic Acid (OCA): The main **_second-line therapy_** for the treatment of **_UDCA non-responders_**. This was the drug which revolutionised the management of high risk PBC. It is licensed for use in PBC (it is the only licensed second-line therapy) in both patients showing an inadequate response to UDCA and in patients unable to tolerate UDCA (around 5% of patients). It is a farnesoid X receptor agonist. It works to both suppress the production of **_bile acids_** and to increase their export from the body. It therefore has a direct action on the **_cholestasis_** process. It is also anti-inflammatory and anti-fibrotic although the role played by these actions in the clinical response in PBC is not, at present, clear. Emerging evidence suggests that it prevents the onset of cellular **_senescence_**, which may be of real importance given the apparent role played by this cellular process in the biology of high risk PBC. The main side-effect with OCA is worsening of, or de novo, **_itch_**. This is relatively uncommon, but when it does occur it shares characteristics with "classical" PBC itch, responding to the same treatments. Our approach is to be proactive with the management of any pre-existing itch before starting OCA therapy. This has proved to be very effective in allowing patients who need it to take OCA without problems. The standard dose of OCA is 5mg per day, increased to 10mg per day if needed, and if it is being tolerated. Unlike UDCA, the dose is not adjusted for weight. It is very important that caution is applied, and the dose adjusted, in its use in cirrhosis. It needs to be avoided completely in advanced cirrhosis because the damaged liver struggles to handle the drug safely.

Osteoporosis: A process of bone thinning that can leave the patient at risk of fractures (especially of the hip and spine). It is a process that happens naturally with age, and which is worsened by female sex, low body weight, smoking and poor diet. There is also a significant familial component (the daughters of mothers with osteoporosis have a significantly higher level of the process themselves). Its relevance to PBC is that the rate is significantly increased in all cholestatic diseases. There are probably a number of factors that contribute to the risk of osteoporosis in PBC. These include lowered levels of vitamin D; a fat soluble vitamin which can be absorbed at reduced levels in cholestasis. There are now effective screening tools and treatments for osteoporosis and with their widespread use the risk of fractures for PBC patients has decreased dramatically.

Overlap: The source of more confusion in PBC than almost anything else! The majority of patients with PBC have a very straightforward disease process with inflammation in the ***portal tract*** and damage to, and eventually loss of, the small ***bile ducts*** in the liver. In a proportion of patients there is a more extensive inflammatory response involving the ***hepatocytes*** themselves. This appearance, termed "***interface hepatitis***" can also be seen in ***autoimmune hepatitis***. This led to the concept that some patients have both conditions (or at least an element of both conditions); a combination that was termed PBC/AIH overlap. The conventional approach to the management of overlap was to combine both PBC and AIH treatment in the form of ***UDCA*** and immuno-suppression respectively. Immuno-suppression was typically in the form of steroids at high doses, reduced to a longer-term maintenance dose, often combined with azathioprine. The problem with this approach was that it often didn't work! In particular, the addition of steroid therapy in the form of prednisolone frequently did not give rise to the rapid and dramatic improvement in ***alanine transaminase*** typically seen in AIH patients treated in the same way. The explanation has come with the discovery that ***UDCA non-responders*** can also, as part of their more aggressive PBC disease process, develop both interface hepatitis and raised ALT. Higher risk PBC does not respond to steroids and needs conventional second-line therapy. Many of the patients diagnosed as having overlap in the past, and who are still being treated with immuno-suppression, are potentially, therefore, on the wrong treatment. Before people look to change treatment, however, it is important to recognise that overlap actually does exist in a small group of patients and for them immuno-suppression is the correct treatment! The question of overlap is, therefore, very complicated and needs to be looked at on a person-by-person basis. The balance between PBC and AIH components in true overlap can vary over time, with people sometimes moving from one predominant component to the other. In all PBC patients, whether or not they are on the correct treatment should be kept under constant review. This is doubly important for patients who are thought to have overlap.

Pancreas: The gland that produces most digestive enzymes. It drains through the pancreatic duct which joins the ***bile duct*** just before it joins the ***duodenum***. The pancreas can be involved in PBC in two ways. The first is through the actions of ***gallstones*** which are seen at increased frequency in PBC patients. A gallstone which blocks the lower bile duct will, typically, also block the pancreatic duct leading to a significant risk of pancreatitis. This is a real medical emergency (but is fortunately uncommon in PBC). More commonly, patients can have reduced pancreatic function. This appears to be part of the PBC process, although it is rarely recognised or commented on. It contributes to the nutritional problems that PBC patients sometimes encounter.

Placebo: A "dummy" tablet given in ***clinical trials*** to one group of the participants. Placebos are designed to fully match the actual drug being investigated in terms of shape size and colour, but to lack the active ingredient. The inclusion of placebo in trials is essential if we are to demonstrate that an effect seen with a new drug is a direct result of the actions of the drug, rather than the extra clinical care (as well as the patient positivity) that can come with a clinical trial.

Platelets: The very small blood cells (or more accurately fragments of cells) that are responsible for blood clotting. Their importance in PBC is that they are a useful blood test measure as to whether there is ***portal hypertension***. In portal hypertension, the spleen swells and pools blood cells including platelets. This leads to a reduced platelet count. A value below 150 is a strong suggestion of the presence of portal hypertension and thus ***cirrhosis***.

Portal Tract: The structures within the liver that contain the ***hepatic artery*** and ***portal vein*** branches as well as the small ***bile duct*** branches. These structures are integral to the functional anatomy of the liver and have been likened to 3-core electric cable because of the triple structure. They are the seat of the disease process in PBC. It is within the portal tracts that the small bile duct damage occurs, accompanied by an infiltration of inflammatory cells (portal tract infiltrate). When the inflammation spreads out from the portal tract into the liver tissue itself this is called ***interface hepatitis*** and is an important feature of both ***UDCA non-responder*** disease and ***overlap***.

Portal Hypertension: A state of increased blood pressure within the *portal vein*. This can arise as a result of injury or obstruction to the portal vein early in life, but is most commonly seen in adults in chronic liver disease. The vast majority of liver disease patients developing portal hypertension do so as a result of cirrhosis. The combination of liver regeneration within a constricted space resulting from fibrosis formation puts pressure on the liver sinusoids (the very small blood vessels in the liver fed by the portal vein and hepatic artery that bathe the *hepatocytes* in blood). Occasionally, and more frequently in PBC than in most other liver diseases, portal hypertension can arise in the absence of cirrhosis. The most important complications of portal hypertension are *varices* and *ascites*. Portal hypertension is detected in practice by a finding of varices on *endoscopy* and strongly suggested by the presence of cirrhosis on *liver biopsy*.

Portal Vein: The large blood vessel that drains blood from the bowel. It enters the liver and all the blood draining from the bowel is therefore "filtered" through the liver. This allows the *hepatocytes* to take up nutrients for processing and the *Kupffer cells* to remove any bacteria or fungi that have crossed the bowel wall to get into the portal vein blood. The portal vein is also an important source of oxygenated blood for the liver, as the level of arterial blood flow into the bowel wall is so high that even the blood draining out through the portal vein is oxygen-rich. The pressure within the portal vein is typically very low (as is the case in all veins); much lower than in arteries. The pressure can, however, rise in chronic liver disease causing complications. This state is known as *portal hypertension*.

PPAR Agonist: A class of drugs that are used as *second-line therapy* in *UDCA non-responders*. Drugs of this class have been in clinical use for decades as lipid lowering treatments (although their application in this setting has rather been replaced by statins). In PBC they reduce *cholestasis* as well as, seemingly, *fibrosis* and *inflammation*. As is the case with *obeticholic acid* they are nuclear receptor agonists, altering protein production by cells. They also, as is the case with OCA, significantly improve *liver function tests*. None of them are, however, as yet approved for use in PBC (although they are widely used in practice "off-label". In contrast to OCA, which can worsen *itch*, they reduce symptom impact and one of the class (*bezafibrate*) is increasingly being used specifically as an anti-itch treatment. There is emerging evidence to suggest that bezafibrate can cause kidney problems so blood tests need to be carefully monitored when it is used in PBC. The class includes, as well as bezafibrate, *fenofibrate*, *elafibranor* and *seladelpar*. All have a slightly different pattern of action, but all appear, in the trials carried out to date, to be effective in high-risk PBC.

Pyruvate Dehydrogenase Complex: An energy generating enzyme complex which is present within the **_mitochondria._** It plays a critical role in conversion of glucose into energy to power cells. It is the target of **_anti-mitochondrial antibodies (AMA)_** in PBC, as well as of the **_T-cell_** response. The response to pyruvate dehydrogenase complex in PBC is a true autoimmune response as the antibodies appear to react completely with the body's own pyruvate dehydrogenase. Why these immune responses come about is a fascinating question in PBC, and lies at the heart of our understanding of the disease. Pyruvate dehydrogenase is essential for cell function, and is highly conserved in evolution (meaning that its sequence and structure is essentially the same in all cell types in all living organisms). It is, therefore, exactly the type of protein that the immune system should be able to ignore. In PBC, however, it doesn't. One theory for how breakdown of immune tolerance to pyruvate dehydrogenase arises is PBC is through lipoic acid, a small additional molecule which is added to allow it to function. The potential to alter the structure via attachment of alternatives to lipoic acid may be the "weak link" in pyruvate dehydrogenase complex.

Rifampicin: An agent commonly used to treat moderate or severe itch in PBC. It is usually only used if **_cholestyramine_** has failed to give adequate itch control. Rifampicin probably works through the PXR nuclear receptor, increasing metabolism of the molecule causing the itch or blocking its production. Rifampicin can sometimes cause nausea and, more significantly, **_liver function test_** abnormality (typically elevation in **_alanine transaminase_**). For this reason, liver function tests should be measured between 2 and 4 weeks after rifampicin is started (and if the dose is increased). If the ALT has increased it should be stopped (after which LFT typically return rapidly to normal). The starting dose is 150mg daily, increased to a maximum of 600mg daily if needed (and if tolerated). Despite these concerns about safety, rifampicin is actually a really useful drug. I have known patients have complete control of their itch for 20 years with it. When using it you do need to be aware it can turn your sweat and urine orange (!) and you will get funny looks from the pharmacist (it is an old TB drug!).

Second-Line Therapy: This is a generic term in PBC, used to describe all the treatments which are used in patients who have shown an inadequate response to first-line treatment with **_UDCA_**. The only licensed second-line therapy in PBC currently is **_obeticholic acid_**. There is trial evidence to suggest that **_bezafibrate_** is beneficial but it is not currently licensed for use in PBC. It is, however, being used increasingly. All other second-line therapies are experimental treatments and should only be used in **_clinical trials._**

Seladelpar: An experimental **second-line therapy** in PBC which is currently undergoing **clinical trial** evaluation in patients who are **UDCA non-responders**. It is one of the family of **PPAR agonist** drugs. It has a slightly different profile of activity to **bezafibrate**, the first PPAR agonist used in PBC. In early phase clinical trials it has been shown to significantly improve both **liver function tests** and **itch**.

Senescence: One of the ways in which a cell responds to injury, and probably a key one in PBC. One way in which the **biliary epithelial cells** in PBC respond to injury is to proliferate (divide to create more BEC in an attempt to regenerate the injured **bile duct**). Injured, proliferating cells can rapidly, however, run out of the ability to replicate and can enter a state called senescence. This has been christened the "zombie cell" state. This is actually not a bad description. The cells don't die but also don't function. They do, however, send out a distress signal in the form of cytokines and chemokines; the chemicals that attract **T-cells** of the immune system. This is probably a protective mechanism of the body to recognise and eliminate the no longer functioning cells. In PBC, senescence of the BEC is a feature of high risk disease and of patients who are **UDCA non-responders**. It is possible that the distress signals sent out by the senescent cells are responsible for the development of **interface hepatitis**, the process of more aggressive inflammation reaching out from the **portal tract** into the plates of **hepatocytes** which is itself a feature of higher risk, UDCA unresponsive PBC. It appears likely that senescence arises as a consequence of aggressive **cholestasis**. It is not clear if, and for how long, senescence is reversible once it arises, and whether any of the drugs we currently use in PBC can reverse it. Research using mouse models of cholestasis suggest that **obeticholic acid**, but not **bezafibrate** may be anti-senescent. This needs to be further studied in PBC patients. The sequence of cholestasis to senescence and then **ductopenia** (the inevitable end-stage of senescence followed by the "clean-up" operation of interface hepatitis) means that treating cholestasis as effectively as we can, as early as we can, has to be the logical approach for the management of PBC.

Setanaxib: A new class of drug that blocks inflammation (through blockade of NADPH oxidase). Early trials suggest that it improves **liver function tests** but has an even more marked effect on **Fibroscan** values, suggesting that it reduces **fibrosis**. It also appears to have a significant effect on fatigue. Further trials in PBC are clearly warranted and are about to commence in early 2023.

Spontaneous Bacterial Peritonitis (SBP): A bacterial infection arising in pre-existing **ascites**. Ascites is a warm, nutrient rich fluid that is relatively inaccessible to the immune system. It is therefore unsurprising that bacteria that get into it thrive and reproduce, leading to active infection. SBP is a recognised complication of ascites in all chronic liver diseases and can contribute to temporary worsening of the liver disease ("disease decompensation" in cirrhosis). The bacteria probably enter the ascites from the bowel, helped by the general leakiness of the bowel wall seen in advanced liver disease. The reduction in the effectiveness of the immune system in cirrhosis also contributes to infection becoming established. SBP should be considered in any patient with ascites if the ascites gets worse quickly, becomes painful, or is accompanied by a worsening in liver function. SBP is diagnosed by taking a small sample of the ascites using a syringe and needle which is then cultured to identify bacteria and analysed for the number of white blood cells. Treatment is with antibiotics.

T-cell: A key part of the immune system. T-cells are lymphocytes (the cells that generate specific immune responses (i.e. those targeted at specific molecules/cells rather than acting more generally)). They split into 2 broad type; helper T-cells and cytotoxic T-cells. The role of helper T-cells is, as their name suggests, to assist the production of targeted immune response by both ***B-cells*** (producing antibodies) and cytotoxic T-cells. They do this both by directly interacting with the cells they are helping via receptors on their surface and by the action of ***cytokines*** (chemicals released by cells which act indirectly to activate or change the nature of other cells of the immune system). Cytotoxic T-cells are the killer cells of the immune response. They recognise cells that are infected with viruses and other pathogens (as well, probably, as cancer cells) and induce them to die. The effect is highly specific (they only kill in response to recognising a particular viral or other "foreign" protein). They are highly potent, so have checks and balances to prevent inappropriate activation (this is at both the level of their recognition of target cells and the need for T-cell help which is itself specific and targeted). PBC patients have both cytotoxic and helper T-cells that react with self-***pyruvate dehydrogenase complex*** (the key immune target in PBC and the target, as well, of course, as ***anti-mitochondrial antibodies.***

UDCA: The first-line treatment for PBC. Ursodeoxycholic acid (UDCA or, as patients frequently call it "urso") is currently the mainstay of treatment for PBC and is recommended by all treatment guidelines for all patients. It is a ***bile acid*** produced naturally by humans (albeit at low levels; in bears it is the major bile acid type giving rise to its name (*ursa* is Latin for bear)). Giving it in tablet form can increase the proportion of UDCA in the human bile acid pool to over 50%. UDCA has a number of potential actions, and it remains unclear which of these are important for its effect in PBC. It is hydrophilic in nature (i.e. is water soluble) which is different to a number of the more toxic bile acids. UDCA replacing these more toxic bile acids in the bile acid pool may significantly reduce their toxicity. UDCA also appears to be anti-apoptotic and antioxidant (i.e. it prevents cell death), which may directly improve the survival of the *biliary epithelial cells (BEC)*. Finally, UDCA is thought to be choloretic (i.e. it leads to the production of a greater volume of more dilute bile). Over the years, there has been argument about the extent of the benefits of UDCA; an argument which led to confusion amongst clinicians about whether it should be used. These debates are largely settled, and the consensus of the experts in the field is that UDCA is almost always of benefit in PBC, and that it should be started in all patients at the point of diagnosis of the disease and continued life-long. It is also now accepted, however, that the degree of benefit from UDCA can vary from patient to patient. In some people there appears to be very significant benefit with normalisation of *liver function tests.* In other patients the benefit seems to be less marked (although almost everyone seems to get some degree of improvement), and there is now an accepted need to identify patients who need additional, *second-line therapy* in a timely fashion. The concept of the *UDCA-responder/non-responder* has, therefore, become integral to how we manage PBC in practice. One legacy of the debates about UDCA is there has been a tendency for patients to be under-dosed. The optimal dose is 13-15mg per day, adjusted over time as peoples' weight changes. For a 70kg person this means a dose range of 910mg-1050mg (which means 1000mg per day in practice given fixed tablet sizes).

UDCA-Responder/Non-Responder: *UDCA* is first-line therapy in PBC, and should be used in all patients. An important minority of patients do not, however, respond sufficiently to UDCA and retain an increased risk of the development of cirrhosis and the need for transplantation. These are termed "UDCA non-responders". The term is actually not helpful as most are, in reality, "partial" or "incomplete" responders rather than "non"-responders. The term has taken hold, however. All patients taking UDCA should be assessed for their response and, if identified as UDCA non-responders, considered for *second line therapy.* One of the complications of this seemingly simple model is that there are number of different criteria that are used to identify UDCA non-response. All are based on combinations of the *liver function tests alkaline phosphatase, alanine transaminase* and *bilirubin,* each expressed as a multiple of the *upper limit of normal* to account for the different reference values in different laboratories (another complication). The two most commonly used criteria sets are "Paris 2" (ALP and ALT less than 1.5 times the upper limit for normal) and "POISE" (named after the pivotal trial of *obeticholic acid* in which they were first used; ALP less than 1.67 times the upper limit of normal and a normal bilirubin). The educational message we use for doctors and nurses is that it matters less which criteria you use in your clinic than that you choose one, use it consistently and, critically, ACT ON THE RESULT WHEN YOU IDENTIFY A UDCA NON-RESPONDER!

UK-PBC: A UK-wide research consortium with over 8000 PBC patient participants. Along with **_Global PBC_** it has been responsible for many of the recent advances in our understanding of PBC and how best to treat it. The main focus of UK-PBC was to understand the mechanism responsible for **_UDCA non-response_** and to support the development, evaluation, approval and implementation into practice of new treatments.

Ultrasound: A quick and easily available approach to imaging the body. It is especially useful for assessing the liver and bile ducts as it allows accurate assessment of liver and spleen size, liver texture (including the presence of any masses) and the integrity of the **_bile duct_**. All PBC patients should have an initial ultrasound to confirm that their **_cholestasis_** is not a result of bile duct obstruction (**_gallstones_** are present at an increased frequency in PBC patients as a result of the changes to bile flow and constitution (although this has been reduced by widespread use of UDCA which dissolves them, albeit very slowly!)). Abnormality on ultrasound, particularly in relation to the bile duct, is usually followed up by **_MRCP_**, another imaging approach using magnetic resonance.

"Upper Limit of Normal": The vast majority of blood tests carried out in the clinic have a range for normal values that reflect normal variability in the population (they are not "black or white", normal or abnormal as, say, a genetic test might be). To complicate things slightly, the assays used by different hospitals can vary, meaning that the range for normal values can be slightly different from centre to centre. For this reason, when looking at whether a test is abnormal or not in PBC, we use the concept of the "upper limit of normal" for tests which are abnormal if elevated such as **_alkaline phosphatase_** (obviously, the reverse applies with use of "lower limit of normal" for tests such as **_albumin_** where a lowering in the value is the abnormality that causes concern). A test value would be described as a multiple of the upper limit of normal. For example, if your alkaline phosphatase was 520 and the upper limit of normal for your local laboratory was 130 your alkaline phosphatase is 4 times the upper limit of normal (4x uln). This is a value that we would be concerned about, and would trigger consideration of a treatment change. The cut-offs used to signify response and non-response to treatment have changed over time as the significance of abnormality becomes better understood. They also differ from centre to centre, and country to country, which is an unhelpful source of confusion for patients. In the UK a good response to treatment is suggested by a bilirubin less than one times the upper limit of normal (< 1x uln) **and** an alkaline phosphatase of less than 1.67 times the supper limit of normal (< 1.67x uln).

Over time it is likely that the target values for treatment will be lowered (as has been the case with cholesterol). I anticipate that within 5 years the target will be completely normal LFT.

Varices: One of the complications of *cirrhosis* of all aetiologies. *Portal hypertension* is a common feature of cirrhosis (and very occasionally chronic liver disease that isn't cirrhotic) because of the impaired flow of the *portal vein* through the distorted anatomy of the cirrhotic liver. The increased pressure can open up residual blood vessels left over from the fetal circulation present in utero and which shuts down, but doesn't completely disappear, when you are born. This can lead to the development of, often high pressure but weak-walled, blood vessels in places where the old fetal and current adult circulations meet. This is most typically in the bowel (although they can also be seen in abdominal wall which is one of the reasons why abdominal surgery in patients with cirrhosis is often high risk). Within the bowel, the commonest site is the lower oesophagus. They can also be a problem in the rectum and stomach. Oesophageal varices can be a particular problem because the passage of food over big varices in a relatively narrow space can probably increase the risk of bleeding through surface trauma. If varices bleed then it is a medical emergency as the blood loss can be significant (because of the relatively high pressure within the vessels). In the setting of an acute bleed the first key step is to give fluid intravenously to support the circulation. After this, we use medicines (such as glypressin) to lower the portal venous pressure to reduce or stop the bleeding and allow the definitive short term treatment which is done at *endoscopy*. The commonest treatment in current practice is to band the varices (to put small rubber bands on them to constrict them and seal them off). Far better than managing a variceal bleed is preventing one in the first place. There are two steps to achieving this. The first is to treat PBC effectively so that cirrhosis doesn't arise in the first place (this comes back to our vision of better, earlier treatment for the disease)! Too often we think of treatments in PBC being about improving *liver function tests*. In reality, we are using them to reduce risks such as those of varices which are much more important, but less easy to see, then blood tests. If someone does develop varices, but those varices haven't bled, then the approach is to lower the pressure in the portal circulation typically using drugs such as propranolol or carvedilol. Having said all this, varices are actually rare in PBC, partly because of the effectiveness of our treatments, and partly because of the nature of the disease itself. PBC patients in whom cirrhosis is suspected should undergo regular check endoscopy to see if propranolol or carvedilol are needed. If a PBC patient has a variceal bleed they normally cope with it well, however it should always lead to the question of: is now the right time to consider liver transplant as an option.

APPENDIX 3: THE NEWCASTLE APPROACH...

......TO MANAGING ITCH IN PBC

Strange as it may seem but whenever I see a patient presenting for the first time with itch in PBC I am pleased. Pleased because I know that we will be able to help them very quickly indeed!! Itch in PBC really is the symptom that should be controllable in everyone. Like all treatment in PBC, we take a stepwise approach. In all the scenarios outlined in this appendix I am describing our local approach in a specialised PBC clinic. Every patient is different and every clinic will have its approaches. You should always discuss your own management with your medical team. If they do things differently to us that is fine, but it is reasonable to discuss why they are taking an approach that is different to the Newcastle approach. It is a question not a criticism as there are different ways of doing it, but it is a useful way to discuss the questions and issues.

Step 1: *Is it PBC itch?* This may seem like a strange question in a PBC patient with itch but, of course, having PBC does not protect people from all the other causes of itch in the population. There are four pointers to the itch being from the PBC

a) *The character of the itch:* PBC itch is very much deep underneath the skin with a frequent sensation of "prickles", little electric shocks or "creepy crawlies" under the skin. Allergic type itch usually feels like it is on the surface of the skin.

b) *The lack of a rash:* Where skin disease is the cause of an itch it is almost always accompanied by a rash. PBC is never accompanied by a rash because the itch is not primarily a result of skin disease. The only catch is the presence of excoriations or scratch marks which can result from prolonged scratching. These very much reflect the severity of the itch, but do not suggest a skin problem.

c) *The body distribution:* PBC itch has an unusual distribution that is unlike any other cause of itch. Particularly characteristic are itch of the palms of the hand and the soles of the feet which are almost never involved in itch of other causes. Other parts of the body typically affected in PBC include the scalp and the back. Remember, however, that itch can affect any part of the body in PBC.

d) *Lack of benefit from antihistamines:* A natural first response to itch amongst the population and GPs is to use anti-histamines. This is a follow-on from the idea that itch is typically a skin issue resulting from allergy. Anti-histamines do not, however, work for PBC itch (normally; there are always exceptions to any rule).

Step 2: *Is there something treatable that is making it worse?* In most PBC patients it is the disease itself giving rise to the itch. Remember, however, that PBC itch is in fact cholestatic itch related to the general disease process rather than PBC per se. Any additional disease with impaired bile flow can make the itch worse in a PBC patient. There are 2 important things to think about

a) *Bile duct obstruction:* PBC is associated with an increased risk of gallstones. They can leave the gallbladder and get into the common bile duct obstructing it. Irritation from a gallstone passing can also lead to scarring or stricturing in the bile duct. Given that UDCA used to be a treatment for gallstones (it dissolves them, albeit very slowly) one scenario is that a gallstone that is too big to leave the gallbladder and get into the bile duct to block it initially is slowly shrunk by the actions of UDCA and, months or years down the line becomes small enough to pass. Because bile duct obstruction (from stones or stricturing) is relatively easy to treat, and itch improvement will never be seen until the blockage is relieved, anyone presenting with PBC itch, or who develops itch or their itch worsens during follow-up, should have an ultrasound scan to check that there is no blockage to bile flow that needs treatment.

b) *Treatment side-effects:* OCA is well known to cause or worsen itch so people are usually alert to this happening. It is less well known that UDCA can (rarely) also cause itch. Female sex hormones in tablet form (the pill or HRT) can also worsen itch. In people presenting with itch, or where itch suddenly worsens, it is important to go through their drug list and just check that it isn't a recently-added treatment that is contributing. If so, the risks and benefits of continuing the particular treatment should be discussed (this is a case-by-case decision). Note that in the case of all these drugs the issue with itch is associated with the starting of the drug or an increase in the dose. Normally, therefore, if you are taking the same dose as you have been for a while it is very unlikely to be the drug. The only caveat is that changes in brand (or in the case of the pill and HRT the type) can sometimes trigger the itch. As with many aspects of PBC if you have found a treatment approach that works for you as much as is possible STICK WITH IT!

Step 3: *Is the itch bad enough to need treatment?* This is actually a really important question. It is a perhaps obvious, but still important, point to make that itch is a symptom. It has no connotations with regard to the disease at all. It therefore doesn't "need" treating. It should be treated if it is bad enough to warrant treatment despite any potential side effects that come with it. Data from UK-PBC suggest that around two thirds of PBC patients will get itch at some point in the disease but only around one third will be getting treatment for it at any time. What makes itch bad enough to warrant treatment? That is entirely a personal decision. In my experience, the following are the sorts of issues that suggest treatment is likely to be beneficial

- Night-time itch that is interfering with sleep
- Constant itch with no days or parts of days without it
- Itch that is getting rapidly worse
- Itch that you are aware of all day (i.e. there aren't any times when you stop noticing it).

Step 4: *Cholestyramine:* Once the decision to treat itch has been taken, we always start off with cholestyramine. The reason is that it is the licensed treatment recommended by guidelines and it is completely safe. We recommend that people either chill it in the fridge overnight (make tomorrow's doses (it is a sachet that is made up into a drink to take) the night before) or add fruit juice to make it more palatable. We recommend that people take it three times a day to start with spaced away from UDCA for the reasons outlined above. It is really important to give it enough time to work (at least 4 weeks) before moving on to another treatment. Everything else that we try has more side effects, and thus greater risk. Colesevelam is a tablet form of bile acid sequestrant (the class of drug that cholestyramine is in) which offers the promise of greater tolerability than cholestyramine given that it is the texture of the suspension that is often the problem with the latter. It is becoming increasingly widely used in this setting. The only trial looking at its use in PBC for the treatment of itch was, however, negative and my own experience is that it does little or nothing to improve itch in PBC. Non-response of itch to colesevelam does **not** mean that the itch is not PBC itch. It just means that colesevelam doesn't work!!

Step 5: *Rifampicin:* If cholestyramine has not worked after 4 weeks, or it is genuinely impossible to take (with my caveat above that it is really important to try to take it) then our next choice drug is currently rifampicin. We start this at a dose of 150mg per day, and check the liver function tests after 2-4 weeks. We also warn people that it will colour their sweat, urine and even tears orange (if they aren't warned people get a shock!!). We need to check the LFTs because rifampicin can sometimes cause liver injury. This is usually mild but is something for people to be aware of. If your LFTs show any deterioration (in particular a rise in ALT) then the rifampicin should be stopped and LFTs monitored until they return to the level they were at before rifampicin was used. If itch control is good, and rifampicin is not causing problems (the other issue beyond orange or pink urine and liver injury is occasional nausea) then we leave people on 150mg per day. If itch control is still not adequate then we increase slowly up to a maximum of 600mg per day. Each time the dose is increased the LFTs need to be checked after 2-4 weeks (remember what I said about cholestyramine being an easier drug to use?). There is no point increasing the dose beyond 600mg as if it is not working at this dose it is not going to work. In our experience, about 70% of people respond to rifampicin making it a very important drug for us in managing itch. If you get a good response to rifampicin **stick with it!** I have patients who have been on it for over 20 years with complete control of their itch. We also have a sense that if people stop it and then re-start it, it is sometimes not as effective as it was originally.......People coming to the clinic are very familiar with my saying "if it ain't broke don't fix it"!!

Step 6: *Bezafibrate:* One of the important developments since the first edition of this book was published has been the emergence of bezafibrate as a treatment for itch (as well, of course as a treatment option for UDCA non-response PBC). A single trial (of relatively short duration) has shown clear benefit and my own experience in clinical practice would mirror it. What we don't have is evidence about long term use (does it continue to benefit itch over months and years) and safety (we already know about potential kidney issues when it is used as a second-line therapy. In my practice I use it after rifampicin in the list of options but other clinics use it after cholestyramine and before rifampicin. Obviously, in higher risk patients bezafibrate is a logical treatment to use earlier as it has a disease-improving as well as an anti-itch effect; something that rifampicin doesn't have.

In this escalating approach to treatment an important question is when non-experts in itch management should seek specialist input. For me it is at this point. Treatments up to and including rifampicin are reasonable for use in a general hepatology clinic. From this point onwards it is starting to get specialised.

Step 7: *Naltrexone:* Naltrexone is an oral opiate antagonist that probably blocks the nerves signalling the sensations in the skin that are interpreted by the brain as itch. It works well in some people (and not at all in others). It can also be difficult to use in practice. There are two issues

- Pain unrelated to PBC (such as toothache or shingles) which is made worse because the body's main natural control system is blocked, and which then can't be treated with opiate drugs (because their actions are blocked).
- An opiate withdrawal-like action ("cold turkey") because the body has become used to high levels of opiates which are suddenly blocked. This can include headaches, shivers, nightmares and loose bowel motions.

The issue of pain can be addressed by non-opiate analgesics but these can be limited, especially as paracetamol may be something that people are keen to avoid because of liver injury. The withdrawal reaction is mitigated by starting on the lowest oral dose possible (12.5mg which is quarter of a tablet) and building up the dose slowly. The withdrawal-type reaction usually settles after a few days but in some people it never settles. The issues with starting naltrexone, and the fact that there are a number of people in whom it doesn't work, mean that we only use it if rifampicin has not had the desired effect.

Step 8: *Experimental Drug Treatments:* These come in two forms.

- New drugs in clinical trial. This is a fast changing landscape with a number of potentially useful treatments under evaluation. The most advanced is the iBAT inhibitor linerixibat, although a number of other drugs are in development. Speak to your consultant about what trials are available.

- Older drugs with some evidence to suggest they work. The obvious example is gabapentin, an anti-epilepsy treatment which has had a new lease of life as a pain-controlling agent. As for pain nerve signals, gabapentin seems to block itch nerve fibres. The only clinical trial of its use in cholestatic itch suggested it wasn't effective. Our experience is very different and we use it a lot! Start at a low dose (say 300mg per day or even lower) and build it up slowly. Too high a dose too quickly can lead to sedation and worsening fatigue.

Step 9: *Physical Approaches:* These are approaches which physically remove the itch causing agent from the blood (rather than blocking its actions through a drug effect). They come in four very different forms:

a) Transplantation: This is perhaps the ultimate physical approach, removing the problematic liver and replacing it with a normal one. Transplant is highly effective at treating itch. However, it is a procedure with risks to life which are difficult to weight up against symptom improvement. This balance can be in favour of transplant in people with the most extreme itch. It is really important, however, that all medical approaches have been attempted properly before transplant is considered.

b) Naso-Biliary Drainage: This is a procedure in which a tube, inserted at endoscopy, is used to drain bile from the liver. This can be highly effective and presumably works because the entity that causes the itch is present in bile (possibly bile acids, possibly something that binds to bile acids) and is removed by the drainage. Although effective the benefit is short term (2 to 3 days for every day the tube is in place) and there is a risk of pancreatitis. This should only, therefore, ever be attempted in specialist centres with experience and as a crisis-intervention (i.e. to give people with the worst itch, potentially on the list for transplantation, some breathing space of itch control).

c) Plasmapheresis/MARS: These are both variants of dialysis in which the blood is, in simple terms, cleaned. In our experience this is less effective than naso-biliary drainage and equally invasive. Again it should only be used for crisis-intervention.

d) Phototherapy: This is, in marked contrast to the three previous interventions, a mild treatment that is potentially usable in lots of patients. Light therapy is used by skin specialists to treat skin disease. It appears that the light energy also breaks down the irritant that causes itch in PBC. Some patients notice that their itch is better in summer. Light therapy is a medical version of this. Where used it needs specialist dermatology input (this is not a conventional sun-bed action!) and there is a limit to how frequently it can be used because of the potential for skin cancer. It works best in small people who have a larger surface area (needed for the light to work) per Kg of body weight.

......TO MANAGING FATIGUE IN PBC

This is a really important issue for patients and a key part of our work in the PBC clinic. It is an area of PBC where taking a structured, long-term approach is really key. In the case of itch there are effective specific therapies. The art is finding the right approach for each patient from a number of available options. In the case of fatigue there is, regrettably, no specific therapy at present. There are many things that we can, and do, do to improve quality of life from fatigue. This needs a comprehensive approach, however, not just a prescription.

Step 1: *Explain, reassure & support:* The first key step is to explain to people that fatigue is part of PBC, that it is "real" and that they are not alone. There are lots of other patients just like them and that we are there to help. We don't sympathise (people don't want our sympathy) but we do empathise; try to understand what it must feel like and to commit to try and help. Most people presenting with PBC fatigue have had, by the time they reach us, a very negative experience of not being believed by clinicians, and being told that they don't have a "proper problem". For some reason, fatigue is an area where doctors feel the need to share and equate their own experience. A PBC patient is not particularly helped by hearing that you were on call last night and are very tired!! Explaining the current understanding of the mechanisms of fatigue is often really useful for patients. This is partly because it helps people to understand the disease process and partly because it reinforces the view that the problem is "real".

Step 2: *Treat treatable causes:* PBC patients frequently have other conditions that are themselves also associated with fatigue, and which may be easier to treat than PBC fatigue. These should be thought about, looked for and, where found, treated. Examples include

- Other autoimmune conditions such as thyroid disease, and the autoimmune causes of anaemia such as celiac disease, haemolytic anaemia and pernicious anaemia. All such conditions are seen at an increased frequency in PBC patients.
- Age-related conditions (i.e. those that are not specifically associated with PBC, but which are common in the typical PBC age group). These include type 2 diabetes, heart failure and kidney disease.

Step 3: *Treat things that make the fatigue worse:* There are a number of clinical processes or problems which are not a direct feature of PBC, but that are seen at an increased frequency in PBC patients, and which appear to contribute to the severity of the fatigue. Reducing their impact can lessen the severity of fatigue. These include

- *Night-time itch:* Itch at night can contribute to poor sleep and thus fatigue the next day. Even if itch is not prominent during the day, if it is present at night then it warrants treating (using the standard itch approach).

- *Sleep-disturbance:* Even in patients without night-time itch poor sleep is common in PBC and, again, contributes to fatigue the following day. Assessment of sleep by the affected individual is notoriously difficult, so the observation of partners is very helpful. If there is a question of poor sleep then the input of a specialist sleep clinic is often really helpful. Simple things that patients can do is avoid simulants (tea, coffee, energy drinks etc) after around 5pm in the day and, wherever possible, avoid sleeping tablets and alcohol. These superficially seem to help sleep but the sleep that you do get is almost always poor quality and therefore of low value.

- *Autonomic disturbance:* Blood pressure regulation seems to be a real issue in PBC with significant ups and downs. Blood pressure can, in particular, fall when people stand up suddenly. These blood flow changes probably result in poor muscle perfusion (and maybe even altered blood supply to the heart) reducing function. This is commonly, in our experience, linked to excessive blood pressure lowering treatment. The scenario is usually that people have been found to have high blood pressure before they were found to have PBC and started on treatment. When they developed PBC the blood pressure drop from the disease occurred, but the treatment was not adjusted, meaning that rather than high blood pressure people had low blood pressure. Re-assessing blood pressure treatment is therefore a very useful thing to look at. DON'T STOP BLOOD PRESSURE TREATMENT WITHOUT DISCUSSING IT WITH YOUR DOCTOR! The things that should make you think about blood pressure regulation as a factor in fatigue in PBC include dizziness when standing up quickly.

- *Depression:* A complex issue. Depression is not a major cause of fatigue in PBC but people with fatigue can sometimes get depressed because of the fatigue, and the depression then makes the fatigue worse. Anti-depressants such as sertraline can help. They don't make the fatigue better but they can help people cope with it.

- *Menopausal Symptoms:* Given the age and gender of the typical PBC patients menopausal symptoms can frequently be an issue. We have, historically, probably under-used HRT because of, probably erroneous, concerns about the potential to worsen cholestasis.

Step 4: *Coping Strategies:* This is really key. At the moment it is not possible to cure fatigue. It is perfectly possible, however, to live a perfectly normal life despite it. The capacity to do this lies IN YOUR HANDS! We can help you cope effectively but, fundamentally, the desire to do so comes from within. Here are some important things that we discuss with patients

- *Owning the problem so you can own the solution:* This is about accepting the reality of the situation. I have several sayings ("you are where you are" and "in life we have to play the hand we are dealt"). There is no point wishing it had not happened or blaming the world. The problem is yours, it is here and you have to get on with making the most of it. It is OK to be fed up for a little bit but after that make a plan and get on with it.

- *Set realistic time scales:* Whatever you do, you will not beat this in a day or a week. I always suggest to people that they take a fixed point in the calendar one year (Christmas, summer holiday, birthday etc) and set the same day next year as the target to be doing more and coping better.

- *Help others to understand:* In the same way that doctors sometimes struggle to understand this so can family members. PBC patients with fatigue normally look very well and people do not understand how you can look well but feel awful. It is just the way the disease works. Explain to partners, children etc what you can and can't do and the importance of their understanding and help. Have a way of being able to flag that you are struggling and need a bit of help without having to go into detail. Getting them to read this book would be a great start!

- *Understand the rhythm of your day:* PBC fatigue is very characteristic in getting worse as the day goes on. People are usually much better in the morning than in the afternoon. Use that information to plan your day. Do important things in the morning. If you are working, and struggle later in the day, discuss with your employer about moving your hours around. These simple changes can make a huge difference without impacting on your effectiveness. One thing that is really critical is avoid doing night shifts if at all possible.

- *Accept there will be good days and bad days:* Again, this is just the way the disease works. If you have a good day enjoy it (but don't overdo it). If you have a bad day then be philosophical. The next day is likely to be better.

- *Exercise:* There are studies showing that even quite low levels of exercise really help with fatigue in PBC. It is just that people struggle with the idea of doing it. The answer is to step it up very gently. Whatever you are doing this week, next week do 10% more. You can't make the disease worse by doing it. Smart phones all have exercise trackers these days which can help you keep an eye on what you are doing.

- *Avoid getting isolated:* THIS IS REALLY IMPORTANT! People can sometimes withdraw from normal activities to save energy (work, social activities etc). This is always a false economy. What you gain from conserved energy you lose in overall life quality. The secret is to keep doing things but to adapt what you do to take account of the limitations.
- *Stay positive:* Treatment is on its way!!

......TO USING UDCA IN PBC

UDCA use in PBC is, at one level, really easy. Use it in everyone and keep using it life-long! There is now very clear evidence that it is safe and has long-term benefits for patients. There are some important things to think about, however.

Dose: It is now clear that the optimal dose is 13-15mg/Kg. Below this dose the effect is less. Above this dose there is no added benefit, and issues around tolerability come into play. It is also really key to get the dose right because to have taken UDCA at the correct dose is usually a requirement for access to second-line therapy. Where within the 13-15mg your dose lies will depend on your weight and the tablet sizes. Anywhere between 13 and 15 is fine. Remember also that your weight can go up and down so adjust the UDCA dose with your doctor if needed.

Timing: We suggest to people that they take UDCA as a single dose at night (although the leaflet in the packs often suggests taking it as split doses during the day; a pattern of use suitable for the old application of UDCA as a tablet to dissolve gallstones). Evening dosing seems to be more effective in PBC, and also gets away from the interaction with cholestyramine (see below) which is take spaced out through the day.

Tolerability: Most people tolerate UDCA fine. Some people get bowel disturbance in the form of either stomach upset or loose bowels. This usually settles with time. If it is a real problem then we suggest starting with a lower dose than your ideal dose and then building up over time. An alternative, if tolerability is still an issue, is to move to split doses given during the day with food. This is a less ideal way of taking it, but better than not taking it at all! Sometimes patients describe weight gain with UDCA. I suspect that this is a result of UDCA working as a bile acid and helping to absorb fat. In essence, it is reversing the fat malabsorption that can occur with PBC because of the bile acid flow abnormalities. Some patients worry about slight hair loss. I am not clear whether this is actually a UDCA effect or an effect of the PBC itself. I would certainly never suggest not taking UDCA because of concern about this. UDCA has no potentially harmful side-effects, which is one of the reasons why it is so useful in PBC.

Drug Interactions: UDCA is very safe and has no harmful interactions with other drugs. The only thing to be aware of is its interaction with cholestyramine. Cholestyramine is first line treatment for itch control and works by binding bile acids in the bowel and carrying them out of the body in the stool. As the bile acids play a role in irritating nerves in the skin causing itch this bile acid elimination effect helps itch. The issue with UDCA is that it is itself a bile acid (as is obeticholic acid for that matter) meaning that it will also bind to cholestyramine and be lost. This binding does not cause any harm, but does mean that the effects of both are lost. We get around this by suggesting that UDCA is taken as a single dose in the evening, and that cholestyramine is taken in spaced doses throughout the day.

Response: The first thing to say about response to UDCA is that it takes several weeks or month to have its maximum effect. This is because it needs to be taken up from the bowel into the bile pool, and to displace the other more toxic bile acids, to have its effect. This takes time. Do not stop taking UDCA if your liver function tests do not improve quickly! The other thing to be aware of is that the symptoms of PBC are unlikely to improve with UDCA. In some people itch can improve a little. The dull-ache abdominal pain over the liver can certainly improve. It is unlikely, however, that fatigue will improve. The main effect of UDCA is on reducing liver injury and risk of fibrosis. This effect is visible through improvement in liver function tests over a number of months rather, regrettably, than through symptom improvement. The degree of liver function test improvement seen will dictate whether or not UDCA is working sufficiently. If not, you should consider second-line therapy. This assessment of degree of response is done after 12 months of UDCA, and the approach is outlined in the section below on second-line therapy.

Stopping: DON'T!! Occasionally people stop UDCA because their liver function tests have returned to normal! This simply shows that the UDCA is working. It does not cure PBC. It just controls it. Once you stop taking it then that control is lost. You would not stop taking blood pressure tablets because your blood pressure was in the normal range would you? Occasionally people have to stop because of tolerability issues (but it is very occasional people in whom the "tricks" described above do not work). If you do need to stop it there is no need to wean it down. You can just stop.

Other situations: These are other situations that arise when UDCA use or discontinuation might be considered. The first is *pregnancy*. If you get pregnant should you continue with UDCA? Our advice is to continue, especially if the disease was at the riskier end of the spectrum before UDCA and has responded well to treatment. People are always cautious about drugs in pregnancy. It is worth remembering two things about UDCA in pregnancy, however. The first is that our bodies naturally produce UDCA. It is just that it is at low levels. All we are doing with UDCA treatment in PBC is boosting the natural levels. The point is that UDCA is not actually foreign at all. The second is that we actually use UDCA as treatment in pregnancy for cholestasis of pregnancy. In 30 years of PBC management I have never encountered anyone with problems from taking UDCA in pregnancy.

The second situation is *transplant*. The evidence is increasingly suggesting that it is really helpful to continue taking UDCA after transplantation. Recurrence of PBC can occur after liver transplant and is a concern for patients. Evidence from the Global PBC group has shown that starting UDCA immediately after transplant (or perhaps more accurately continuing it) is associated with a significantly reduced risk of recurrent PBC, and reduced disease severity if it does recur. This is logical, as we now know that UDCA works most effectively when used early in the disease. The day of the transplant in someone who goes on to get recurrence of the disease is the earliest point there is! The evidence also suggests that you should not wait for recurrence to develop post-transplant as UDCA is less effective used in that way. Our current practice is, therefore, to start all transplanted patients back on UDCA and to continue it life-long.

The third situation is people with **AMA and normal LFTs**. This is a group of people who are increasingly being recognised. Assuming a person has not had a biopsy showing PBC (an unlikely scenario) then this is not, by definition, PBC (only one out of the three key tests, the AMA, is positive and at least two need to be present for the diagnosis). The presence of AMA is associated with a small risk of developing PBC in the future, but current experience is that when PBC presents itself in this way it tends to be very mild. The guideline advice is, therefore, to check LFTs ever year and if they become abnormal (i.e. the person has reached a diagnosis of PBC by developing the second diagnostic feature) start UDCA. In our experience, the rate of starting UDCA in this group is actually very low. Our rule of thumb is not to start UDCA until LFT abnormality is seen. There are, however, a couple of settings where we don't follow this rule. The first is in people who appear to have the symptoms of PBC (itch or fatigue) even though their LFTs are normal. Frequently, AMA was detected when these people were investigated for their symptoms, suggesting a real association. We know that neither itch nor fatigue severity is associated with degree of LFT abnormality. Taken to its logical conclusion, this could include PBC patients with normal LFTs. In this setting, we discuss the issues and leave people to make their own decision. Around 50% go on to take up UDCA. The other setting is the relatives of patients with very aggressive PBC. If someone presents with AMA, whose mother had a transplant at 40, it is very difficult to reassure them that PBC is normally a very mild disease. Given the familial risk, and the fact that UDCA works best when given early in the disease, we again discuss the option for UDCA. In this setting, the take up is very high. For what it's worth, if I was in the first group of symptomatic patients I wouldn't take UDCA, but if I had the high risk family member I would. Remember, UDCA is cheap and very safe which makes it a low risk decision to take it.

......TO SECOND-LINE THERAPY IN PBC

Second-line therapy is now a standard part of our management approach for PBC. It should be considered in everyone (although the majority of people won't need it). The following is the Newcastle approach. This is a rapidly changing area and is one where practice will differ from centre to centre.

Step 1: *Check that UDCA has been used at the correct dose:* Second-line therapy is typically used in PBC in patients who have shown an inadequate response to UDCA given at the correct dose. Clearly, therefore, to meet second-line therapy criteria primary therapy (UDCA) needs to have been tried. Around 95% of PBC patients in the UK have received UDCA, with the vast majority continuing on it. There are 3 aspects to UDCA to consider in the context of second-line therapy

- *Is the dose correct?* The optimal dose is 13-15mg/Kg. Is the dose you are taking still correct for you (remembering that body weight can go up over time meaning that the UDCA dose needs to be adjusted)? If you are not on 13-15mg/Kg of UDCA discuss with your doctor about increasing the dose.

- *Have you been treated for long enough?* UDCA takes time to get into the system and, therefore, needs to be given time to work. The long-term response pattern will be reached after about 3 months, although formal response assessment needs 12 months of therapy. This is likely to come down over time. If you have had UDCA for less than around 6 months you need to give it a little more time

- *If you are not on UDCA, why not?* Second-line therapy for PBC almost certainly does not work as well in people not taking UDCA. If you have struggled taking it in the past try again. If your doctor has not offered it to you ask for it. If you struggle with nausea try some of the tricks suggested in the section on UDCA use above. If you are really struggling to take the full dose, remember that some is better than none.

Step 2: *Is second-line therapy indicated?* We currently use cut-offs for Alkaline Phosphatase of around 200 and Bilirubin of 20. If either of the tests is above the line then you fall into the group that could benefit from second-line therapy. Below the line for both and your risk from PBC is very low. Note that the blood level cut-offs are not defined nationally (the instructions for OCA, the main second-line therapy, say that it should be used in people "showing an inadequate response to UDCA" without defining cut-offs). What this also means is that there is some latitude about use. OCA is also appropriate for use in people who are unable to tolerate UDCA.

Step 3: *Is it suitable for you?* This is a slightly different question. Not everyone reaching the blood values for second-line therapy will end up taking it. There are two main reasons why you might not take it

- *Very advanced disease:* All the second-line therapy drugs can make very advanced disease worse rather than better, and transplant is a much better option. This is only a very small group but an important one. The sorts of things that should make people worry are jaundice, a history of variceal bleeding, a history of ascites or a history of encephalopathy. If you have cirrhosis, but don't have these complications, then you may well need to reduce the dose that you take.

- *Personal choice:* Not everyone with an alkaline phosphatase over 200 and/or a bilirubin over 20 is the same. At the end of the day there is a personal balance to be struck between risks and benefits, which needs to take account of age, severity of disease and other health problems. If I were 30, with a bilirubin of 40 and an alkaline phosphatase of 1000 (we see people like this) then I would take it without hesitation. If I were 105 with an alkaline phosphatase of 201 and cancer I wouldn't. Most people are somewhere in between. The really important thing is that if the decision is not to take second-line therapy **this must be your decision!**

Step 4: *Which Agent?* There are currently 3 options.

- *Obeticholic Acid (OCA):* This is the licensed therapy and our default first choice. The starting dose is 5mg per day, increased to 10mg per day after 3 months if the effect seen is insufficient. If you have cirrhosis, then in many cases a lower dose must be used (5mg once a week increased over time to a maximum of 10mg twice a week). This dose increase must be discussed with your doctor. OCA is very safe in PBC (provided caution is applied in using it in patients with very advanced disease). Its major side effect is itch. Our approach to itch management is outlined below.

- *Bezafibrate:* This is a drug with trial evidence to support its use in PBC, although it is not licensed for use in this setting. If it is used in PBC in place of OCA it must be for a specific reason (other than cost). We use it in place of (or increasingly in addition to) OCA in people showing an inadequate response to OCA. We also use it in some patients in preference to OCA where the risk is low (bilirubin under 20 and alkaline phosphatase below 250), and where the patient has significant itch that we worry will be worsened by OCA.

Fenofibrate is used as alternative in countries where bezafibrate is not licensed and is, thus, not available.

- *Clinical Trials:* There are a number of ongoing trials of second-line agents in people showing an inadequate response to UDCA. Interest in clinical trials in PBC is, in my experience, very high.

Step 5: *Follow-Up:* At present, there are no hard and fast rules for how we approach patients on second-line therapy longer-term. The following represents our practical approach

- All patients should be followed-up long-term. By definition, they are in the high risk group and need to be monitored as such.
- We assess response to the second-line agent at 1 year using the same alkaline phosphatase of 200 and bilirubin of 20 cut-offs as for UDCA response.
- In patients who are still showing an inadequate response swapping second-line agent and, increasingly, adding a second agent should be considered.
- At present, we are not stopping second-line agents for lack of response. All patients seem to derive some benefit, even if it is not of the degree we would ideally like to see.

ITCH WITH OCA: A PRACTICAL GUIDE

The trials have suggested that pruritus with OCA is quite common. Our experience in routine use is that itch is only rarely an issue. This is largely because of the practical steps we take to mitigate it

Step 1: *Warn patients:* Forewarned is forearmed. If people are aware that they may get some itch which is typically mild then it tends to be much better tolerated than if it were an unexpected development

Step 2: *Pre-OCA management:* We assess all patients in whom we are considering OCA for itch before we start OCA. If itch is present we treat it, even if the severity is such that it wouldn't otherwise need treating

Step 3: *Post-OCA management:* We assess people early after the start of OCA and if they are developing itch treat it aggressively. Rifampicin is usually the agent of choice

Step 4: *Dose adjust:* If, despite these steps, there is still a problem with itch then we discontinue the OCA (but continue the itch treatment) and wait for the itch to resolve. We would then re-start OCA at a very low dose (5 mg every second or third day). Once established on a regular small dose then people are normally able to increase the dose over time

Step 5: *Consider OCA and bezafibrate combination therapy:* OCA and bezafibrate are probably synergistic in terms of their PBC actions and therefore make a logical combination. Furthermore, bezafibrate appears to have an anti-itch action. We have experience of treating people with the combination who were unable to tolerate OCA alone because of itch.

APPENDIX 4: KNOWING YOUR NUMBERS

A critical part of "owning the problem and owning the solution" in PBC is for you to know and understand your test values so that you can ask your doctor or nurse what their future management plans are. This way you can make sure you get the best possible care. I have devised this simple table to help you collate your results. I suggest you copy it and take a version every time you go to the clinic. A downloadable version will be developed and made available later in 2023.

Test	Target Value in 2023	Likely Future Target Value	YOUR Values Today in Clinic
Blood Tests _Alkaline Phosphatase_	Under 217	Under 130	
Bilirubin	Under 20	Under 12	
Alanine Transaminase	NA	Under 40	
Fibroscan	Under 15.1	Under 7.7	
Symptoms _Itch (Scale 0-10)_	Under 4	Under 4	
Fatigue (Scale 0-10)	Under 4	Under 4	

Explanation: For the **_Blood tests_** the "target values in 2023" are the values that clinics should be working towards based on current treatment guidelines. The alkaline phosphatase and bilirubin thresholds are the POISE criteria which were used in the key trial which led to the licensing of obeticholic acid. Alanine transaminase currently doesn't form part of these criteria. It is likely that, over the next few years, the treatment target will move to normalization of alkaline phosphatase, alanine transaminase and bilirubin. This change will occur because it is increasingly clear that anything other than normal blood test values (the thresholds given for future use in the table) is associated with some ongoing disease activity. We can and must be more ambitious about our goals for treatment in PBC. Note that the values given are for the Newcastle laboratory. There may be small differences between different labs so check with your clinician as to your local values.

Fibroscan should now be a routine part of follow-up for everyone with PBC. The suggested 2023 threshold is the value for increased risk. A value above this suggests a high risk of presence already of, or progression in the future to, cirrhosis. In the future we should aim for the lower threshold of 7.7. Below this value PBC is very low risk indeed. That is what we should all be aiming for.

For *Symptoms* it is difficult to given accurate cut-offs because symptoms are all about individual impact. For both the symptom types the scales are 0-10 ("where zero is no symptom and 10 is the worst severity you can imagine"). Conventional wisdom is that a value below 4 is associated with low (or at least tolerable) symptom impact.

ABOUT THE AUTHOR

Professor Jones has treated people with PBC for over 30 years. He runs the specialist PBC clinic at the Freeman Hospital in Newcastle upon Tyne in the UK and leads the UK-PBC research programme that has done much to transform the care of PBC patients around the world. He was awarded an OBE in the 2018 Queen's Birthday Honours List for services to patients with liver disease.

Printed in Great Britain
by Amazon

20147895R00159